BASIC MATERNITY NURSING

BASIC MATERNITY NURSING

PERSIS MARY HAMILTON R.N., Ed.D.

SIXTH EDITION

with **198** illustrations

The C. V. Mosby Company

ST. LOUIS • BALTIMORE • TORONTO   1989

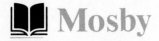

Editor: Linda L. Duncan
Assistant editor: Joanna May
Project manager: Mark Spann
Book and cover design: Gail Morey Hudson

SIXTH EDITION

The C.V. Mosby Company
11830 Westline Industrial Drive, St. Louis, Missouri 63146

Library of Congress Cataloging in Publication Data

Hamilton, Persis Mary.
  Basic maternity nursing/Persis Mary Hamilton.—6th ed.
    p. cm.
  Includes bibliographies and index.
  ISBN 0-8016-2700-1
  1. Obstetrical nursing.   I. Title.
  [DNLM: 1. Obstetrical Nursing.   2. Pregnancy—nurses' instruction.
WY 157.3 H219b]
RG951.H32 1989
610.73'678—dc19
DNLM/DLC
for Library of Congress   88-13544
                                                      CIP

GW/RRD/RRD   9 8 7 6 5 4 3

Preface

An understanding of childbearing as it affects the family unit is essential to an effective maternity nurse. This understanding and its implications for care are the essence of family-centered maternity nursing. The original purpose of this text was to fill the need for a textbook in family-centered maternity nursing. The need for such a basic text has not changed since that time. In fact, it has expanded. More and more persons are becoming involved in maternal-child care as parents assume increasing responsibility for their reproductive lives, their health, and the health of their children. Planning-for-parenthood classes, husband-coached childbirth, and alternate birthing centers are a few examples of the family-centered maternity care being practiced today.

In addition to the expanded need for a basic maternity nursing text, there has been an enormous increase in knowledge about safe maternal-child care. To meet these changing needs, this sixth edition has been completely revised and updated.

The plan of this book, as indicated by the unit titles, is family centered. Normal conditions are followed by abnormal ones.

Unit I, "The Childbearing Family," has two chapters: "Sexuality and Reproduction," and "The Expectant Couple." These chapters serve as a foundation for the book. In them are discussed the anatomy and physiology of human sexuality and reproduction, the history of maternal-child care, and the family as a social unit.

Unit II, "The Mother, Father, and Developing Child," focuses on pregnancy and includes chapters on embryonic and fetal development, the psychological and physiological changes that occur during pregnancy, prenatal care, and possible complications of pregnancy.

Unit III, "Labor and Birth," includes chapters on the mechanism of labor, nursing care during labor, nursing care during the birth, and possible complications of the labor and birth process.

Unit IV, "The Newborn Baby," describes nursing care for normal newborns and newborns with special needs. Some of the most recent developments of the care of normal and high-risk infants have been included in these chapters.

Unit V, "Postpartum Care," describes the needs of mothers and nursing interventions in three chapters: "Nursing Care of the Mother," "Complications and Surgery," and "Care of the New Family."

As additional aids to students and instructors, each chapter is preceded by a list of learning objectives and a vocabulary list of important terms and is followed by an annotated summary, a list of key concepts covered in the chapter, study questions, and a reference list. Nursing care is framed in the steps of the nursing process, and a list of NANDA diagnoses is provided. A glossary and index complete the text.

Rather than presenting a catalog of scientific information, it has been my desire to convey scientific facts and principles in such a way that readers will relate them to the families they serve in human terms of kindness, warmth, and understanding.

Delore Veenstra, RN, MS, served as my consultant for this revision. Her expertise in both maternity nursing and education, her thoroughness, and her sensitivity have been invaluable aids for this revision.

Many other persons have contributed to this revision, both professionally and personally. I especially appreciate the numerous nurse-educators who took time to critique the last edition and portions of this one.

It is my hope that the additions and changes made in this edition will make the book even more valuable to the nurses and families for whom it was written.

Persis Mary Hamilton

Contents

UNIT ONE
THE CHILDBEARING FAMILY

CHAPTER 1

Sexuality and Reproduction

VOCABULARY

Adolescence
Climacteric
Colostrum
Menarche
Menstruation
Mittelschmerz
Ovulation
Puberty
Sexual response cycle

LEARNING OBJECTIVES

- Describe human sexuality from birth to old age.

- Describe the male and female generative structures and products, and explain their functions.

- List the six categories of complications that affect male reproductive system functioning.

- Discuss fertility, infertility, and sterility in men and women.

- Describe five methods used to estimate the time of ovulation in women.

HUMAN SEXUALITY THROUGHOUT LIFE

One of the first questions a parent asks when a baby is born is "What is it, a boy or a girl?" The answer is critical. Knowledge of the baby's sex sets in motion a constellation of actions and reactions by the parents, society, and the new individual. Maleness or femaleness is a pivotal fact about which a person develops, both psychosocially and physically. A person's sex is an important factor throughout life.

Childhood

Although the reproductive organs are immature and the body contours of boys and girls are similar during childhood, sexual identity, or gender, is developing. Boys learn their gender role, that is, to talk, dress, and act as men. Girls learn to talk, dress, and act as women. Problems arise only when the gender role is different from the chromosomal sex as a result of congenital or developmental abnormalities.

Adolescence

Adolescence is a period of transition from childhood to adulthood. It is characterized by the dramatic physical changes of puberty and the complex emotional and social adjustments necessary to become an adult. Gender identity is normally completed as the reproductive organs reach maturity.

Puberty

Puberty is that time of life when the reproductive system matures. Puberty is marked by a preliminary period of a year or more called *prepubescence*, when the secondary sex characteristics appear. At this time the endocrine glands, particularly the pituitary gland and the gonads, begin to produce greater quantities of their hormones. These powerful chemicals are distributed to every part of the body by means of the bloodstream, causing changes in body contour, rate of growth, and body organ development. In girls these changes appear between the ages of 10 and 15 years. In boys such changes appear between the ages of 12 and 17 years.

Typical changes in boys are increased size of the testes and penis; growth of pubic, facial, axillary, and chest hair; broadening of the chest, narrowing of the hips; height and weight increases; production of sperm; and nocturnal emissions (wet dreams).

Typical changes in girls are growth of the nipples and breasts, growth of pubic and axillary hair, broadening of the hips and pelvis, menarche (onset of menstruation), and ovulation following menarche by 6 to 12 months.

Both boys and girls experience skin changes. The oil glands become more active, which causes pimples and blackheads. The sweat glands produce more perspiration, which causes body odor. The blood vessels of the skin respond to emotions by dilating, which causes blushing.

In addition to the physical changes of puberty, adolescents must solve profound psychosocial problems, including responsiveness to the opposite sex, exaggerated self-consciousness, and growing needs for independence. These drives often conflict with the values they have accepted from their parents, and they may feel confused and frightened. In healthy situations and with time, experience, and reasoning, these conflicts are resolved, and adulthood is attained.

Adulthood and maturity

Maturity is the full development of one's potential. Physical maturity occurs spontaneously when there is adequate nutrition and exercise and when illness is prevented or treated. Psychological maturity can be expected to occur in a mentally healthy setting, where needs are met and illness is prevented or treated. Sexual maturity includes the physical development of the reproductive organs and an acceptance and appreciation of one's sexual identity, sexual responsiveness, and ability to use reproductive capacities responsibly.

Climacteric

It was once believed that the body went through a climax every 9 years. The *menopause*, when menses cease in women, was viewed as one of the climaxes. The *climacteric* has come to signify the entire period of life when the reproductive organs become inactive. It includes the cessation of menses in women and reduced fertility in men.

HUMAN SEXUAL RESPONSE

Humans have a constant need for tenderness, closeness, and acceptance by others. The intensity of this drive fluctuates from time to time depending on the situation. The most intense expression of this drive has been termed the *sexual response cycle*.

Two researchers, Masters and Johnson, objectively observed 10,000 such cycles in healthy men and women of all ages. They found that in the typical cycle there are four phases: excitement, plateau, orgasm, and resolution. In general, the body reacts to psychic and physical stimulation by increased muscle tension and vasocongestion of certain areas of the body. With age, these responses are diminished but do not disappear, nor does the need for or pleasure in them disappear. Specific sexual response cycles of men and women will be discussed in the following section.

REPRODUCTIVE SYSTEMS
Male
Generative structures of the male

The reproductive system of the male includes the testes, seminal ducts, seminal vesicles, prostate and bulbourethral glands, urethra, scrotum, and penis. Together these structures yield three unique products: sperm, seminal fluid, and androgens (Fig. 1-1).

Testes. The primary male sex organs are called *testes*. These small oval structures are supported in a saclike pouch called the scrotum. Within the testes are a number of wedge-shaped lobes, each containing the convoluted, "seed-bearing" seminiferous tubules. The *Sertoli cells,* found along with the tubules, are where the sperm grow. These tubules also secrete the major part of the seminal fluid, or semen, in which the sperm are transported. The *interstitial cells* of testes are the source of the male hormone testosterone.

The tiny seminiferous tubules of the testes unite to form a plexus from which a few ducts (eight to fifteen) emerge and enter a single, large convoluted duct called the *epididymis*. The epididymis is attached to the body of the testes, and yet is a part of the system of ducts by which the sperm and semen leave the body. From the seminiferous tubules semen flows into the epididymis, where the sperm develop tadpolelike tails and are stored until ejaculation, their forcible ejection from the body.

Seminal ducts. From the epididymis of each testicle the semen passes up through the seminal duct. This duct, called the *ductus (vas) deferens,* is about 18 inches long and carries the semen to the urethra. The ductus and testicular vessels, nerves, and lymphatics are enclosed in a fibrous sheath, the *spermatic cord*.

Glands. Surrounding the urethra, the duct that leaves the urinary bladder, is the *prostate gland*. Just behind the prostate gland and on the base of the bladder are two *seminal vesicle glands*. Their ducts join the ductus deferens to form *ejaculatory ducts*. The two ejaculatory ducts then empty into the urethra. Just below the prostate gland lie two small glands called Cowper's or *bulbourethral glands*. These add their secretions in the seminal fluid through ducts that open into the urethra. The semen then passes to the outside of the body through the *urethra.*

External genitalia. The external genitalia are the scrotum and penis. The *scrotum* is divided into two sacs by a septum. Each sac contains a testis, an epididymis, and the lower part of the spermatic cord. About the seventh month of gestation, the testes descend into the scrotum, where they remain at a cooler-than-body temperature throughout life. If they do not descend spontaneously, surgical intervention may be necessary to prevent infertility, since sperm do not thrive at body temperature.

The *penis* is a cylindrical organ through which the urethra passes. It is composed chiefly of highly vascular, spongelike erectile tissue. When in a relaxed state, the penis is dependent and flaccid. When there is mental and physical stimulation of the autonomic nervous system, the blood spaces become engorged, causing rigidity, enlargement, and erection. The glans penis is the structure at the distal end over which skin is folded double to form a retractable casing called the foreskin or prepuce.

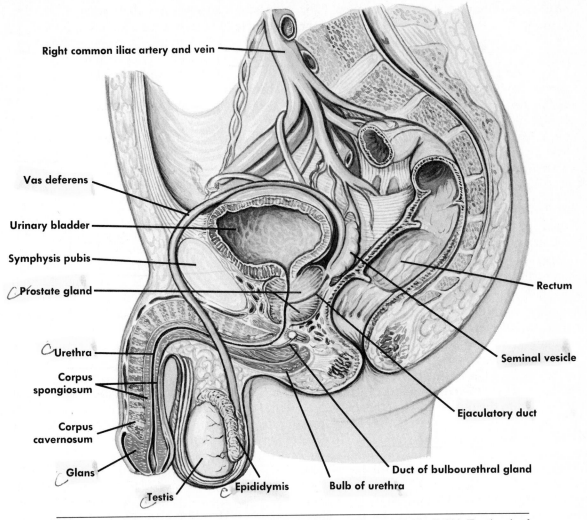

Fig. 1-1   Male reproductive structures. (From Anthony, CP, and Kolthoff, NJ: Textbook of anatomy and physiology, ed 9, St. Louis, 1975, the CV Mosby Co.)

Generative products of the male

Sperm. The germ cells, or *sperm*, that are formed in the testes have the appearance of microscopic tadpoles. Each sperm consists of three parts: a compact head (cell nucleus), a neck and midsection (middle piece), and a tail (flagellum) with which it propels itself (Fig. 1-2). The nucleus, or head, of the sperm contains the chromosomes that are responsible for inherited traits. There are two types of sperm, androsperm and gynosperm. *Androsperm* contain the Y chromosome that produces boys. Androsperm survive better in alkaline than in acid secretions; live about 1 day; have a smaller, round head; and are more numerous than gynosperm. *Gynosperm* contain

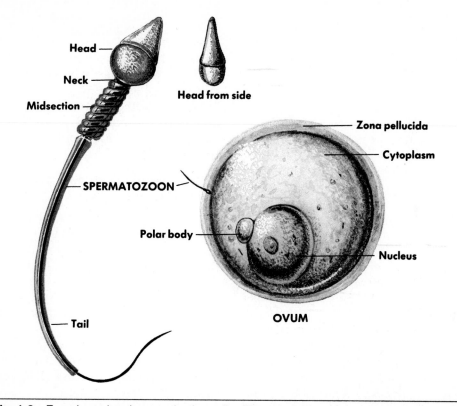

Fig. 1-2 Female and male reproductive cells. (From Anthony, CP, and Kolthoff, NJ: Textbook of anatomy and physiology, ed 9, St. Louis, 1975, The CV Mosby Co.)

the X chromosome that produces girls. Gynosperm survive 2 to 3 days in acidic secretions and are larger and have more oval heads than androsperm.

Seminal fluid. The collected secretions from the testes, epididymides, seminal vesicles, and prostate and bulbourethral glands are called *seminal fluid* or *semen.*

Androgens. The third product of the male reproductive system is a group of hormones collectively called *androgens.* The chief one, testosterone, is related chemically to progesterone. Androgens are secreted by the interstitial cells of the testes into the bloodstream. Androgens are necessary for the development of male reproductive organs and sec-

ondary sex characteristics. Together with the follicle-stimulating hormone made by the pituitary gland, androgens maintain sperm production. They inhibit the pituitary gland, stimulate protein synthesis, and cause phosphate and potassium retention. When injected into the female, androgens suppress lactation and menstruation and reduce uterine activity.

In the fetus, androgen production is stimulated by the chorionic gonadotropin secreted by the placenta. After birth the testes remain dormant until puberty, when the interstitial cell–stimulating hormone (ICSH) of the adenohypophysis stimulates them to produce androgens. ICSH is identical to the luteinizing hormone of females. Without enough ICSH, male characteristics fail to develop. If castration (orchidectomy) occurs before puberty, atrophy of male reproductive structures occurs.

Generative functions of the male

Coitus. The biological purpose of the male reproductive system is to manufacture and deliver the male gamete to the mouth of the female uterus. Delivery is accomplished through the act of copulation, or coitus, when the erect penis, inserted in the vagina, ejaculates semen.

Ejaculation is the forcible expulsion of semen from the body. Ejaculation occurs during sleep irregularly (wet dreams), during sexual intercourse or as a result of masturbation. The amount of semen varies from 1 to 7 ml per ejaculation.

Male sexual response cycle. The sexual response cycle generally follows a standard pattern in men (Fig. 1-3). This cycle consists of the four phases mentioned earlier:

1. The *excitement phase* develops as a result of physical or mental stimulation. The penis responds from higher centers in the brain and from reflex nerves in the spinal cord. Vasocongestion of the blood spaces of the penile shaft causes enlargement and erection. The muscles of the hands, feet, and rectum may contract. A generalized body rash called a "sex flush" may appear. The heart and respiration rates may double, and the blood pressure rises 67% above resting levels. Psychosensory diversion such as sudden loud noises and fears may interfere with erection.

2. A high level of sexual tension is maintained during the *plateau phase*, which some men learn to prolong.

3. The *orgasmic phase* develops involuntarily from recurring contractions of the muscles of the penis and deep perineum, causing forceful ejaculation of the seminal fluid in three or four contractions, followed by minor, irregular ones.

4. The *resolution phase* occurs in two stages: the initial stage, called the refractory period, when the penis reduces 50% in size; and the second stage, when the penis returns to its normal, unstimulated size.

After the initial refractory period, the entire cycle may be repeated again. The plateau phase may be prolonged or hastened with conscious effort.

Complications of the male sexual response cycle

Complications that affect the functioning of the male reproductive system fall into six general categories: (1) impotence, (2) ejaculatory disorders, (3) dyspareunia, (4) aging, (5) infertility, and (6) sterility.

Impotence. Impotence refers to the inability of a man to have and maintain a penile erection.

Primary impotence means that the man has never been able to achieve or maintain an erection sufficient to enter the vagina. This primary type may be caused by a severe mental block or by endocrine or neurological disorders.

Secondary impotence means that the man has had coitus in the past but cannot do so now. The many physical causes for secondary impotence include anatomical abnormalities; cardiorespiratory, endocrine, genitourinary, neurological, vascular, and hematological diseases; surgical intervention; and various medications. Regardless of the cause, once the man experiences difficulty in erection, fear becomes a major part of the problem. Treatment may involve both sexual partners and consists of concentrating on mutual enjoyment of the physical sensations and deemphasizing goal-oriented (orgasm) performance, thus permitting the man to allow involuntary responses to take place.

Ejaculatory disorders. Ejaculatory disorders include ejaculatory incompetence and premature ejaculation.

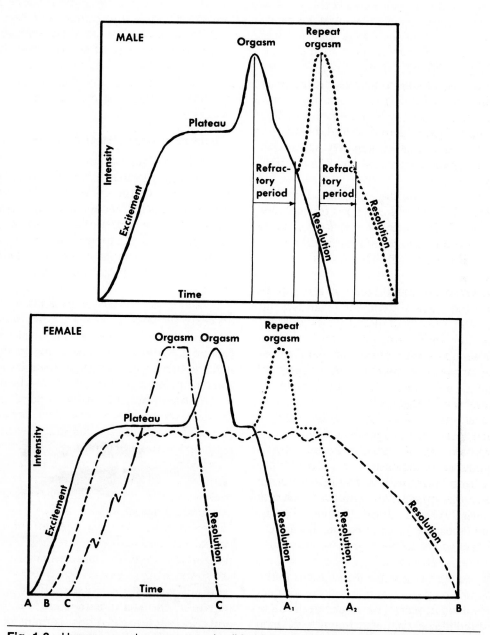

Fig. 1-3 Human sexual response cycle. (Modified from Masters, WH, and Johnson, VE: Human sexual response, Boston, 1966, Little, Brown & Co.)

Ejaculatory incompetence occurs when the man is unable to ejaculate inside the vagina, usually because of a severe mental aversion. Treatment consists of encouraging the partner to stimulate the man manually to ejaculation. Once he has ejaculated in response to her stimulation, he is able to identify with her as a pleasure symbol rather than as a threat or a form of contamination. She then stimulates him to the point of ejaculation and inserts the penis into the vagina immediately. Once this is accomplished, the mental block is neutralized and the condition cured.

Premature ejaculation is defined by researchers Masters and Johnson as the inability to control the ejaculatory process long enough during vaginal penetration to satisfy the partner 50% of the time when coitus occurs. The treatment they devised is a technique called the "squeeze technique," whereby the woman squeezes the penis at the coronal ridge of the glans just before ejaculation, thereby helping the man to learn control.

Dyspareunia. Dyspareunia, or painful coitus, occurs in men for a variety of reasons, including:

Infections of the glans

Phimosis (constriction of the foreskin)

Hypersensitivity to vaginal secretions

Peyronie's disease, which causes inflammation and scar tissue

Traumatic injury with resulting scar tissue

Vasocongestion caused by prolonged sexual stimulation without ejaculation

Various prostatic infections and tumors

Diagnosis and treatment of the specific cause usually relieve the pain.

Aging. Aging causes specific changes in the male sexual response cycle but does not necessarily cause impairment. If a man does not understand these changes, he may develop impotence because of fear of sexual performance.

In general, each of the phases of the response cycle is slowed or diminished in aging

men. Masters and Johnson indicated that if the man is encouraged to ejaculate on his own demand schedule and to have intercourse as it fits both partners' needs, the average couple is able to function sexually well into the 80-year age group. Sexual dysfunction in the older male is believed to be caused largely by fear and false expectations.

Female
Generative structures of the female

The female reproductive system includes the ovaries, uterine tubes, uterus, vagina, vulva, and breasts. Together these structures produce the female gamete (ovum) and hormones. The structures provide a repository for the male semen, a nesting place for the fertilized egg to grow into an infant, and milk to nourish the newborn baby (Figs. 1-4 and 1-5).

Ovaries. The primary sex glands of the female are the two *ovaries*. They are about the size and shape of almonds and are situated on each side of the uterus, below and behind the uterine tubes. The ovaries are anchored in place by ligaments, through which the ovaries receive the nerves and blood supply. The ovaries contain small secretory sacs, or follicles, embedded in connective tissue. Each follicle contains an ovum that matures and is discharged from the ovary into the pelvic cavity by a process called *ovulation*. The ovaries also produce the two major female hormones: progesterone and estrogen.

Uterine tubes. The two uterine tubes (also called *fallopian tubes* or *oviducts*) are small muscular structures almost 5 inches long that are attached to either side of the upper body of the uterus. These tubes carry ova to the uterus by the combined action of peristalsis and cilia that line the tubes. There is no direct connection between the ovaries and the uterine tubes, but fingerlike projections called fimbriae extend from the ends of the tubes. The movement of fimbriae causes a current in the

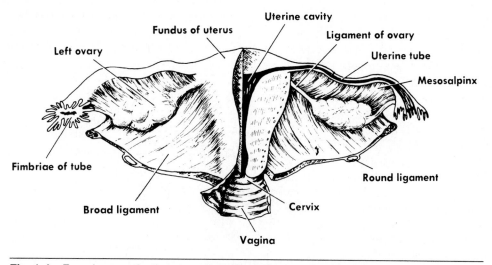

Fig. 1-4 Female reproductive structures. (From Brooks, SM: Basic science and the human body: anatomy and physiology, St. Louis, 1975, The CV Mosby Co.)

peritoneal fluid that sweeps the ovum into the tube, where it takes about 5 days to travel to the uterus.

If free-swimming sperm are traveling up the tube and an ovum is moving down the tube, fertilization may occur whenever they meet. Usually the fertilized egg continues down into the uterine cavity before embedding itself. Occasionally, the egg embeds itself in the lining of the tube; this is called a *tubal pregnancy.* Rarely, a fertilized egg that fails to find its way into the tube may attach itself to the peritoneal cavity; this causes an *abdominal pregnancy.* A pregnancy outside the uterus is known as an *ectopic* or *extrauterine pregnancy* (see Fig. 6-1).

Uterus. The uterus is a hollow, pear-shaped, muscular organ about the size of a closed fist. The uterus is normally tipped forward, or anteflexed, and is located in the pelvis between the urinary bladder and rectum. The uterus is held in place by ligaments:

The *broad ligaments* attach to either side of the uterus. Uterine blood vessels and

nerves pass through these ligaments.
The *uterosacral ligaments* connect the uterus to the sacrum on either side of the rectum.
The *cardinal ligament* extends below the base of the broad ligament and keeps the uterus from dropping down into the vagina.
The *round ligaments* extend from the uterus near the uterine tubes through the inguinal canal to the labia majora.

The uterus is divided into three areas: (1) the lower, smaller part called the neck or *cervix,* (2) the central part called the body or *corpus,* and (3) the uppermost, rounded part called the _fundus,_ which is above the level where the uterine tubes enter the uterus. The two prolongations of the uterus into which uterine tubes open are termed the horns or *cornua.*

The cervix is divided into three parts: (1) the *internal os,* which opens into the uterus, (2) the *external os,* which opens into the va-

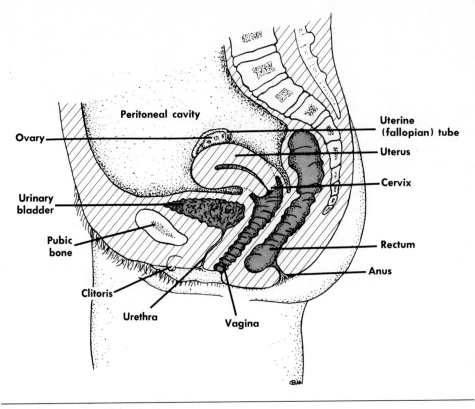

Fig. 1-5   Female pelvic structures.

gina, and (3) the *cervical canal,* which is the area between the two openings.

The outside of the uterus is covered by connective tissue called the *perimetrium.* The inside surface, called the *endometrium,* is made up of secretory tissue that contains blood vessels and glands. The endometrium is the layer that is sloughed each month at menstruation. The wall of the uterus, called the *myometrium,* is the largest part of the three layers (Fig. 1-6).

The thick wall of myometrium is made up of a network of muscle fibers that grow and stretch as the uterus changes during pregnancy. The fibers of the inner layer run in a circular direction, those of the middle layer run in a figure-eight pattern, and those of the outer layer run primarily in a lengthwise direction. Since the blood vessels of the uterus pass through these interlaced patterns, the contraction of the fibers after childbirth constricts the vessels and controls uterine bleeding.

Vagina. The vagina is the muscular membranous canal about 3 inches long that connects the uterus with the vulva. The vagina receives the penis and semen at coitus, discharges menstrual flow, and forms the passage through which birth takes place. The cervix projects down into the upper vagina so that spaces are formed between the cervix and the walls of the vagina. These spaces are called

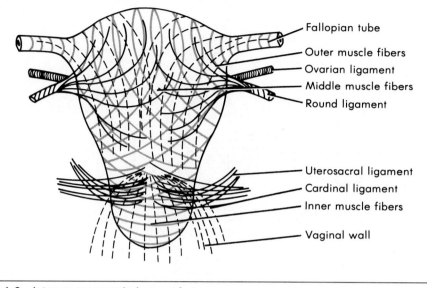

Fig. 1-6 Interwoven muscle layers of uterus.

fornices, and the deepest one, the *posterior fornix,* is found behind the cervix. The walls of the vagina have many folds, or *rugae,* that allow it to stretch during coitus and child-birth.

Pelvic floor. The pelvic floor is made up of several layers of muscles, including the sphincter and levator ani groups. The sphincters are relatively weak, ringlike muscles that close the outer openings of the vagina, rectum, and urinary meatus. Of note is the *bulbocavernosus muscle,* which surrounds the vagina; together with the external sphincter, this muscle makes a figure eight around the vagina and rectum. The powerful levator ani group includes the *pubococcygeal, iliococcygeal,* and *puborectal* muscles. These muscles, termed the *pelvic diaphragm,* form a hammock above which the uterus, vagina, rectum, and bladder are suspended by ligaments and fasciae (Fig. 1-7).

Vulva. The external genitalia of the female are called the vulva (Fig. 1-8) include the mons pubis, labia majora, labia minora, clitoris, vestibule, and perineum. Closely associated and located nearby are the urinary meatus, vaginal opening, rectum, and Bartholin's and Skene's glands.

The *mons pubis,* also called the mons veneris ("Mt. Venus"), is a skin-covered mound of fat that pads the pubic bone. After puberty, coarse hair grows over the mons and down over the labia majora.

The *labia majora,* or larger lips, are the large folds of skin and fatty tissue that extend backward and down from the mons to about 1 inch from the rectum. Hair and sebaceous glands are located in this skin. Sometimes painful, hard-to-cure infections invade these glands, requiring intensive medical treatment.

The *labia minora,* or small lips, lie within the labia majora. These two small folds of mod-

13

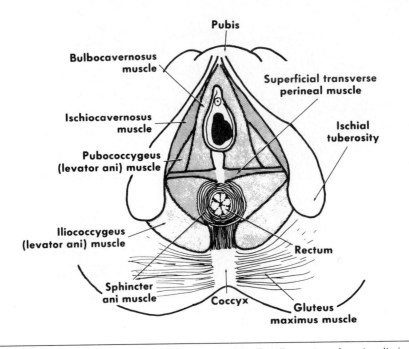

Fig. 1-7 Muscles of perineum. (From Phillips, CR: Family-centered maternity/newborn care: a basic text, ed 2 St. Louis, 1987, The CV Mosby Co.)

ified skin extend back from the clitoris. These lips have no hair but many glands.

The *clitoris* is a small elongated body of erectile tissue located just above the anterior angle of the labia minora corresponding to the penis in the male. The clitoris responds to sexual stimulation by erecting and is probably the most erotic area of the female body. Nurses should note the relationship of the clitoris to the urinary meatus and vagina. If nurses force a urinary catheter into the clitoris by mistake, they cause great pain because so many sensory nerves are found there.

The *vestibule* is the triangular space between the labia. The urethra, vagina, and Bartholin's glands open into the vestibule.

The ducts of two *Skene's glands* empty their lubricating secretions through openings on each side of the urinary meatus. On each side

of the vaginal orifice are the ducts of *Bartholin's glands*. The secretions from these and from Skene's glands are normally alkaline. These secretions maintain the constant moisture necessary for healthy mucous membranes. Aging women occasionally experience vaginitis from lack of adequate lubricants. Skene's and Bartholin's glands also are important clinically because they sometimes harbor stubborn pathogens such as yeast or *Neisseria gonorrhoeae*.

Although nurses often refer to the whole area of the external genitalia as the *perineum,* strictly speaking the perineum is the region between the vaginal orifice and the anus. The perineum is composed of muscle covered with skin and is important because it may be torn during childbirth. A deep tear may extend all the way through the perineum to the anal

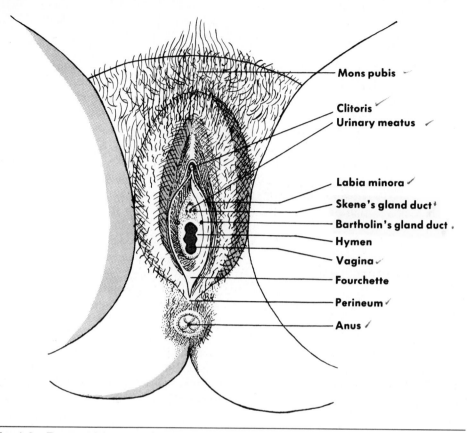

- Mons pubis
- Clitoris
- Urinary meatus
- Labia minora
- Skene's gland duct
- Bartholin's gland duct
- Hymen
- Vagina
- Fourchette
- Perineum
- Anus

Fig. 1-8 External female genitalia.

sphincter. To avoid this possibility, a controlled incision called an *episiotomy* may be made in the perineum late in labor and then repaired after childbirth.

Generative products of the female

Ova. When a girl is born, she has within her ovaries all the potential *ova* that she will ever produce. The ova lie dormant within the graafian follicles, awaiting their turn to mature. When the time comes, each ovum in its follicle grows and migrates toward the surface of the ovary. By the time the mature ovum ruptures out into the abdominal cavity, it is the largest cell in the body, about 1/125 of an inch in diameter.

The ovum consists of a mass of protoplasm with a large *nucleus* surrounded by a crown of projecting fibers called *corona radiata*. Between the corona radiata and the cytoplasm is a clear zone called the *zona pellucida* (Fig. 1-2). The large nucleus in each ovum contains 23 chromosomes, half the total number in human beings. If the ovum is not fertilized within 24 hours, it disintegrates and passes out of the uterus as waste.

Hormones. The female reproductive system is regulated by several hormones, including estrogen, progesterone, the pituitary hormones, and the prostaglandins.

Estrogen is secreted by the graafian follicles

15

of the ovary and by the placenta during pregnancy. Estrogen acts to promote female secondary sex characteristics, breast and uterine tissue growth, and uterine contractions. Estrogen inhibits lactation.

Progesterone is secreted by the corpus luteum and the placenta. Progesterone works with estrogen to prepare the endometrium for the ovum. Progesterone also promotes the growth and development of breast tissue. Unlike estrogen, progesterone helps to quiet uterine contractions. For this reason, supplementary dosages may be given to halt premature labor.

Pituitary hormones are secreted in the pituitary gland located deep in the cranium. As with other hormones, pituitary hormones are distributed by way of the blood. The three that exert powerful influence on the female reproductive system are *follicle-stimulating hormone, lutenizing hormone,* and *prolactin,* or *lactogenic hormone.* The actions of these hormones will be described in the discussion of the menstrual cycle. Progesterone and estrogen inhibit the pituitary gland from releasing these three hormones. Thus follicle growth and ovulation are prevented from occurring out of sequence. This fact provides a method of ovulation control. Most birth control pills (oral contraceptives) work on the principle that progesterone and estrogen prevent ovulation.

Prostaglandins (PG) are a recently recognized group of hormones classified as PGA, PGB, PGE, and PGF. Prostaglandins are secreted by many body tissues, most notably the prostate gland in men and the endometrium of the uterus in women. In women they affect ovulation, tubal and uterine contractions, sloughing of the endometrium, and onset of abortion and labor.

Generative functions of the female

Coitus. The purpose of the female reproductive system is to provide a suitable receptacle for the male penis at coitus and a nesting place where the fertilized ovum can grow into a baby.

During the female sexual response cycle, changes occur in the vagina that enhances fertilization. Secretions act as chemical buffers to increase sperm motility, and vaginal shape is altered to trap semen in a pool into which the cervix is immersed after orgasm.

Female sexual response cycle. The sexual response cycle in women, as in men, includes four phases: The excitement phase, plateau phase, orgasmic phase, and resolution phase (Fig. 1-3).

1. The *excitement phase* develops from any source of physical or mental stimulation. Vasocongestion of the clitoris and labia minora and majora occurs, causing the vagina to weep a serumlike lubricant within seconds of stimulation. The nipples become erect, and breast size increases.

2. During the *plateau phase,* a sudden redness of the skin, the "sex flush," appears. The clitoris swells and retracts under the clitoral sheath. The vagina lengthens and enlarges, and the outer third swells closed, forming the so-called orgasmic platform. The uterus draws up in a "tenting effect" that produces additional space near the cervix.

3. During the *orgasmic phase,* blood pressure, respiration, and heart rates are greatly increased. The clitoris, vagina, and rectum pulsate rhythmically; and the uterus contracts strongly. There may be widespread perspiration.

4. As the *resolution phase* proceeds, the uterus relaxes, allowing the cervix to dip into the seminal pool in the vaginal depths.

After organsm and with continued stimulation, the woman may return to plateau levels of response immediately and is capable of multiple orgasms.

Pregnancy. The second and most obvious function of the female reproductive system is to carry a pregnancy to term. Since this is the primary subject of this text, we simply men-tion the fact here and move on to the third function of the reproductive system: preparing the body for pregnancy.

Menstrual cycle. The menstrual cycle is a periodic series of changes that recur in the uterus and associated organs beginning at puberty and ending at menopause. The cycle varies in length from 18 to 40 days, averaging 28 days (mense means "month"). The menstrual cycle is divided into four phases that are characterized by changes in the uterine endometrium: (1) menstruation, (2) the proliferative phase, (3) the secretory or luteal phase, and (4) the premenstrual or ischemic phase.

The onset of menstruation is considered day 1 of the cycle, which is temporarily suspended during pregnancy and is affected by hormonal and emotional disturbances and a variety of diseases. The menstrual cycle is sometimes described in terms of an ovarian and a uterine cycle because of the simultaneous changes that take place in those organs. These changes occur in response to two powerful gonadotropic hormones of the anterior pituitary gland, follicle-stimulating hormone (FSH) and luteinizing hormone (LH) (Fig. 1-9).

Menstruation is the periodic discharge of a bloody fluid from the uterus, which is caused by the shedding of the endometrium. The discharge consists of disintegrated endometrial and stromal cells, old blood cells, and secretions of glands. The length of the flow averages about 5 days. At the beginning of menstruation, estrogen, progesterone, and LH blood levels are falling or are at their lowest during the cycle, and the level of FSH has just begun to rise. In the ovary, an ovum has just begun to mature in a vesicle or ovisac called the *graafian follicle.*

During the *proliferative phase,* the uterine lining grows and thickens at an eight- to tenfold rate, leveling off at ovulation. This growth is a result of an increasing level of estrogen produced by the graafian follicle as it grows

in the ovary. The proliferative phase lasts about 9 days, or until day 14 of the 28-day cycle.

The *secretory* or *luteal phase* is initiated by ovulation in response to a surge of LH from the pituitary gland. With the rupture of the ovum from the graafian follicle, a corpus luteum forms and produces great quantities of progesterone and estrogen. These hormones cause the glands in the uterine lining to widen and become tortuous. Progesterone and estrogen cause the cells of these glands to secrete thin fluid containing glycogen. The three layers of the fully mature uterine lining thus are prepared to receive and nourish a fertilized ovum should one become available. Such implantation generally occurs about 7 to 10 days after ovulation, or on day 23 of the 28-day cycle. The fertilized ovum, now a trophoblast, produces human chorionic gonadotropin, which stimulates continued production of progesterone and estrogen by the corpus luteum. These hormones help maintain the uterine lining.

If the ovum is not fertilized, the *premenstrual* or *ischemic phase* follows. The corpus luteum regresses, progesterone and estrogen levels drop, the arteries in the endometrium constrict, and the uterine lining shrinks and dies from ischemia (lack of blood). This process takes about 3 to 5 days, lasting between days 24 and 28 of the 28-day cycle. With the breaking off of small patches of necrotic endometrium and exposure of blood vessels, menstruation begins, and the cycle is repeated.

Menstrual cycle complications. The menstrual cycle is a normal process that does not have to interfere with a woman's mental or physical functioning. Ovulation results in a rather wide fluctuation of levels of powerful hormones, however, and together with the recurring menstrual periods, this may produce other effects in some women.

At ovulation some women experience *mit-*

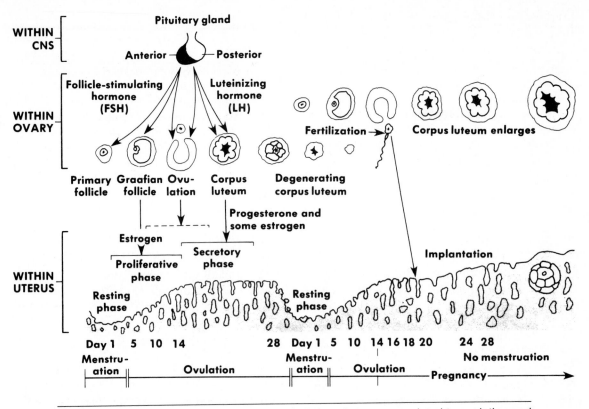

Fig. 1-9 Menstrual cycle. Cyclical changes in lining of uterus are related to ovulation and pregnancy.

telschmerz ("middle pain") caused by bleeding from the graafian follicle. The pain disappears in a few hours and serves as a signal of fertility for such women. Most women have a slight variation in body temperature and a change in cervical mucus before and after ovulation. By recording these changes, women can estimate their time of ovulation (Table 1-1).

In recent years physicians have recognized a disorder called *premenstrual tension* or *syndrome (PMS)*. The syndrome is caused by the high blood levels of progesterone that are present during the secretory phase of the menstrual cycle. Progesterone promotes sodium retention, and sodium holds water in the tis-

sue, causing weight gain, edema, and a feeling of "logginess." Low sodium intake and diuretics may be prescribed to reduce such fluid retention.

During menstruation, personal hygiene is especially important to reduce body odor and maintain a feeling of well-being. Normal activities can and should be carried on without interruption. It is not "normal" for a woman to be "sick" during menstruation. Some women, however, do experience uterine cramping, low back pain, and fatigue. Painful menstruation is termed *dysmenorrhea* and heavy, prolonged flow is termed *menorrhagia*. When these symptoms are severe

Table 1-1 Estimation of the time of ovulation

Data	Preovulation	Ovulation	2 days postovulation until menstruation
Basal body temperature (BBT)	36.2°-36.3° C (97.2°-97.4° F)	Drop of 0.1°-0.2° C (0.2°-0.3° F), followed by a rise of 0.4°-0.5° C (0.7°-0.8° F)	36.7° C (98° F)
Cervical mucus	Dry, no mucus; then clear, watery, slippery mucus with increasing *spinnbarkheit* (elasticity test)	Abundant, egg white–like mucus with spinnbarkheit, 12-24 cm, that dries in fern pattern	Cloudy, sticky, impenetrable to sperm, dries in a granular pattern

enough to interfere with normal activities, women should consult a gynecologist, a physician who specializes in disorders of the female reproductive system.

Accessory structures, function, and products

Mammary glands. The mammary glands are the milk-secreting or lactating organs of the female body and serve an important role in sexual stimulation and response (Fig. 1-10). Although breasts are present in both sexes, they normally develop and function only in the female. Breast size varies according to age and inherited characteristics and depends on the amount of fat deposited in them. There is no relation between breast size and ability to produce milk.

Each breast is composed of 16 to 20 lobes that develop embryonically as modified sweat glands. The lobes are composed of glandular tissue and fat and are separated from each other by connective tissue called *septa.* Each lobe consists of several lobules arranged in grapelike clusters around tiny ducts. Fig. 1-10 shows these clusters, which are called either *alveoli* or *acini.*

The lactating cells of the alveoli produce milk, which flows toward the nipple through the tiny ducts of the lobules and then through the larger ducts of the lobes. These ducts en-

large to form *ampullae,* which open individually through tiny holes in the nipples. The *nipple* is made of especially adapted skin surrounded by a pigmented area called the *areola.* The tiny nubs that stand out on the areola are sebaceous glands. These glands, known as *Montgomery's glands,* provide oil to protect the moistened nipple skin.

Lactation. At puberty, estrogen and progesterone cause the breasts to develop. Thus, if pregnancy occurs, the alveolar tissue is ready to produce milk. During pregnancy, the increase of these hormones further stimulates the tissue. As a result, the woman notices breast tenderness, enlargement, and oozing of a yellow liquid called *colostrum.*

Immediately after birth, the amount of progesterone and estrogen suddenly drops, triggering the pituitary gland to produce large amounts of *prolactin.* As a result, on about the third day after birth, the breasts become warm, tender, and swollen. This initial engorgement is caused by an infilling of blood and lymph, not by milk retention. In about 8 to 12 hours, the milk-secreting alveoli cells begin to function, and free-flowing, bluish white milk replaces the colostrum. During the next week, vascular engorgement gradually subsides, and milk production increases.

There are no large storage areas in the breasts. Milk is secreted in response to the

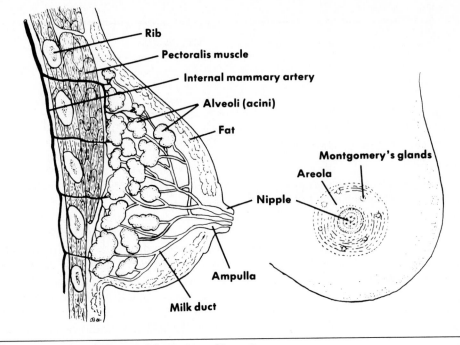

- Rib
- Pectoralis muscle
- Internal mammary artery
- Alveoli (acini)
- Fat
- Montgomery's glands
- Areola
- Nipple
- Ampulla
- Milk duct

Fig. 1-10   Cross section and front view of breast.

stimulus of nursing. After about 2 weeks, milk production averages about 120 to 180 ml per feeding. Both quantity and quality of milk are affected by the mother's diet, activities, and emotions.

Once the milk-producing cells have begun functioning, the stimulation of sucking and the regular emptying of the ducts keep them producing for many months or even years. The mother's reproductive organs, however, return to the menstrual cycle, which was suspended by the pregnancy. This means that ovulation will occur at regular intervals, and the nursing mother could become pregnant again. Many women do not know this fact, and they erroneously believe that nursing prevents pregnancy.

Products. Colostrum is the thin, golden fluid secreted by the breasts during the later months of pregnancy. This fluid is chiefly composed of serum and white blood cells from the mother's blood. Colostrum is rich in salt, protein, and fat and has a laxative effect in newborn infants. Colostrum helps infants expel the thick, sticky matter called *meconium* that fills their bowels in utero.

The composition of 100 ml of mature human milk is as follows:

75 calories
1.1 gm protein
4.0 gm fat
9.5 gm carbohydrate
87.1 ml water
0.21 gm ash
Sodium (Na)
Potassium (K)
Calcium (Ca)
Phosphorus (P)
Magnesium (Mg)
Iron (Fe)

Zinc (Zn)
Vitamin A
Vitamin B$_1$ (thiamine)
Vitamin B$_2$ (Riboflavin)
Niacin
Vitamin C (ascorbic acid)
Vitamin D
Vitamin E (alpha tocopherol)

Complications of the female sexual response cycle

Complications that affect the functioning of the female reproductive system fall into six categories: (1) orgasmic dysfunction, (2) vaginismus, (3) dyspareunia, (4) aging, (5) infertility, and (6) sterility. Infertility and sterility will be discussed in the next section.

Orgasmic dysfunction. *Primary orgasmic dysfunction* is defined as the consistent nonorgasmic response to any type of stimuli. *Situational orgasmic dysfunction* means that a woman has had at least one orgasmic response but is not presently orgasmic.

Research has established that women have a natural capacity to function sexually as well or better than men, and yet many do not. Instead they deny, repress, or distort their normal sexual responsiveness. Early social and cultural training seems to be the root cause, including neglect, ignorance, shame, denial, and occasionally actual mental or physical trauma. Rigid religious orthodoxy, prior homosexual experiences, masturbatory guilt, bad feelings about the sexual partner, or a dysfunctional partner is often part of the history.

Treatment involves both partners working with cotherapists. Therapy consists of a detailed sex history, identification of the cause, education concerning female anatomy and physiology, and individualized nondemanding exercises with concentration on mutual sensate enjoyment and deemphasis on attaining orgasm. The couple is guided toward increasing acceptance of and pleasure in their normal

sexual capacities. With anxiety gone, a high percentage of women become orgasmic.

Vaginismus. Vaginismus is a psychophysical condition in which the muscles surrounding the vagina go into involuntary spastic contraction, effectively closing the vagina, thus preventing penile entrance. A high percentage of women with this disorder have mates who are impotent. Religious orthodoxy is a major cause, but it may follow serious mental or physical trauma, fear of childbirth, painful intercourse, or homosexual orientation.

Treatment begins with identifying the cause. If there is pain caused by unrepaired tears or scar tissue, surgery may be indicated. When a physical cause of pain is ruled out, treatment consists of educating the couple about the anatomy of the female pelvis by means of charts, self-examination, and partner examination. Then the couple is provided with a set of dilating probes. In privacy and with gentleness, increasingly larger probes are introduced into the vagina until penile entrance is possible. Once coitus occurs, the condition is cured.

Dyspareunia. Dyspareunia, or painful coitus, may occur from many causes, including vaginal scarring, infection, clitoral irritation, sensitivity, broad ligament tears, pelvic inflammatory disease, endometriosis, senile or radiation vaginitis, insufficient vaginal lubrication, tumors, and mental aversion or fear. Accurate assessment of the cause or causes must be made if treatment is to be effective. When all physical causes for pain have been eliminated, the woman may need help to identify the source of her negative feelings toward coitus. Exercises that promote mutual sensate awareness may then be of value to help restore the woman's natural capacity for sexual response.

Aging. Aging is a normal part of life. Although it does cause specific changes in the female sexual response cycle, it does not necessarily impair it. This is especially true if estrogen is given to supply the deficiency caused by normal ovarian atrophy and if childbirth injuries have been properly repaired.

In general, each phase of the sexual response cycle is slowed or diminished in the aging female. There is less vaginal lubrication, less vasocongestion, and less muscle tension; vaginal size also is decreased. The clitoris continues to function as receptor and transformer of impulses, and there seems to be no reduction in sensitivity. Because women live longer than men, masturbation for sexual release is commonly practiced by older women.

FERTILITY, INFERTILITY, AND STERILITY
Fertility

Fertility is the ability to procreate. In men fertility is highest between 24 and 35 years of age who are at high levels of physical and mental health. These men have no abnormalities of the reproductive organs and have sperm counts of 90 to 300 million per milliliter, with at least 75% normal sperm forms and active sperm motility. In women fertility is highest between 20 to 30 years of age who are at high levels of physical and mental health. These women have no abnormalities of the reproductive organs or menstrual cycle and produce ova regularly.

Infertility

Infertility is the probable inability to procreate. The inability to conceive and bear children comes as a tragedy to otherwise healthy adults. For these individuals, childbearing, nurturing, and parenting are normal expectations of adult sexuality, personal fulfillment, and family responsibility. Current knowledge of infertility has increased greatly as a result of extensive research.

Normally, 65% of couples can achieve pregnancy within 6 months and 80% within 1 year. Infertility is defined as the inability to conceive after at least 1 year of adequate exposure when no contraceptive method is used. The causes of infertility are many. Male factors account totally or partly for 40% to 50% of infertility problems, female factors account for 40% to 50%, and unknown factors account for 10% to 20% of cases.

Male factors include frequency of coitus, penile insertion problems, anatomical abnormalities of the reproductive system, abnormalities of sperm or antibodies, severe nutritional deficiencies, psychological disorders, and social habits such as alcohol or drug abuse.

Female factors include anything that interferes with the development of a healthy ovum, its passage into the uterine tube, its fertilization, its implantation in the uterus, and the growth and safe delivery of the baby. Other factors involve anything that interferes with the deposit of sperm in the vagina or their passage through the vagina, cervix, uterus, and tubes to the ovum. These factors may be developmental, vaginal-cervical, uterine, tubal, ovarian, or general. General factors include serious nutritional deficiencies, endocrine disorders, psychological problems, coital problems, chronic disease states, immunological reactions to sperm, and social habits such as alcohol and drug abuse.

With so many causes for infertility, it is necessary for couples who desire to bear children to undergo extensive diagnostic study. A careful history is taken, and a complete physical examination is made of both partners. Semen is analyzed early in the diagnostic process, and the woman is asked to keep a basal body temperature record and evaluation of cervical mucus (Table 1-1). Various other tests are performed to try to identify the cause of the couple's infertility, and appropriate therapy is prescribed. Because of the complexity of the diagnosis and treatment of infertility, it has become a subspecialty of obstetrics and gynecology. Couples can be referred to local physicians or to infertility clinics found in major medical centers.

Sterility

Despite the tremendous strides that have been made in the treatment of infertility, in 5% to 10% of medically healthy couples no cause for barrenness can be found. They are said to be sterile. Sterility is the absolute inability to procreate. The irradiation or surgical removal of the reproductive organs causes sterility, as does ligation of the vas deferens in men or the uterine tubes in women. At present, ligation is not considered a reversible procedure, although plastic reconstruction may be attempted.

Sterility only refers to procreation, not to hormone production or sexual responsiveness. For example, in *vasectomy* the vas deferens is severed near the testes. This blocks the passage of sperm but does not interfere with the movement of other secretions along the seminal path nor reduce the blood level of hormones. In *tubal ligation* the uterine tubes are severed. This blocks the passage of ova or sperm but does not interfere with the production of estrogen and progesterone, which continue to enter the bloodstream. As a result, secondary sex characteristics are maintained, and the menstrual cycle continues without interruption.

▶ KEY CONCEPTS

1. Human sexuality affects both physical and psychosocial development throughout the life span.
2. Male generative products are sperm, semen, and the androgen hormones.
3. The sexual response cycle is a patterned response to sexual stimulation.
4. Complications that affect the male sexual system are impotence, ejaculatory disorders, dyspareunia, aging, infertility, and sterility.
5. Female generative products are ova and the hormones estrogen and progesterone.

6. Uterine phases of the menstrual cycle are resting, proliferation, and secretion.
7. Ovarian changes during the menstrual cycle include:
   a. Development of a primary follicle, which becomes a graafian follicle as the ova ripen
   b. Ovulation
   c. Change of the follicle into the corpus luteum, which continues on during pregnancy or disintegrates if no pregnancy occurs
8. Breast growth during pregnancy occurs in response to estrogen and progesterone. After birth, the sudden drop in these hormones triggers the pituitary gland to produce prolactin, which stimulates lactation.
9. Infertility is the probable inability to procreate. Sterility is the absolute inability to procreate.

■ ANNOTATED SUMMARY

I. Human sexuality throughout life—maleness and femaleness are pivotal factors around which people develop
   A. Childhood—sexual identity (gender role) is learned from people around child
   B. Adolescence—the period of transition from childhood to adulthood, including puberty
   C. Puberty—time reproductive system matures; typical secondary sex characteristics involve growth, hair, body odor, and menstruation or nocturnal emissions
   D. Adulthood and maturity—full development of one's potential
   E. Climacteric—the period when the reproductive organs become inactive
II. Human sexual response—typical cycle: excitement, plateau, orgasm, and resolution
III. Reproductive systems
   A. Male
      1. Generative structures of the male
         a. Testes—primary male sex organs
         b. Seminal ducts
         c. Glands—prostate gland, seminal vesicles, and bulbourethral gland
         d. External genitalia—scrotum and penis
      2. Generative products of the male
         a. Sperm—androsperm and gynosperm

b. Seminal fluid—collected secretions of the glands

c. Androgens—including testosterone

3. Generative functions of the male
   a. Coitus—copulation
   b. Male sexual response cycle

4. Complications of the male sexual response cycle
   a. Impotence—inability to maintain an erection; may be primary or secondary
   b. Ejaculatory disorders—incompetence and premature ejaculation
   c. Dyspareunia—painful coitus
   d. Aging—slows sexual response cycle but should not prevent it

B. Female
   1. Generative structures of the female
      a. Ovaries—primary female sex organs
      b. Uterine tubes—carry ova from ovaries to uterus
      c. Uterus—muscular organ divided into cervix, corpus, and fundus
      d. Vagina—canal for coitus and birth
      e. Pelvic floor—made of layers of muscles
      f. Vulva—external genitalia
   2. Generative products of the female
      a. Ova
      b. Hormones—estrogen, progesterone, and pituitary hormones
   3. Generative functions of the female
      a. Coitus—and nesting place for baby to grow
      b. Female sexual response cycle
      c. Pregnancy
      d. Menstrual cycle—consists of menstruation, proliferative phase, secretory phase, and premenstrual phase
      e. Menstrual cycle complications— mittelschmerz, premenstrual tension, dysmenorrhea, and menorrhagia
   4. Accessory structures, functions, and products
      a. Mammary glands—composed of fat, glands, and connective tissue
      b. Lactation—occurs in response to prolactin

c. Products—colostrum, then milk

5. Complications of the female sexual response cycle
   a. Orgasmic dysfunction—primary or situational nonorgasmic response
   b. Vaginismus—involuntary spastic contraction
   c. Dyspareunia—painful coitus
   d. Aging—sexual response cycle slows and secretions lessen

IV. Fertility, infertility, and sterility
   A. Fertility—ability to procreate
   B. Infertility—probable inability to procreate; the problem originates equally between men and women (40%-50%); special diagnostic workups and treatment protocols exist
   C. Sterility—absolute inability to procreate; does not affect sexual response or secondary sex characteristics

● STUDY QUESTIONS AND LEARNING ACTIVITIES

1. Cover the labels of Figs. 1-4 and 1-7 with paper and identify the parts.
2. Using a lifelike model of female pelvic anatomical parts, locate the ovaries, uterine tubes, uterus, urinary bladder, urinary meatus, clitoris, and openings of Bartholin's and Skene's glands.
3. Compare the four phases of the sexual response cycle of men and women.
4. Summarize the events of the menstrual cycle.
5. Of what is colostrum composed? What action does it have in the newborn infant?
6. Describe the sequence of events that occurs in the breasts from before pregnancy to full lactation. What hormones influence these changes?
7. Discuss infertility in men and women. Give the definition, causes, and treatment.

REFERENCES

Anthony, CP, and Thibodeau, GA: Textbook of anatomy and physiology, ed 12, St. Louis, 1988, The CV Mosby Co.

Brooks, SM, and Paynton-Brooks, N: The human body: structure and function in health and disease, ed 3, St. Louis, 1980, The CV Mosby Co.

Masters, WH, and Johnson, VE: Human sexual response, Boston, 1966, Little, Brown & Co.

CHAPTER 2

Changing Patterns of Maternal-Child Care

VOCABULARY

Cesarean birth
Childbed fever
Culture
Family
Midwives
Nurse-practitioner
Obstetrics

LEARNING OBJECTIVES

- Briefly describe some historical event in maternal-child care during the following periods: early societies, ancient Greece, the Roman Empire, Medieval Europe, the Renaissance, the early modern period, and the twentieth century.

- Define the family and describe five types of families.

- Discuss adolescent pregnancy and patients' rights.

- Define the role in maternal-child care of nurse-practitioners, childbirth educators, midwives, and obstetricians.

For the first time in history, women have control of their reproductive lives. This control affects their educational, vocational, coupling, and parenting choices. It makes possible a true partnership between men and women in planning the timing and size of their families. This sense of control profoundly affects the expectations of couples as they seek health care services for the childbearing experience. As a result, the services offered by health care providers have changed dramatically in recent years. To understand the present status of maternal-child care, it is helpful to look briefly into the past.

Obstetrics is a branch of medicine defined as the art and science of caring for the childbearing woman and her unborn baby. The word is derived from the Latin verb *obstare*, which means "to stand by." In the past, obstetric health care giving was confined to standing by the mother and adapting care to her medical treatment. The new emphasis is reflected in the term *maternal-child care*, a branch of nursing that is family centered and that assumes responsibility for the whole cycle of life, emphasizing healthful living for the entire family. Regardless of the term used or the emphasis given, some form of maternity care is as old as the human race.

HISTORY OF MATERNAL-CHILD CARE
Earliest societies

In the earliest societies, mothers naturally helped their own daughters give birth to the grandchildren. As societies became more complex, specialization increasingly grew common. Some mothers specialized in giving obstetric care, not only to their own families, but also to all who wished to employ these mothers' services because of their experience and skill. These women were called *midwives*, and their activities are mentioned in some of the oldest historical records from ancient Egypt, Mesopotamia, Palestine, Greece, and Rome.

Midwives were distinguished from physicians through ancient and medieval history because they were always women, whereas physicians were nearly always men. Midwives were concerned only with childbirth, whereas physicians were concerned with treating the sick. Physicians were rarely called to join a midwife in a maternity case unless the expectant mother was ill. In this case the physician simply treated the mother's illness while the midwife supervised delivery of the baby.

Ancient obstetrics differed from modern maternity care in its general lack of prenatal care. Unless complications of pregnancy made it necessary for a physician to treat her illness, the expectant mother usually went without any medical attention until labor began and the midwife was called. For normal deliveries this was quite satisfactory, but for abnormal ones often it was too late. Mothers with difficult deliveries usually labored hopelessly until they died.

Lack of prenatal care was caused by a lack of knowledge of the anatomy and physiology of pregnancy. Growth of such knowledge has been by slow, painstaking addition over the centuries.

Ancient Greece

The first person to attempt a study of anatomy and physiology with anything approaching a scientific attitude was Hippocrates, a Greek physician of 400 BC, who has been called "the father of medicine." In addition to setting high standards of unselfish public service for physicians, as reflected in the "Hippocratic oath," he studied many diseases and illnesses, including complications of pregnancy. In cases of breech presentation, Hippocrates advised internal cephalic version, or turning the fetus by hand while it was still in the uterus. He believed that babies could not live unless delivered head down.

The Roman Empire

Centuries later, in the Roman Empire, the work begun by Hippocrates was continued and advanced by Celsus in the early first century AD and by Soranus a century later. These men described removal of the baby through an incision in the woman's abdomen. It was a *lex caesarea*, or law of Caesar's land, that the operation be performed as a last resort to save the baby of all dying mothers; thus the procedure became known as the *cesarean birth*. Since the operation was performed on nearly exhausted women and nothing was known about aseptic technique or suturing the uterus, infection and hemorrhage caused a high maternal death rate. To help avoid this in the case of very small women, Soranus introduced a method of inducing premature labor a month or two early, while the fetus was still small enough to pass through a contracted pelvis. Soranus wrote the oldest known textbook for midwives about 120 AD. With the decline of the Roman Empire, however, his ideas were lost, and similar techniques were not rediscovered until the seventeenth century.

Medieval Europe

The medieval period in Europe was almost barren of progress in medical knowledge. Rare exceptions occurred where Europe came in contact with the more progressive Arab world. In southern Italy, where Arab influence was felt, an educated woman of Salerno named Trotula became noted as a teacher of midwives. About 1050 AD she wrote a book entitled *Diseases of Women, Before, During and After Delivery*. In Spain, too, there was some progress in medicine under Arab influence. Bishop Paulus of Merida is said to have performed a cesarean birth about 1300 AD. Elsewhere in Europe, the science of medicine languished. Speculation, superstition, and folk myths were accepted without question.

The Renaissance

A new interest in gaining scientific information by observation and experimentation came with the Renaissance. This attitude led to modern scientific methods. Dissection was introduced into the study of anatomy in the fourteenth century at the University of Bologna, Italy. Thus great progress was made during the next 2 centuries, resulting in the first careful anatomical textbook with diagrams of the entire body produced by Vesalius and such discoveries as the *fallopian tubes*, by Fallopio.

Progress was slow and costly. Advances were made against the church and other elements of society that were opposed to change. The use of human bodies for study was forbidden. Medical students and professors at Bologna had to rob graves to get bodies to dissect. Prejudice ran to such extremes that a Dr. Wertt of Hamburg, Germany, was burned at the stake in 1522 because he had disguised himself as a woman and attended a delivery to study the process of birth.

Despite such obstacles, medical science and education advanced. The first school for midwives in Germany was established in Munich in 1589; the first one in France was started in Paris in 1629. There were no professional nurses at this time; midwives performed nursing functions for their maternity patients.

Early modern period
Physiology

Fetal heart tones were discovered in 1650 by Legout, and fetal blood circulation was described in a theory advanced in 1651 by William Harvey. In 1701 van Deventer began the study of the mechanism of labor. Franz Naegele continued the study of labor in 1812, giving his name to the method of descent of the baby's head through the pelvis. He also developed *Naegele's rule* for calculating the expected date of delivery.

Forceps

Forceps for pulling the baby through the birth canal in difficult deliveries were first invented in 1580 by Peter Chamberlen in England, but the instrument was kept a family secret for over a century. Forceps were first made public in France in 1720, but many decades passed before they came into general use by the medical profession. Then, in 1860, John Braxton Hicks taught his method of pulling the baby out feet first by grasping it with the fingers instead of forceps.

Asepsis

Until the mid-nineteenth century, nothing was known of infectious microbes or the need for aseptic procedure. Physicians and other attendants spread diseases by moving directly from one patient to another. All too frequently epidemics of puerperal sepsis called *childbed fever* swept through maternity wards, causing a tragically high death rate. As a result, home delivery was preferred to hospital delivery by anyone who could afford it.

The first moves to block this scourge of infant mortality were taken in 1843 by an American doctor, Oliver Wendell Holmes, followed in 1847 by Ignaz Semmelweis in Vienna. These two men suspected that cross infection was spreading puerperal sepsis, and they required all hospital personnel to wash and disinfect their hands before they touched each patient. Both men were ridiculed, but the death rate went down dramatically in their wards. A few years later these men were vindicated by Louis Pasteur's discovery that puerperal sepsis was caused by the streptococcus bacillus. In following decades, aseptic technique became standard.

Anesthesia

Anesthesia was first introduced in obstetrics by Sir James Simpson of England in 1847 when he employed ether and chloroform to ease the mother's pain during delivery. He was bitterly attacked for this by his fellow surgeons and by the clergy. The church believed that pain in childbirth was God's punishment to woman for her part in original sin, and that to attempt to remove pain was to tamper with God's plan. Despite such prejudice, progress in anesthetics continued until pain control became an accepted practice of modern obstetrics.

The twentieth century in the United States

The dramatic expansion of medical, social, and psychological knowledge since 1900 has significantly affected maternal-child health throughout the world. Programs aimed at primary prevention of disorders, secondary prevention (treatment), and tertiary prevention (rehabilitation) have resulted.

1900 to 1918

In 1900 the Instructive Nursing Association in Boston began sending nurses to visit expectant mothers who were scheduled for delivery in the Boston Lying-In Hospital. The idea caught on elsewhere; in 1907 two visiting nurses were employed in New York by the Association for Improving Conditions of the Poor for the purpose of visiting expectant mothers in their homes. From these modest beginnings, public health prenatal care has grown to nationwide proportions.

In 1909 Theodore Roosevelt called the first White House Conference on Children and Youth. Since then, U.S. presidents have called similar conferences every 10 years to review the status of maternal-child health. Many agencies, some private and some tax supported, contributed to the growth of interest in maternal-child health care. For example, the American Association for the Study and Prevention of Infant Mortality was founded in 1910 and has held annual conferences since then. In 1912 Congress created the Children's Bureau. The bureau's research and broad responsibilities have been a major influence in improving the health and general welfare of mothers and children. The bureau has distributed millions of copies of its book *Infant Care* since it was first published in 1914.

1918 to 1941

The Maternity Center Association, a voluntary agency in New York City, was founded in 1918. This association set an example for the United States in establishing public health maternity centers for prenatal care and in making hospital care and visiting nurses available to all classes of people. The first midwifery school and clinic in the United States opened in New York City in 1931. The clinic was taken over in 1934 by the Maternity Center Association, which has continued to sponsor it to the present day. This first school was designed to educate nurse-midwives to high professional standards, as well as provide maternity care to women who preferred delivery at home and whose condition indicated that a normal birth could be expected. The association served many poorer residents of the city who could not afford the high cost of hospitals and many of the foreign-born women who were afraid to go to American hospitals for childbirth.

One of the pioneers in providing maternity

care to women in isolated areas was Mary Breckenridge, a public health nurse who went to England to obtain professional training in midwifery. In 1925 she organized the Frontier Nursing Service at Hyden, Kentucky, to provide care for the neglected people in the Appalachian Mountains. With two other nurse-midwives, she rode horseback to remote mountain areas to deliver babies and provide other nursing needs. This service continues to this day; in addition, the Frontier Nursing Service has operated a school of midwifery since 1939.

In 1925 the Joint Committee on Maternal Welfare was established. In 1935 Title V of the Social Security Act, this committee provided grants to improve the health and welfare of mothers and infants.

1941 to the present

Obstetrics in the United States began as a physician-oriented specialty, with obstetric nurses providing hospital care and public health nurses providing home care. Midwives practiced in poor and remote areas where physicians did not wish to go. Even during World War II (1941-1945), when physicians were scarce and the birthrate was high, midwifery was not widely accepted. In 1955 the American College of Nurse-Midwives was formed, setting up standards of practice and education and a national certification examination. Not until the pediatric practitioner (a relatively new role for nurses) was accepted by physicians, however, was the historical role of the nurse-midwife recognized. In 1970 the American College of Obstetricians and Gynecologists recognized the American College of Nurse-Midwives. By 1977 there were about 2,000 nurse-midwives in the United States, and midwifery was recognized legally in all but three states.

Midwifery. Despite this official recognition, midwives have not been accepted widely by the medical community. The public, however, is seeking the services of midwives in increasing numbers. Midwives provide screening and supervision during the entire pregnancy cycle: the prenatal period, birth, and the postpartum and interpregnancy periods. They manage normal pregnancies, and when complications arise, midwives call for an obstetrician. In general, there are two categories of midwives, lay and nurse midwives. Lay midwives are self-taught or have taken brief courses of study. Nurse-midwives are registered nurses, usually with master's degrees earned in one of several accredited programs in the United States and Canada. Those who qualify may seek certification from the American College of Nurse-Midwives.

Maternal-child nursing. The changing expectations of couples today are reflected in the new roles and functions of nurses who work within the medical community in hospitals, clinics, and public health agencies. These nurses include nurse-practitioners, childbirth educators, obstetric technicians, and home health aides.

Nurse-practitioners. The new nursing role that has developed to meet the need for expanded health care services is the nurse-practitioner. The term originated in 1965 with the establishment of the pediatric nurse-practitioner program at the University of Colorado. The functions of nurse-practitioners include health maintenance and disease prevention. Their duties range from taking health histories and doing physical assessments to ordering laboratory tests and prescribing medications approved by a physician.

By 1980 there were about 260 nurse-practitioner programs in the United States, some offering advanced degrees. Many nurse-practitioners are employed by private physicians, many others by clinics and community agencies, and some are in private practice. Maternal-child care nurse-practitioners provide continuity of care to mothers and infants throughout pregnancy. After delivery, they provide child health and development supervision. Their function during the pregnancy cycle is much like a midwife's except that nurse-practitioners do not deliver infants. National standards for nurse-practitioners, have not yet been established.

Childbirth educators. Childbirth educators provide educational courses for men and women in subject areas relative to the pregnancy cycle, such as Lamaze preparation for childbirth and breast-feeding techniques. These educators learn the subject matter of the courses and become certified to instruct by organizations such as The American Society for Psychoprophylaxis in Obstetrics, Inc., and LaLeche League International, Inc.

Other team members. Two new members have been added to the maternal-child health team: obstetric technicians and home health aides.

Obstetric technicians are licensed practical-vocational nurses who have received intensive education in maternity nursing beyond the basic program. These technicians are prepared to give supportive care to families in the childbearing cycle within hospitals and birth centers.

Home health aides are nurse's aides who have received special instruction in the home care of mothers and infants. These aides provide valuable assistance to new families as they move from the hospital to the home when there is no extended family to help.

Physicians, midwives, maternal-child care nurse-practitioners, registered nurses, childbirth educators, obstetric technicians, and home health aides all function within their scope of practice to provide maternity care. Their reward is the joy and challenge of develop a helping relationship with mothers and families in the experience of childbearing.

THE FAMILY

The term *family-centered maternity care* means that the focus of maternal-child services is on the family and its members.

Definition

A *family,* by definition, is a group of persons bound together by ties of blood or ideology. Each family has a *history, goals,* and accepted ways of attaining those goals called *procedures* or *norms.* The family develops certain values and beliefs on which its members base decisions. If members differ from the family-approved values, they are censured or disciplined. At least five types of families have been identified in our society: nuclear, extended, single-parent, communal, and expanded.

Types

The *nuclear family* consists of parents and their dependent children, occupying a separate dwelling from others and subsisting on the occupational earnings of the parents.

The *extended family* consists of three generations living in the same dwelling. Family centered rather than individual centered, the extended family provides acceptance and security for its members but restricts mobility and prescribes behavior.

The *single-parent family* consists of a mother or father and the dependent children. An increasingly common phenomenon of modern life, these families are socially and economically vulnerable. Tremendous burdens are placed on the responsible parent; however, unique opportunities result for the development of child-adult relationships.

The *expanded family* resembles the extended family except that more than three generations of kin may live together. These modern-day tribes have many of the same advantages and disadvantages of extended families.

The *communal family* consists of a group of persons who are not necessarily blood related and who live together for common ideological or economic purposes. The kibbutz of Israel and collective farms of China are examples. The success of communes depends on the commitment of individual members to group goals, beliefs, and norms.

Family members are connected by powerful bonds, which become even stronger during stressful events such as pregnancy. Anything that affects one member of a family affects all of the members to some degree. This interdependency and interconnectedness can be used to increase the effectiveness of health care or can be ignored, which decreases the value of the health care.

Culture

Culture is the sum of the history, goals, norms, values, and beliefs of families. In her helpful book, *Community, Culture, and Care: a Cross-Cultural Guide for Health Workers,* Ann Brownlee provides a list of questions health workers can ask to deepen their understanding of the social and cultural heritage of various groups. The questions are clustered into four categories:
1. Forms of activities
2. Forms of social relations
3. Perceptions of the world
4. Perceptions of the individual and the self
Knowledge of these aspects of a culture can give maternal-child nurses the necessary means for providing effective, nonjudgemental care.

Fathers

The father used to be the "forgotten man" during pregnancy, at the birth, and during the postpartum period. No longer is this the rule. To the modern couple, the father is a full partner with the mother in the entire childbearing and child-rearing experience. Because of this partnership, the man's perception of the event of fatherhood and his role and functions throughout the pregnancy cycle will be discussed in this text.

ADOLESCENT PREGNANCY

The teenage pregnancy rate has reached crisis proportions in the last decade, with one in ten young women becoming pregnant each year. This increase has occurred despite widespread availability of contraceptive information and services. These pregnancies are of special concern because of the consequences for young mothers and their babies.

Adolescent women are a high-risk population for complications in pregnancy. These complications occur because of inadequate nutrition, late and minimal prenatal care, and inconsistency in following medical prescriptions. As a result, perinatal mortality and maternal morbidity are much higher in teenage pregnancies than in pregnancies of women in their twenties. Early and adequate prenatal care is the best way to reduce complications of pregnancy.

Adolescents may be sexually mature, but they are not emotionally or socially mature. Adolescence is normally a stage of development in which individuals work out their own value systems and master certain major tasks. Erikson called these tasks "identity vs. intimacy." Pregnancy greatly complicates mastery of these tasks.

Pregnancy during adolescence is frequently unwanted and therefore represents a crisis of considerable proportion. Fortunately, counseling is available in many communities. Many adolescent girls decide to keep their babies instead of relinquishing them for adoption or having an abortion. The decision is legally theirs. Many young women are quite capable of child care, and others have much difficulty. All need a stable support person to help them succeed in whatever decision they make.

The single adolescent father is often forgotten, blamed, or discounted. It is a mistake to assume that he is unconcerned about the pregnant girl or the baby. If the father wants to be involved, it is important to include him in the planning of alternative solutions regarding the future of the child. By being involved in the planning, prenatal care, labor, and birth, the father may be able to understand the privileges and responsibilities of sexuality.

PATIENTS' RIGHTS

Expectant couples and individuals are beginning to realize that the rights they expect and enjoy as guests in a hotel or any other public place are not abridged when they enter a hospital as a patient. This expectation is relatively new. In 1972 the American Hospital Association adopted a "Patient's Bill of Rights" as a national standard for care. The statement was intended to give consumers of hospital services an understanding of their rights and responsibilities. Soon after, the Childbirth Education Association published the "Pregnant Patient's Bill of Rights," which is reproduced on pp. 33-34. These rights represent the point of view of modern couples who are expecting a child.

▶ *KEY CONCEPTS*

1. In the earliest societies, midwives attended women during childbirth; physicians were called on only to treat illness. No formal prenatal care was given.
2. In ancient Greece, Hippocrates advised cephalic version to avoid breech deliveries. In ancient Rome, Soranus wrote the oldest known textbook for midwives. He described induction of premature labor when a woman had a contracted pelvis. The law of Caesar required an abdominal incision as a last resort to save infants of dying mothers. The procedure is still called a cesarean birth.
3. The medieval period was barren of progress in maternal-child care. With the Renaissance, the study of anatomy and physiology brought such knowledge as fallopian tubes, fetal blood circulation, and the mechanism of labor. Forceps were used first in England, and asepsis was introduced by Holmes, an American. Anesthesia

was introduced in 1847 in England but was denounced as against God's will.
4. In the United States, home care of mothers and infants began in 1900 in Boston. The Maternity Center Association was founded in New York in 1918 and the first school of midwifery in 1931. Maternal-child care was taken over by physicians. Only recently has midwifery gained legal and profession status in response to popular demand for personal rights. Now new roles are emerging, including maternal-child nurse practitioners, childbirth educators, obstetric technicians, and home health aides.
5. A family is a group of persons bound together by ties of blood or ideology. The family has a history, goals, procedures, and norms; culture is the sum of all these factors. Families may be nuclear, extended, single-parent, expanded, or communal.
6. Today the father is included in all phases of the pregnancy cycle.
7. Adolescent pregnancy is of epidemic proportions in the United States today, occurring in one of every ten adolescents. Teenage pregnancy produces serious physical, psychological, and social consequences.
8. In 1972 the American Hospital Association published a "Patient's Bill of Rights" and the Childbirth Education Association published the "Pregnant Patient's Bill of Rights."

■ *ANNOTATED SUMMARY*

Control of reproduction has affected expectations of young adults as they seek health care services.
Obstetrics is a branch of medicine; maternal-child care is a branch of nursing.
  I. History of maternal-child care
    A. Earliest societies—midwifery developed from need, but lack of knowledge of anatomy and physiology and prenatal care cost lives when there were complications.
    B. Ancient Greece—Hippocrates studied anatomy and physiology; set high standards for medical practice; and advised internal cephalic version for breech presentations.
    C. The Roman Empire—cesarean birth was a legal requirement to save babies of dying mothers; Soranus recommended induction

The Pregnant Patient's Bill of Rights

1. *The Pregnant Patient has the right,* prior to the administration of any drug or procedure, to be informed by the health professional caring for her of any potential direct or indirect effects, risks or hazards to herself or her unborn or newborn infant which may result from the use of a drug or procedure prescribed for or administered to her during pregnancy, labor, birth or lactation.

2. *The Pregnant Patient has the right,* prior to the proposed therapy, to be informed, not only of the benefits, risks and hazards of the proposed therapy but also of known alternative therapy, such as available childbirth education classes which could help to prepare the Pregnant Patient physically and mentally to cope with the discomfort or stress of pregnancy and the experience of childbirth, thereby reducing or eliminating her need for drugs and obstetric intervention. She should be offered such information early in her pregnancy in order that she may make a reasoned decision.

3. *The Pregnant Patient has the right,* prior to the administration of any drug, to be informed by the health professional who is prescribing or administering the drug to her that any drug which she receives during pregnancy, labor and birth, no matter how or when the drug is taken or administered, may adversely affect her unborn baby, directly or indirectly, and that there is no drug or chemical which has been proven safe for the unborn child.

4. *The Pregnant Patient has the right* if Cesarean section is anticipated, to be informed prior to the administration of any drug, and preferably prior to her hospitalization, that minimizing her and, in turn, her baby's intake of nonessential pre-operative medicine will benefit her baby.

5. *The Pregnant Patient has the right,* prior to the administration of a drug or procedure, to be informed if there is NO properly controlled follow-up research which has established the safety of the drug or procedure with regard to its direct and/or indirect effects on the physiological, mental and neurological development of the child exposed, via the mother, to the drug or procedure during pregnancy, labor, birth or lactation—(this would apply to virtually all drugs and the vast majority of obstetric procedures).

6. *The Pregnant Patient has the right,* prior to the administration of any drug, to be informed of the brand name and generic name of the drug in order that she may advise the health professional of any past adverse reaction to the drug.

continued.

of labor in mothers with contracted pelvises and wrote a textbook for midwives.

D. Medieval Europe—progress occurred only where Arab influence was felt; Trotula, teacher of midwives, wrote a book about diseases related to childbearing.

E. The Renaissance—anatomy studied at University of Bologna; Fallopio discovered uterine tubes; a German male physician was executed for observing a birth; the first school for midwives was established in Munich in 1589.

F. Early modern period
   1. Physiology—Legout discovered fetal heart tones; Harvey described fetal blood circulation; van Deventer began study of the mechanism of labor; Naegele named descent of head through pelvic and devised a rule for calculating expected date of delivery.
   2. Forceps—invented in England in 1580; kept secret until 1720.
   3. Asepsis—childbed fever (puerperal sepsis) spread reduced by handwashing, which was initiated by Holmes in the

---

The Pregnant Patient's Bill of Rights—cont'd

7. *The Pregnant Patient has the right* to determine for herself, without pressure from her attendant, whether she will accept the risks inherent in the proposed therapy or refuse a drug or procedure.
8. *The Pregnant Patient has the right* to know the name and qualifications of the individual administering a medication or procedure to her during labor or birth.
9. *The Pregnant Patient has the right* to be informed, prior to the administration of any procedure, whether the procedure is being administered to her for her or her baby's benefit (medically indicated) or as an elective procedure (for convenience or teaching purposes).
10. *The Pregnant Patient has the right* to be accompanied during the stress of labor and birth by someone she cares for, and to whom she looks for emotional comfort and encouragement.
11. *The Pregnant Patient has the right* after appropriate medical consultation to choose a position for labor and for birth which is least stressful to her baby and to herself.
12. *The Obstetric Patient has the right* to have her baby cared for at her bedside if her baby is normal, and to feed her baby according to her baby's needs rather than according to the hospital regimen.
13. *The Obstetric Patient has the right* to be informed in writing of the name of the person who actually delivered her baby and the professional qualifications of that person. This information should also be on the birth certificate.
14. The Obstetric Patient has the right to be informed if there is any known or indicated aspect of her or her baby's care or condition which may cause her or her baby later difficulty or problems.
15. *The Obstetric Patient has the right* to have her and her baby's hospital medical records complete, accurate, and legible and to have these records, including Nurses' Notes, retained by the hospital until the child reaches at least the age of majority, or, alternatively, to have the records offered to her before they are destroyed.
16. *The Obstetric Patient,* both during and after her hospital stay, *has the right* to have access to her complete hospital medical records, including Nurses' Notes, and to receive a copy upon payment of a reasonable fee and without incurring the expense of retaining an attorney.

Prepared by Doris Haire, Chairperson, Committee on Health Law and Regulation, International Childbirth Education Association.

U.S. and Semmelweis in Vienna; Pasteur discovered streptococcus bacillus as cause.
4. Anesthesia—first introduced by Simpson in England in 1847 to ease pain of childbirth.
G. The twentieth century in the United States—dramatic expansion of medical, social, and psychological knowledge occurred.
   1. 1900 to 1918—Instructive Nursing Association in Boston initiated visiting nurse services to expectant mothers; first White House Conference on Children and Youth in 1909; Children's Bureau created in 1912.
   2. 1918 to 1941—Maternity Center Association founded in New York City to give prenatal care; first school for midwives in the U.S.; Mary Breckenridge organized Frontier Nursing Service in Hyden, KY.; Social Security begun in 1935, provided grants to improve conditions for mothers and infants.
   3. 1941 to the present—scarcity of medical care for women during WWII, but no acceptance of midwifery; American college of Nurse-Midwives founded in

1955, recognized by American College of Obstetricians and Gynecologists in 1970; rapid in public acceptance and use.

   a. Midwifery—provides screening and supervision during entire pregnancy cycle, including birth; two types—lay-midwife and nurse-midwife; American College of Nurse-Midwives grants certification.

   b. Maternal-child nursing—emphasis on family; nurses working within traditional medical agencies.

     (1) Nurse-practitioners—new role for registered nurses with advance study in specialty area; same as midwives, except do not deliver babies

     (2) Childbirth educators—instructors of special courses for parents such as Lamaze and breast-feeding techniques

     (3) Other team members—obstetric technicians who are LVNs or LPNs with additional education; home health aides who provide home care

     (4) Whole team works together to foster healthy family members

II. The family

   A. Definition—a group of persons bound together by ties of blood or ideology, having a common history, goals, and norms; the family is characterized by interdependency and interconnectedness.

   B. Types

     1. Nuclear—parents and dependent children

     2. Extended—three generations living together

     3. Single-parent—a mother or father and dependent children

     4. Expanded—more than three generations living together

     5. Communal—a group of persons not necessarily related by blood

   C. Culture—the sum of the history, goals, norms, values, and beliefs of families; health workers need to ask four categories of questions to understand a culture more fully—forms of activities, forms of social relations, perceptions of the world, and perceptions of the self and individual.

   D. Fathers—once forgotten during pregnancy, they are now active participants.

III. Adolescent pregnancy—incidence has doubled in last 10 years; adolescent mothers and their babies are high-risk patients; fathers need to be included if they choose.

IV. Patients' rights—no longer content to be treated as objects, patients now have many rights.

● **STUDY QUESTIONS AND LEARNING ACTIVITIES**

1. Many of today's common terms or events stem from persons or events in history. Define the following terms and identify the historical predecessor of each: Hippocratic oath, cesarean birth, fallopian tubes, Naegele's rule, Braxton Hicks' contractions.

2. Compare the parenting expectations of young couples today to those of your parents and grandparents.

3. Discuss the problems and privileges of child rearing in a single-parent, nuclear, and communal family.

4. List some of the special hazards of adolescent pregnancy.

5. Investigate your local hospital's policies on the rights of maternity patients. How do they compare with those identified by the International Childbirth Education Association?

REFERENCES

Anderson GD: Comprehensive management of the pregnant teenager, Contemp Obstet Gynecol 7:75, 1976.

Anderson S, Bauwens E, and Warner E: The choice of home birth in a metropolitan county in Arizona, JOGN Nurs 7:41, 1978.

Anisfeld E, and Lipper E: Early contact, social support, and mother-infant bonding, Pediatrics 72(1):79, 1983.

Brownlee AT: Community, culture, and care: a cross-cultural guide for health workers, St. Louis, 1978, The CV Mosby Co.

Erikson EH: Childhood and society, ed 2, New York, 1963, WW Norton.

Haire DB: The pregnant patients' bill of rights, J Nurse-Midwifery 20:29, 1975.

Horn M, and Manion J: Creative grandparenting, bonding the generations, JOGN Nurs 3:233, 1984.

Klaus MH, and Kennell JH: Parent-infant bonding, ed 2, St. Louis, 1981, The CV Mosby Co.

Miller MA, and Brooten DA: The childbearing family: a nursing perspective, Boston, 1977, Little, Brown & Co.

Phillips CR, and Anzalone JT: Fathering: participation in labor and birth, St. Louis, 1982, The CV Mosby Co.

UNIT TWO

THE MOTHER, FATHER, AND DEVELOPING CHILD

CHAPTER 3
Embryonic and Fetal Growth

VOCABULARY

Chromosomes
Embryo
Fetal death
Fetus
Gestation
Mitosis
Nidation

LEARNING OBJECTIVES

- Describe the processes of ovulation, insemination, and conception.

- Describe the stages of growth of the fertilized ovum from conception to fetus.

- Describe the growth of the placenta from its embryonic beginnings.

- Describe the hormones produced by the placenta.

- Discuss placental transfer, amniotic fluid, and fetal circulation.

- Explain how inherited characteristics are passed on from generation to generation.

- Define Mendel's law.

- Discuss how and when sex is determined.

- Explain the difference between identical and fraternal twins, and state how frequently twins occur in the population.

- Define an ovum, embryo, and fetus.

- Define live birth, stillbirth, and fetal death, and identify the gestational age that is considered legal "life."

GERMINAL STAGE (1 TO 10 DAYS)
Conception

Conception is the union of an ovum and a sperm. However, for conception to occur, two other events must happen first: ovulation and insemination.

Ovulation is the rupture of the ovum from its follicle in the ovary (Fig. 3-1). The liberated ovum usually passes into the uterine tube. Undulation of the tube and ciliary action move the ovum along the tube. If the ovum fails to meet sperm within 48 hours, the ovum dies and dissolves.

Insemination is the expulsion of semen from the male urethra into the female vagina. Several million sperm enter the female reproductive tract with each ejaculation of semen. By lashing their tails, and with some assistance from muscular contractions of surrounding structures, the sperm travel through the uterus and into the fallopian tubes at a rate of about 1 foot per hour. The sperm live for several days, swimming about like a school of fish. If ovulation occurs during those days, the ovum will be fertilized soon after leaving the ovary.

Some evidence suggests that at least 50 million sperm are needed to secrete enough of

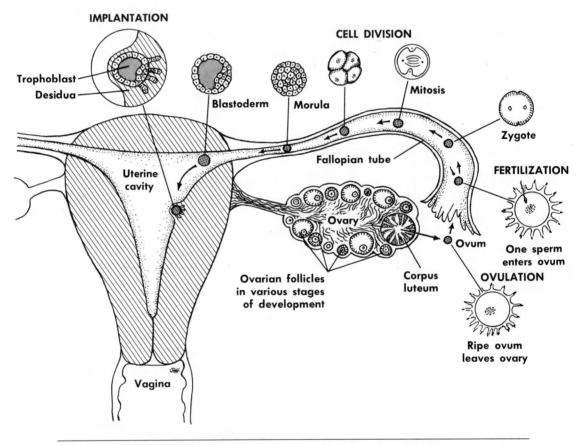

Fig. 3-1 Ovulation, fertilization, and implantation sequence.

the enzyme hyaluronidase to dissolve the corona radiata ("radiate crown") that surrounds the ovum. Once this barrier is removed, a single sperm may enter the ovum. In a process as yet unexplained, the surface of the ovum immediately changes and seals out any more sperm, thus preventing an abnormal chromosome number.

Zygote formation

As the single sperm enters the ovum, the tail drops off, and the head swells to form the male pronucleus. The nucleus of the ovum is the female pronucleus. The two nuclei, with their 23 chromosomes each, fuse and form the first cell, which will later divide into trillions. Each of these cells contains 46 chromosomes. Together these cells form the new individual. This first new cell is called the *zygote*.

Cell division (cleavage)

List new cell.

About 24 hours after conception, the zygote undergoes division, or cleavage, by an interesting process called *mitosis*. The nucleus of the zygote contains 46 chromosomes. These chromosomes line up in pairs; each splits lengthwise and then divides in half, making two identical sets of 46 chromosomes for the two new cells that are formed from the first. All future cell division of the body follows this fascinating process.

Morula to blastula

The ovum divides and divides again every 12 to 15 hours as it slowly moves down the fallopian tube. Soon the ovum resembles a mulberry, or *morula*, as it is called. About 6 days later, when the ovum reaches the uterine cavity, considerable change has occurred inside. The cells have arranged themselves into an outer layer and an inner cluster of cells that projects into the cavity. Fluid fills the space between this layer and cluster. This structure is now called the blastoderm, or *blastula*.

Implantation (nidation)

As the blastula tumbles into the uterine cavity, it loses its outer membrane, which is called the zona pellucida. The blastula then prepares to undergo *nidation*, or implantation, in the endometrium. The outer layer of cells, the *trophoblast*, secretes proteolytic enzyme, which dissolves some of the endometrium. Trophoblastic cells then absorb the product. In this way the ovum buries itself in the uterine lining and is nourished by it.

Endometrial nest

By the time nidation occurs, the mother's uterus has reached the premenstrual-secretory stage and is at the height of its vascularity. Such an environment is ideal for the embedding of the ovum, which is like a tiny parasite. The endometrium is now called the *decidua,* and the area directly under the trophoblast is called the *decidua basalis*. Normally the implantation site is in the anterior or posterior fundal region of the uterus.

EMBRYONIC STAGE (10 DAYS TO 8 WEEKS)

By the end of the second week of gestation, the ovum is completely buried, and trophoblastic cells surrounding it begin to form the *chorion,* or outermost sac. The chorion sends out thousands of projections called *villi*, which invade the decidua and lay the groundwork for the placenta. Villi function as minute roots in the rich "soil" of maternal tissue. Cytotrophoblastic cells in the chorion produce *human chorionic gonadotropin (hCG)*. This hormone is excreted in the woman's urine and serves as the basis for most tests for pregnancy.

While these changes are going on outside, tremendous changes are taking place inside the ovum. Two cavities have appeared in the ball of cells. A new layer of cells called the *mesoderm* (middle skin) has grown over the original lining, passing between the two new cavities. The more central cavity, the *yolk sac,*

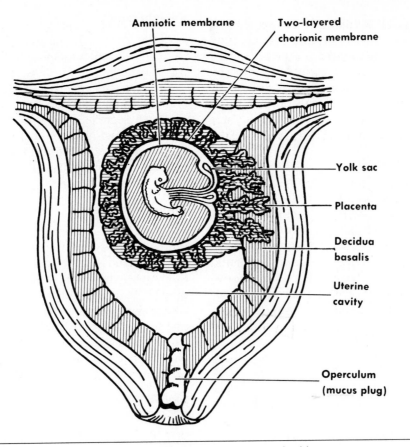

Fig. 3-2 Developing embryo 1 month old.

will ultimately disappear, since it serves no useful purpose in humans. The other cavity, the *amniotic cavity,* will soon enclose the embryo.

Embryonic disc

Now there are three layers of cells lying between the yolk sac and the amniotic cavity. Together these layers form the *embryonic disc,* from which the entire body is ultimately formed. The *ectoderm* (the outermost layer of the amniotic cavity) will become the skin, the nervous system, and the sense organs. The *mesoderm* (the middle layer) primarily will become the musculoskeletal, circulatory, and genitourinary systems. The *entoderm* or *endoderm* (the innermost layer) will become the respiratory and gastrointestinal tracts as well as the urinary bladder and part of other body systems. All the body systems are the result of complex embryonic infoldings of one layer of tissue on another.

Chorionic vesicle growth

The embryo develops from the body stalk within the amniotic cavity. A membrane, the *amnion,* lines the cavity, which normally contains a watery liquid called *amniotic fluid,* in which the embryo safely floats. A second membrane, the *chorion,* is completely covered by an outer layer of villi. All these structures are buried beneath the uterine decidua and are now called the *chorionic vesicle*. As the embryo and chorion increase in size, they grow toward the uterine cavity, pushing aside the decidua that covered them (Fig. 3-2). The chorionic villi on that side also disappear, leaving only the villi on the original implantation site. This area will become the placenta.

By the end of the seventh week of gestation, all the essential body systems are present. The fetal stage involves growth and maturity of structures begun in the embryonic stage.

Umbilical vessels and placenta

The chorionic projections become numerous and branched, dipping into large maternal blood spaces or sinuses. Each projection is covered by millions of microscopic villi that contain blood capillaries. The capillaries unite to form larger and larger veins until finally they join to form one large vessel, the *umbilical vein*. Fetal blood is sent back to the placenta through two *umbilical arteries*. In 1%

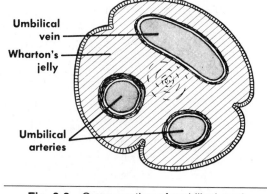

Fig. 3-3 Cross section of umbilical cord.

of infants there is only one umbilical artery; a high percentage of these infants fail to survive or have serious defects.

The umbilical vein and arteries are enclosed in the umbilical cord. The cord is filled with a gelatinous substance called *Wharton's jelly*, which helps prevent kinking. The cord is an elongation of the body stalk of early embryonic development and is about 2 feet long at term (Fig. 3-3).

The *placenta* consists of a maternal portion (decidua basalis) and a fetal portion (chorionic

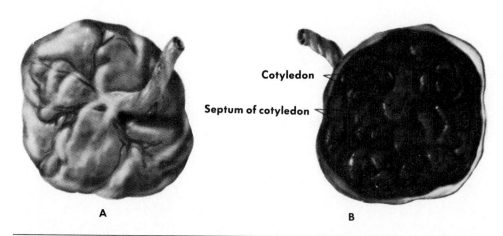

A

B

Fig. 3-4 Placenta. **A,** Fetal surface. **B,** Maternal surface. (From Placental circulation, Nursing Education Aid No 2, Ross Laboratories, Columbus, Ohio.)

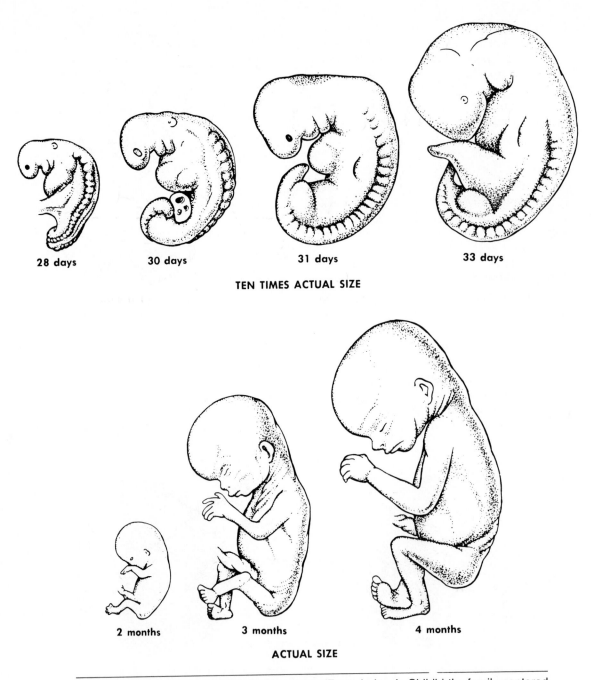

28 days   30 days   31 days   33 days

TEN TIMES ACTUAL SIZE

2 months   3 months   4 months

ACTUAL SIZE

Fig. 3-5 Embryonic and fetal development. (From Iorio, J: Childbirth: family-centered nursing, ed 3, St. Louis, 1975, The CV Mosby Co.)

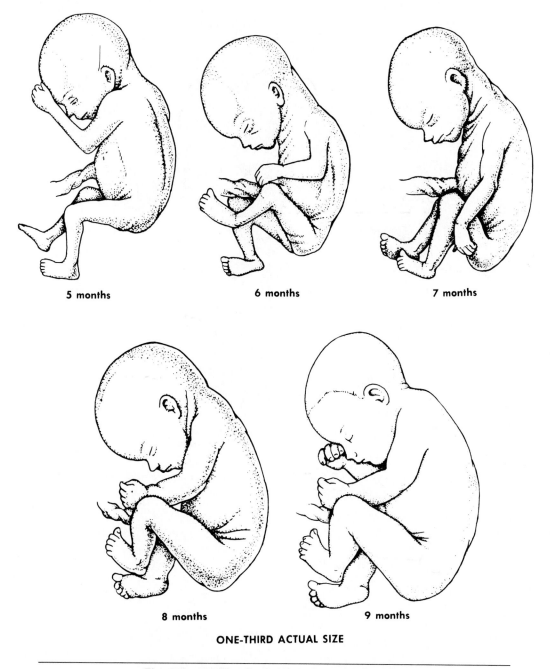

5 months   6 months   7 months

8 months   9 months

ONE-THIRD ACTUAL SIZE

Fig. 3-5, cont'd. For legend see opposite page.

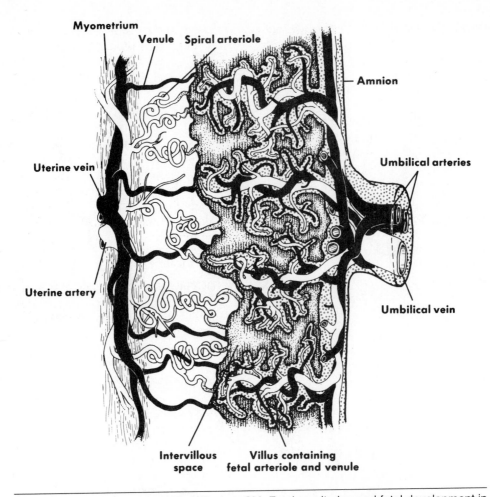

Myometrium

Venule   Spiral arteriole

Amnion

Uterine vein

Umbilical arteries

Uterine artery

Umbilical vein

Intervillous   Villus containing
space   fetal arteriole and venule

Fig. 3-6   Placental transfer. (From Tucker, SM: Fetal monitoring and fetal development in high-risk pregnancy, St. Louis, 1978, The CV Mosby Co.)

villi). The maternal surface is deep red and divided into sections (*cotyledons*). The fetal surface is covered with the amniotic membrane and is smooth and grayish in color with prominent blood vessels. Usually the umbilical cord comes from the center of the placenta (Fig. 3-4).

At term the placenta weighs about 1 pound. The placenta is getting "old" by term, and areas of dead tissue, called *infarcts*, appear in it. The function of this amazing organ during pregnancy is to provide hormones for the mother and nutrients and oxygen for the infant. At birth that function is complete. Soon after birth the placenta separates from the endometrium and slips out of the uterus, its essential role fulfilled.

PROGRESSIVE DEVELOPMENT

The progressive development of the embryo from the fourth week to birth is illustrated in Fig. 3-5 and described in Table 3-1. Growth and development continue from conception in an orderly sequence, as a total process, and in a predictable pattern.

Postmaturity (pregnancy beyond 42 weeks)

About one in eight babies is not born when he or she is "ready" but stays on beyond the normal time. Surprisingly, these babies are not better off for having remained in their watery prison. They appear "wasted" because of loss of subcutaneous fat. Their skin is dry and parchmentlike; the vernix caseosa is gone. Their fingernails and hair are long, and skin may be stained with meconium. Postmature infants typically appear alert and wide-eyed, an ominous indication of chronic need for intrauterine oxygen.

Perinatal mortality is higher in postmature infants than those born at term. Approximately 75% to 85% die during labor. Their poor condition is caused by progressive dysfunction of the aging placenta. The placenta has become less and less efficient in providing the fetus with necessary food and oxygen. Postmature infants are cared for as high-risk babies.

To prevent such risk, when the calculated length of the pregnancy seems accurate, after 42 weeks the physician may elect to induce labor or perform a cesarean delivery.

RELATED FACTS
Placental transfer

Maternal and fetal blood flow through two different systems; they do not freely mix. Three tissue layers separate these two blood flows: (1) fetal trophoblastic tissue, (2) connective tissue, and (3) endothelial tissue of fetal capillaries (Fig. 3-6). Any substance that passes between mother and fetus must cross these permeable tissue layers. Although called the *placental barrier,* these tissues do not stop all harmful substances from entering fetal cir-

culation, as was once believed. Rather, the tissues serve as a filter through which all substances move. Oxygen passes from the maternal side to the fetal side, that is, from the area of higher concentration to the area of lower concentration. Nutrients pass from the mother to the fetus and waste products from the fetus to the mother.

On the maternal side of the barrier, uterine arteries bring blood into the intervillous spaces and uterine veins carry blood away. On the fetal side, umbilical arteries bring blood into the area and the umbilical vein returns blood to the fetus.

Placental hormones

The placenta, which develops from the chorionic projections, is not only the food source and purifier of the fetus. The placenta is also a temporary endocrine gland, secreting hormones essential for maintenance of the pregnancy. By the end of the second week of gestation, as mentioned earlier, cytotrophoblastic cells in the chorion secrete human chorionic gonadotropin (hCG), which helps maintain the corpus luteum.

About the fourth month of gestation, the developing pregnancy requires more progesterone and estrogen than the corpus luteum can supply. At that time the placenta takes over and produces more than 50 times the nonpregnant levels of these hormones. The corpus luteum then shrivels and ceases to function.

By the fourth week of gestation, *human placental lactogen (hPL)* can be detected. This hormone continues to be produced throughout pregnancy, preparing the mother's body for lactation.

Estrogen and progesterone are of major importance during pregnancy. The *estrogens:*
1. Thicken the uterine muscle wall
2. Greatly enhance uterine blood supply
3. Enlarge the breasts
4. Facilitate embryonic development.

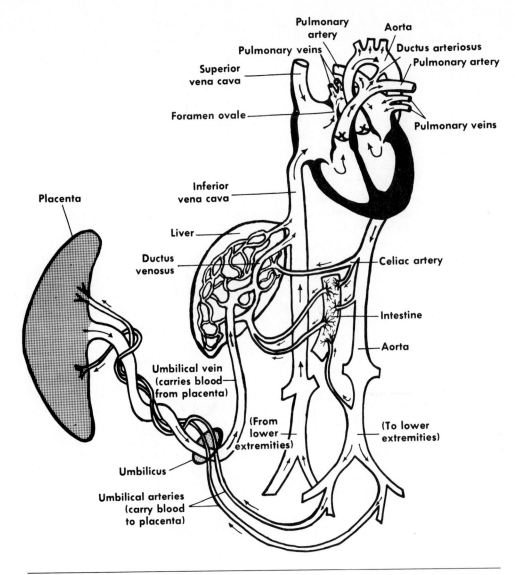

Fig. 3-7 Fetal circulation.

Progesterone:
1. Prevents ovulation
2. Aids in the development of the endometrium

3. Relaxes the uterine musculature until labor begins
4. Readies specialized cells of the breasts for milk production.

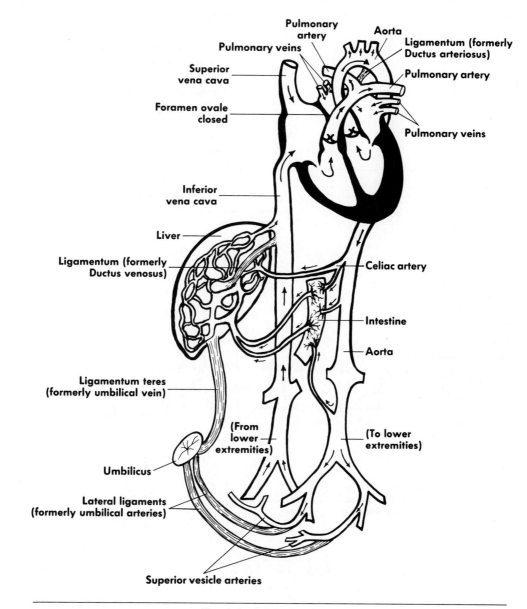

Fig. 3-8 Adult circulation.

Amniotic fluid

The amount of amniotic fluid gradually increases until at full term the fetus is immersed in about 1,000 ml. This fluid is slightly alkaline and composed of 98% water and numerous other elements during pregnancy, including urea, epithelial cells, fat, bilirubin, fructose, and albumin. Amniotic fluid:

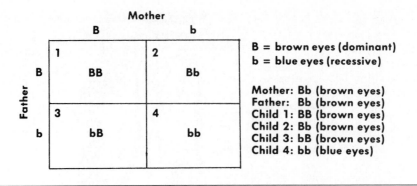

Mother

	B	b
B	**1** BB	**2** Bb
b	**3** bB	**4** bb

Father

B = brown eyes (dominant)
b = blue eyes (recessive)

Mother: Bb (brown eyes)
Father: Bb (brown eyes)
Child 1: BB (brown eyes)
Child 2: Bb (brown eyes)
Child 3: bB (brown eyes)
Child 4: bb (blue eyes)

Fig. 3-9 Punnett square demonstrating the application of Mendel's law of inheritance to recessive trait that causes blue eyes when both parents carry trait.

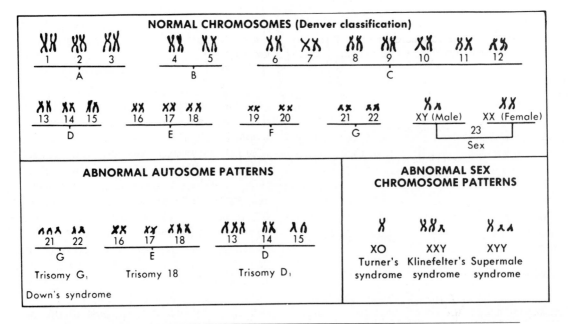

Fig. 3-10 Idiogram of normal chromosomes and some abnormal autosome and sex chromosome patterns. (From Hamilton, PM: Basic pediatric nursing, ed 5, St. Louis, 1987, The CV Mosby Co.)

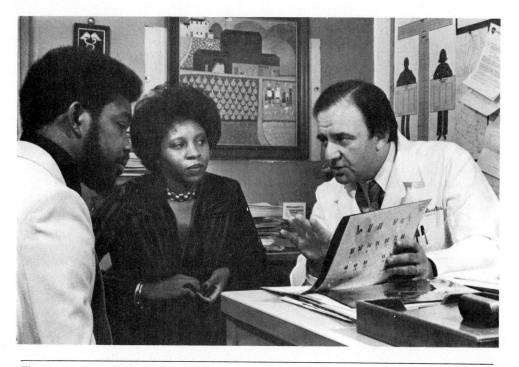

Fig. 3-11 A young married couple, who have had an infant with a major birth defect, confer with a genetic counselor physician over the advisability of having another child. (Courtesy The National Foundation–March of Dimes.)

1. Protects the fetus from trauma and heat loss
2. Allows freedom of movement, permitting symmetrical growth and musculoskeletal development
3. Acts as an excretion-secretion system
4. Is a source of oral fluid for the fetus

Analysis of this amazing fluid by amniocentesis has made prenatal detection of some disorders possible. (See Chapter 6.)

Fetal circulation

The fetus does not need the liver (a nutrition factory) or lungs (an oxygen exchange center) but instead uses the mother's. Three specially provided shunts route most fetal blood past these organs: (1) the ductus venosus, which runs straight through the liver; and (2) the foramen ovale and(3) ductus arteriosus, which bypass the lungs (Fig. 3-7).

Blood, rich with oxygen and nutrients, leaves the placenta through the umbilical vein. The blood is then diverted through the liver to the inferior vena cava by way of the *ductus venosus*. This diversion avoids the portal system of the liver. On reaching the heart, the blood next bypasses the nonfunctioning lungs by flowing through the *foramen ovale*, an opening between the left and right atria. A third shunt is a short vessel called the *ductus arteriosus*, which diverts most of the blood from the pulmonary arteries directly into the aorta.

The fetal heart pumps the blood at a rate of

120 to 160 beats per minute to the body. The blood pressure in the arteries is approximately 60/35 mm Hg.

At birth, atmospheric pressure forces air into the infant's lungs. The umbilical cord is severed and tied, and the umbilical vessels within the infant wither from disuse. The three shunts that controlled fetal circulation close because of the changes in blood pressure. Fetal circulation then becomes the same as adult circulation (Fig. 3-8).

Heredity and sex determination
Transmission of traits

All the inherited characteristics and sex of a baby are fixed at the moment of conception when the male sex cell, the sperm, enters the female sex cell, the ovum. At that time the two cells, with their 23 chromosomes each, fuse to form the first cell. This cell will divide later into trillions of differentiated cells that together will make a new individual.

Each one of those trillions of cells, whatever its function, will contain a nucleus with 46 chromosomes that are exactly like the original 46. These chromosomes are composed of nucleoprotein, a compound consisting of protein, ribonucleic acid (RNA), and deoxyribonucleic acid (DNA). These substances are the means whereby inherited traits pass from generation to generation.

Genes

The basic units of the chromosomes are genes, a portion of a DNA molecule. Genes are arranged along the chromosomes like beads on a string, each occupying a definite and constant position called a *locus*. Each human trait is produced by a gene from the mother and one from the father.

Dominance

At cell division the 23 chromosomes from the mother pair off with the corresponding 23 chromosomes from the father, causing the pairs of genes to lie opposite each other.

If two genes produce exactly the same characteristic, such as blue eyes, the genes are called *homozygous*. The child then will have blue eyes. If the genes are contrasting, such as one for blue and one for brown, the genes are called *heterozygous*. The brown one will assert itself as dominant over the recessive one, thus causing the child's eyes to be brown. However, the child will be a carrier of the recessive blue-eye gene and can pass on that gene.

In this manner a defect may be passed from generation to generation, never appearing until, by chance, it is paired with a similar gene from the other parent.

Mendel's law

The phenomenon that genes remain unchanged and are passed on in a predictable pattern was first reported by Gregor Johannes Mendel (1822-1884), an abbot in a monastery in Moravia. According to Mendel's law, when the father and mother carry a recessive gene, one fourth of their children will have a trait, two fourths will be carriers but not exhibit the trait, and one fourth will not carry the gene (or trait) at all. A later geneticist, R.C. Punnett, developed a square to portray graphically Mendel's law (Fig. 3-9).

Sex determination

The sex of an individual is determined by the type of spermatozoon that fertilizes the ovum. If an ovum is fertilized by a gynosperm containing a X chromosome, the zygote will have two X chromosomes and will be female. If an ovum is fertilized by an androsperm containing a Y chromosome, the zygote will have a Y and an X chromosome and will be male.

Father	Mother
X (gynosperm) + X (ovum)	= XX = girl
Y (androsperm) + X (ovum)	= YX = boy

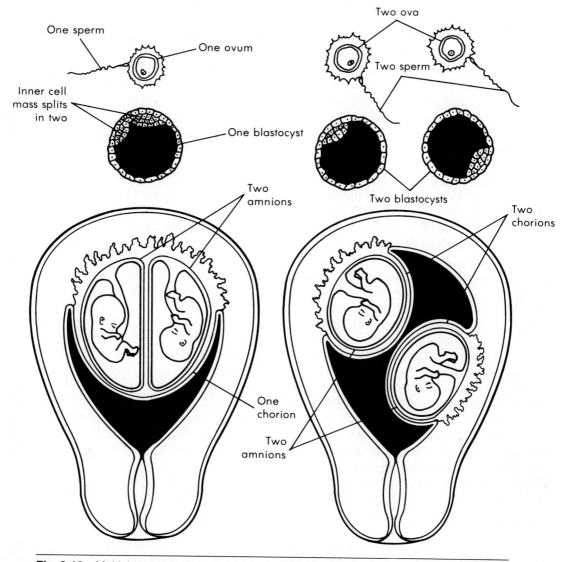

One sperm

One ovum

Two ova

Two sperm

Inner cell mass splits in two

One blastocyst

Two blastocysts

Two amnions

Two chorions

One chorion

Two amnions

Fig. 3-12 Multiple pregnancies. **A,** Identical twins develop from one ovum and one sperm. **B,** Fraternal twins develop from two ova and two sperm.

Karyotyping

In recent years geneticists have been able to photograph the nuclei of human cells and to enlarge them sufficiently to visualize the 46 chromosomes. This technique is called *karyotyping,* or "nucleus picturing." When the scrambled 46 chromosomes are clipped from the photograph and arranged into matching pairs from the largest to the smallest, the resulting picture is called a *karyotype.* An artist's drawing of this picture is called an *idiogram* (Fig. 3-10).

A normal person has a karyogram that shows 22 pairs of chromosomes called *autosomes* and one pair of *sex chromosomes*. In the female, pair 23 appears as XX. In the male, pair 23 consists of one X about the size of pair 12 and one Y, and the pair is designated XY.

Abnormalities

Karyotyping has demonstrated that several serious birth defects are caused by abnormal forms or numbers of chromosomes (Fig. 3-10). One of the first autosome or nonsex chromosomes defects to be identified was a disorder called *trisomy 21*. This name means that three chromosomes occur in the twenty-first place instead of two. Trisomy 21 causes a condition characterized by mental retardation and a flat facial appearance, called Down's syndrome, or mongolism. Other autosomal defects have been identified, including trisomy 18, trisomy D_1, and mosaicism, a mixture of abnormal forms. All these cause severe developmental defects.

Defects of the sex chromosomes are numerous. Among them is Turner's syndrome, a condition in which the second sex chromosome is missing. The person has a total of 45 instead of the normal 46 chromosomes. In these persons the sex chromosomes are neither XX as in girls, nor XY as in boys, but just one X. As a result, the person has the body of a prepubescent girl throughout life, never maturing sexually.

Another well-known sex chromosome defect is called Klinefelter's syndrome. In this condition there may be a variety of abnormal sex chromosomes, including XYY, XXY, XXYY, XXXYY, and so forth. The individual seems to have a male physique but does not develop normally. Many other defects of the reproductive system are caused by abnormal forms of sex chromosomes.

Sex-linked characteristics

Another type of inherited characteristic is sex linked, which means the genes that cause these characteristics are carried on the sex chromosomes. Researchers have found that the X sex chromosome carries many genes, whereas the Y of the male carries almost none. As a result, recessive traits carried by the mother could appear in a son because he does not have a matching X chromosome to carry a dominant gene. Hemophilia and color blindness are examples of sex-linked defects.

Genetic counseling

Knowledge about genetically caused birth defects has increased significantly in recent years. Many disorders such as Down's syndrome now can be diagnosed early in pregnancy. When there is high risk of genetic defects, as with older mothers or those with a family history of birth defects, amniocentesis may be done and the fetal cells karyotyped. If the fetus is defective, genetic counseling may help the parents decide whether to allow a pregnancy to go to term or to abort the fetus (Fig. 3-11).

Multiple pregnancy

Occasionally more than one fetus develops at a time. The incidence of multiple pregnancies is as follows:

Twins—1 in 89 pregnancies
Triplets—1 in 89^2 (7,921) pregnancies
Quadruplets—1 in 89^3 (704,969) pregnancies
Quintuplets—1 in 89^4 (62,742,241) pregnancies

Two basic mechanisms produce multiple pregnancy: (1) unusual division of a single fertilized ovum and (2) fertilization of more than one ovum at the same time or almost the same time (Fig. 3-12).

Identical twins

When a single ovum divides to produce more than one baby, all the infants will have the same pattern of chromosomes and will therefore be identical. About 25% of twins are identical. They have one common placenta and one chorion, although each has his or her own amniotic sac. The incidence of identical twinning is not related to maternal age, heredity, and number of previous children.

Fraternal twins

When two ova are released and are fertilized by separate sperm, the infants will be different and will be called fraternal. Each will have his or her own placenta, chorion, and amniotic sac. About 75% of twins are fraternal. The incidence is higher in older mothers, those with more than two prior pregnancies, and those with an inherited twinning trait. Drugs used to promote ovulation in infertile women may cause release of several ova at the same time. If fertilization occurs under these circumstances, multiple pregnancy results.

STANDARDIZED MEASUREMENTS AND TERMINOLOGY

Never again do persons grow at the rate they do in utero! In 9 months' time, one cell becomes legion; weight increases geometrically; and cells are arranged in fantastic complexity. And wonder of all, cells are in just the right kinds and numbers to form a baby—one who is unique from, but similar to, all others.

To provide a means to assess an infant's growth and development, certain standards are used to categorize measurements and terminology.

Length of the fetus is usually measured from crown (of the head) to heel (of the foot). Embryo measurements are crown to rump. It may be helpful to refer to a centimeter-inch ruler while reading about the growing fetus. Remember the following approximations:

1 inch	=	2.5 centimeters
2 inches	=	5 centimeters
4 inches	=	10 centimeters
8 inches	=	20 centimeters
12 inches	=	30 centimeters
20 inches	=	50 centimeters

Weight is usually expressed in grams while the fetus is tiny and in pounds or kilograms when it grows larger. Some gram-ounce-pound equivalents are as follows:

28.35 grams	=	1 ounce	
226.80 grams	=	8 ounces	
453.60 grams	=	16 ounces	= 1 pound
1,361 grams	= 1.36 kilograms	= 3	pounds
2,382 grams	= 2.82 kilograms	= 5½	pounds
3,171 grams	= 3.17 kilograms	= 7	pounds

Age is expressed in days, weeks, calendar months, and lunar months. A lunar month is 29½ days. Normal gestation in human beings varies from 266 to 280 days (38 to 40 weeks).

The developing baby is called by different terms during various stages of growth.

ovum From conception to 2 weeks' gestation (until embryonic shield evolves).

embryo From 2 to 8 weeks (until human form develops).

fetus From 8 weeks to birth.

newborn infant or baby (neonate) From birth to walking alone (about 1 year of age).

MEDICAL-LEGAL CLASSIFICATION
Legal identity

The complex social structure of our modern world demands a legal identity for each citizen. Birth registration is required in more organized societies to provide unique identification for each member.

In the United States, each state has its own laws governing birth registration. The U.S. Public Health Service has suggested guidelines that should eventually help standardize the laws. For the present, however, nurses must know the laws in the state where they practice. The general definitions given here are provided as guides for better understanding of the specific laws within the various states.

Live birth

An infant born alive is a live birth. *Live* means that after separation from the mother, the baby breathes or shows other evidence of life such as heartbeat, umbilical cord pulsation, or movement of voluntary muscles. The

Table 3-1 Fetal development

	4 weeks	8 weeks	12 weeks	16 weeks	20 weeks
EXTERNAL APPEARANCE					
	Body flexed, C shaped Arm and leg buds present Head at right angles to body	Body fairly well formed Nose flat, eyes far apart Digits well formed Head elevating Tail almost disappeared Eyes, ears, nose, and mouth recognizable	Nails appearing Resembles a human Head erect but disproportionately large Skin pink, delicate	Head still dominant Face looks human Eye, ear, and nose look typical Arm-leg ratio proportionate Scalp hair appears Motor activity present	Vernix caseosa appears Lanugo appears Legs lengthen considerably Sebaceous glands appear
CROWN-TO-RUMP MEASUREMENT (CM)					
	0.4-0.5	2.5-3	6-8	11.5-13.5	16-18.5
APPROXIMATE WEIGHT (GM)					
	0.4	2	19	100	300
MUSCULOSKELETAL SYSTEM					
	All segments that give rise to muscle masses present	First indication of ossification—occiput, mandible, and humerus Fetus capable of some movement; definitive muscles of trunk, limbs, and head well represented	Some bones well outlined; ossification spreading Upper cervical to lower sacral arches and bodies ossify Smooth muscle layers indicated in hollow viscera	Most bones distinctly indicated throughout body Joint cavities appear Muscular movements can be detected	Sternum ossifies Fetal movements strong enough for mother to feel
CIRCULATORY SYSTEM					
	Heart develops; double chambers visible; heart begins to beat Aortic arches and major veins completed	Main blood vessels assume final plan Enucleated red cells predominate in blood	Blood forming in marrow	Heart muscle well developed Blood formation active in spleen	

Adapted from Whaley, LF, and Wong, DL: Nursing care of infants and children, ed. 3, St. Louis, 1987, The CV Mosby Co.

24 weeks	28 weeks	32 weeks	36 weeks	40 weeks
Body lean but fairly well proportioned Skin red and wrinkled Vernix caseosa present Sweat glands forming	Lean body, less wrinkled and red Nails appear	Subcutaneous fat beginning to collect More rounded appearance Skin pink and smooth Has assumed delivery position	Skin pink, body rounded General lanugo disappearing Body usually plump	Skin smooth and pink; copious vernix caseosa Moderate to profuse hair Lanugo on shoulders and upper body only Nasal cartilage apparent
23	27	31	35	40
600	1,100	1,800-2,100	2,200-2,900	3,200+
	Astragalus (talus, ankle bone) ossifies	Middle fourth phalanges ossify Permanent teeth primordia (first traces) indicated	Distal femoral ossification centers present	
Blood formation increases in bone marrow and decreases in liver				

Table 3-1   Fetal development—cont'd

4 weeks	8 weeks	12 weeks	16 weeks	20 weeks
GASTROINTESTINAL SYSTEM				
Stomach at midline and fusiform Conspicuous liver Esophagus short Intestine a short tube	Intestinal villi developing Small intestines coil within umbilical cord Palatal folds present Liver very large	Bile secreted Palatal fusion complete Intestines have withdrawn from cord and assume characteristic positions	Meconium in bowel Some enzyme secretion Anus open	Enamel and dentin depositing Ascending colon recognizable
RESPIRATORY SYSTEM				
Primary lung buds appear	Pleural and pericardial cavities forming Branching bronchioles Nostrils closed by epithelial plugs	Lungs acquire definite shape Vocal cords appear	Elastic fibers appear in lungs Terminal and respiratory bronchioles appear	Nostrils reopen
RENAL SYSTEM				
Rudimentary ureteral buds appear	Earliest secretory tubules Bladder-urethra separates from rectum	Kidney able to secrete urine Bladder expands as a sac	Kidney in position Attains typical shape	
NERVOUS SYSTEM				
Well-marked midbrain flexure No hindbrain or cervical flexures Neural groove closed	Cerebral cortex begins to acquire typical cells Differentiation of cerebral cortex, meninges, ventricular foramina, cerebrospinal fluid circulation Spinal cord extends entire length of spine	Brain structural configuration roughly complete Cord shows cervical and lumbar enlargements Fourth ventricle foramina developed	Cerebral lobes delineated Cerebellum assumes some prominence	Brain grossly formed Cord myelination begins Spinal cord ends at level of S-1

24 weeks	28 weeks	32 weeks	36 weeks	40 weeks
Alveolar ducts and sacs present Respiratory-like movements begin Lecithin appears in amniotic fluid	Surfactant forming on alveolar surfaces	Lecithin/sphingo-myelin (L/S) ratio = 1.2:1	L/S ratio $\geq$ 2:1 (indicates adequate surfactant for lung expansion)	Pulmonary branching only two-thirds complete
			Formation of new nephrons ceases	
Cerebral cortex layered typically Neuronal proliferation in cerebral cortex ends	Appearance of cerebral fissures; convolutions rapidly appearing		End of spinal cord at level L-3	Myelination of brain begins

Table 3-1 Fetal development—cont'd

4 weeks	8 weeks	12 weeks	16 weeks	20 weeks
SENSE ORGANS				
Eye and ear appearing as optic vessel and otocyst	Primordial choroid plexuses Internal ear developing Ventricles large relative to cortex Development progressing Eyes converging rapidly	Earliest taste buds indicated Characteristic organization of eye attained	General sense organs differentiated	Nose and ear ossify
GENITAL SYSTEM				
Genital ridge appears (fifth week)	Testes and ovaries distinguishable External genitals sexless but begin to differentiate	Sex recognizable Internal and external sex organs specific	Testes in position for descent into scrotum Vagina open	

apparent age of the infant is of no consequence in most states. If the baby is alive at birth, a birth certificate is issued. If the infant later dies, a death certificate is issued, just as if he or she had lived a full lifetime.

Fetal death (stillbirth)

The term *stillbirth* is a general one that focuses on the mother. The legal term *fetal death* focuses on the baby. The law usually considers that an unborn fetus arrives at legal *life* when it is gestationally 20 to 22 weeks old. Most authorities define 20 weeks' gestation as a fetus whose length is 25 cm or weight is 500 gm. Any lifeless embryo or fetus that is expelled when it is smaller than this size is not considered to have ever been alive legally, and no legal certificate need be recorded. If, however, a lifeless fetus larger than 25 cm or 500 gm is delivered, a fetal death certificate is required by most states.

SIGNIFICANCE OF EMBRYONIC AND FETAL DEVELOPMENT

A working knowledge of the marvelous development of the human baby from conception to birth is essential to nurses practicing maternal-child nursing. They use this knowledge to counsel and teach parents, fulfill legal responsibilities, care for parents and infants, and provide inspiration for themselves.

Counseling and teaching

Knowledge dispels fear. The pregnant woman may have many fears about her unborn child. She may have heard terrible old wives' tales about "marking" the baby or how raising her arms above her head may strangle the baby on the cord. Such fears can be allayed by accurate information. The nurse is often the one parents go to with questions. The nurse should be prepared to offer simple, positive, scientifically accurate answers about the developing fetus.

24 weeks	28 weeks	32 weeks	36 weeks	40 weeks

	Eyelids reopen
	Retinal layers
	  completed; light
	  receptive
	Pupils capable of
	  reacting to light
		Sense of taste
		  present
		Aware of sounds
		  outside mother's
		  body		

Testes at inguinal ring in descent to scrotum		Testes descending to scrotum		Testes in scrotum Labia majora well developed

Modern expectant parents will want to follow the size and development of their baby. They will wonder about the placenta, about the cord, when the mother will "feel" the baby move, how the fetus can "breathe," and much more. These questions are not caused by fear but by interest. The nurse should be prepared to answer these questions simply and clearly.

Legal responsibility

The significance of embryonic development to the nurse comes into sharp focus with legal requirements for a death or birth certificate. Nurses should know the simple requirements of the law and cooperate to fulfill them. When questions of legal requirements arise, medical record specialists employed by most hospitals usually are able to answer. The nurse must see that the questions are properly referred and not ignored.

Caring for parents

Nurses should know about the normal development of the fetus so that they will be alert to abnormal symptoms. Parents may report or nurses may observe such symptoms. This knowledge is especially essential during labor and birth because the infant's life may be in peril.

Caring for infants

Nursery nurses care for infants at various stages of development—from tiny, immature infants to well-developed, full-term babies. When nurses have a working knowledge of fetal development, they can better understand the handicaps of the immature and premature infant.

Source of inspiration

"Such knowledge is too wonderful for me" said the psalmist of old (Psalms 139:6).

61

Nurses, too, stand in awe at the marvel of life. They never can reduce their study of things medical and their contact with human beings to cold science, even though they use scientific information constantly. Nurses must have warmth and wonder. To be a source of strength to others, nurses must continually renew their own souls. A knowledge of the marvel of human development from a single cell to a full-term infant provides nurses with an illuminating source of joy that they can then transmit to patients.

▶ *KEY CONCEPTS*

1. Conception is the union of an ovum and sperm. After rupture from the ovary, ova live 48 hours, then die unless fertilized. One sperm, among millions, swims up the fallopian tubes to fertilize an ovum. The enzyme hyaluronidase dissolves the corona radiata to permit a sperm to penetrate the ovum.

2. A fertilized ovum (zygote) has 46 chromosomes. Cells then divide by mitosis to form the morula, then the blastula. Implantation (nidation) of the blastula occurs because trophoblasts secrete a proteolytic enzyme that dissolves the endometrium, providing nourishment and burying the ovum in the uterine lining.

3. In the embryonic stage (10 days to 8 weeks), the chorion sends out villi into the endometrium and produces human chorionic gonadotropin (hCG). Two cavities are formed inside the ovum: the yolk sac and amniotic cavity, with the embryonic disc between the cavities. This disc has three cell layers from which all body parts form. The embryo forms from the body stalk within the amniotic cavity, which is filled with amniotic fluid.

4. The placenta develops from chorionic villi. Blood moves from the fetus to placenta in two arteries and from placenta to fetus in one vein. Wharton's jelly insulates these vessels within the umbilical cord. The placenta weighs about 1 pound at term. After 42 weeks of gestation, the fetus may be damaged because of infarcts in the aging placenta.

5. Fetal circulation has three unique features to shunt blood past the unused liver and lungs: the foramen ovale, ductus venosus, and ductus arteriosus. These structures normally close after birth.

6. Inherited traits are transmitted by genes on 23 chromosomes (22 autosomes, 1 sex chromosome) from each parent. Genes (traits) follow Mendel's law of dominance. Sex is determined by X and Y chromosomes: boys, XY; girls, XX. Karyotyping is nucleus picturing. Sex-linked disorders occur because the Y chromosome has few genes; therefore the X chromosome dominates, causing a defect. Chromosomal abnormalities include trisomy 21, or Down's syndrome. Genetic counseling is indicated for at-risk parents.

7. Multiple births occur in two ways: from one ovum (identical twins) and from more than one ovum (fraternal twins).

8. Birth registration is essential. A live birth indicates the infant shows signs of life, such as breathing or moving. Fetal death means the fetus was at least at 20 to 22 weeks' gestation (length: 25 cm; weight: 500 gm).

■ *ANNOTATED SUMMARY*

I. Germinal stage (1 to 10 days)
   A. Conception—the union of an ovum and sperm; requires ovulation and insemination
   B. Zygote formation—first cell
   C. Cell division (cleavage)—occurs through process of mitosis
   D. Morula to blastula—ovum becomes morula for about 6 days, then a fluid-filled blastula
   E. Implantation (nidation)—occurs because trophoblast secretes enzyme that dissolves endometrium and allows ovum to be buried
   F. Endometrial nest—formed in the endometrium

II. Embryonic stage (10 days to 8 weeks)—the chorion, or outer sac, sends out villi that invade the decidua and form the roots of the placenta; produces hCG; yolk sac and amniotic cavity formed
   A. Embryonic disc—three layers of cells, ectoderm, mesoderm, and endoderm, lie between two cavities

B. Chorionic vesicle growth—embryo develops from body stalk within amniotic cavity

C. Umbilical vessels and placenta—umbilical vessels enclosed in umbilical cord, two arteries, one vein; placenta, decidua basalis, and chorionic villi

III. Progressive development—occurs in orderly sequence as a total process, in a predictable pattern from embryo to fetus to birth at 40 to 41 weeks

A. Postmaturity (pregnancy beyond 42 weeks)—postmature infants have higher mortality because of progressive placental dysfunction

IV. Related facts

A. Placental transfer—maternal and fetal blood flow through two systems separated by three tissue layers; nutrients, wastes, and some harmful substances pass

B. Placental hormones—estrogen and progesterone important to maintenance of pregnancy

C. Amniotic fluid—amount increases throughout pregnancy to 1,000 ml at birth; serves many useful functions

D. Fetal circulation—three special structures shunt blood: ductus venosus, foramen ovale, ductus arteriosus; all close after birth

E. Heredity and sex determination

1. Transmission of traits—23 chromosomes from mother and 23 from father; chromosomes are made of nucleoproteins composed of protein, RNA, and DNA

2. Genes—arranged along chromosomes in pairs

3. Dominance—dominant genes assert their characteristics over recessive genes

4. Mendel's law—genes remain unchanged and follow predictable pattern; Punnett square demonstrates Mendel's law with recessive and dominant genes

5. Sex determination—gynosperm (X) produce girls; androsperm (Y) produce boys

6. Karyotyping—nucleus picturing permits study of genetic makeup of individuals

7. Abnormalities—a variety of aberrant patterns of autosomes and sex chromosomes

8. Sex-linked characteristics—those characteristics (genes) attached to X or Y chromosomes

9. Genetic counseling—helpful function when defects are likely or diagnosed by karyography

F. Multiple pregnancy—two mechanisms; unusual division of one ovum, and more than one fertilized ova

1. Identical twins—25% of twins; share one placenta and one chorion, but have own amniotic sacs

2. Fraternal twins—75% of twins; have own placentas, chorions, and amniotic sacs; higher incidence in older mothers and those who take fertility drugs

V. Standardized measurements and terminology (ovum, embryo, fetus, neonate)

VI. Medical-legal classification

A. Legal identity—birth registration is required

B. Live birth—life signs evident after birth

C. Fetal death (stillbirth)—when fetus is beyond 20 weeks' gestation and born without life

VII. Significance of embryonic and fetal development

A. Counseling and teaching—needed by parents

B. Legal responsibility

C. Caring for parents

D. Caring for infants

E. Source of inspiration

● **STUDY QUESTIONS**

1. Describe the products of conception as they appear by the third month of pregnancy.

2. Fetal circulation largely bypasses what two major body organs? Where and what are the three special shunts that cause these bypasses?

3. State the special obstetrical names given a developing baby during the following periods of development: (a) from conception to 2 weeks'

gestation, (b) from 2 to 8 weeks' gestation, (c) from 8 weeks' gestation to birth, (d) from birth until the child is walking.

4. Describe a fetus of 24 weeks' gestation.
5. Under what circumstances would the following certificates be issued: fetal death certificate, live birth certificate, death certificate?
6. How many chromosomes come from each parent? Explain why the sex of a baby is determined by the father rather than the mother. What is a sex-linked characteristic?
7. Describe the two basic mechanisms that produce multiple pregnancy. Which mechanism produces more twins?

REFERENCES

Anthony, CP, and Thibodeau, GA: Textbook of anatomy and physiology, ed 12, St. Louis, 1987, The CV Mosby Co.

Brooks, SM, and Paynton-Brooks, N: The human body: structure and function in health and disease, ed 2, St. Louis, 1980, The CV Mosby Co.

Francis, CC, and Martin, AH: Introduction to human anatomy, ed 7, St. Louis, 1975, The CV Mosby Co.

Hamilton, PM: Basic pediatric nursing, ed 5, St. Louis, 1987, The CV Mosby Co.

Whaley, LL, and Wong, DL: Nursing care of infants and children, ed 3, St. Louis, 1987, The CV Mosby Co.

CHAPTER 4

Psychological and Physiological Changes

VOCABULARY

Crisis intervention
Hegar's sign
Leukorrhea
Spontaneous abortion
Striae gravidarum
Trimester
Urinary frequency

LEARNING OBJECTIVES

- Define a crisis and what three factors influence how people react to a crisis

- List the steps of crisis intervention

- Discuss the legal and moral considerations of induced abortion

- Describe the typical psychological adjustments of a woman during the initial weeks of pregnancy, the second and third trimesters, and the immediate postpartum period

- Describe the physical changes in various body systems brought about by pregnancy

- List normal weight gain during pregnancy by trimester

Pregnancy is a momentous event in the life of a woman and her family. Although the profound changes that occur affect the whole person, for the sake of study we will first discuss the psychological effects and then the physical effects of pregnancy.

PSYCHOLOGICAL CHANGES

Pregnancy is a time of crisis, a time of disruption, of changing identities and roles for everyone: the mother, father, and family members. The psychological effects of pregnancy can be understood more fully when considered within the framework of crisis theory.

Crisis theory

People respond to crisis in a typical manner, regardless of the nature of the event that disrupts their lives. Indeed, the definition of a crisis is a state of psychological disequilibrium that may be caused by a situation or by a developmental stage. Initially, there is a period of *shock* and *denial*, then *confusion* and *preoccupation* with the problem as various alternatives are considered. This is followed by *action* to effect a solution, and finally there is *learning from experience*. How people react to crisis depends on three factors: their *perception of the event*, their *situational supports*, and their *coping mechanisms. Crisis in-*

65

tervention is the help offered by an outside person to facilitate the return of equilibrium to the disrupted lives.

Crisis resolution usually takes 1 to 6 weeks and is a time in which those affected are most receptive to outside suggestion. Although pregnancy spans 9 months, it is the initial news of pregnancy that may create a crisis for everyone concerned.

Initial adjustment to pregnancy

When a woman first learns she is or might be pregnant, she reacts with shock and denial. A common response is: "Some day, but not now." Her emotions range from elation to despair. Even when the pregnancy is planned, an initial period of disbelief is common.

A man's first reaction to the news that he is to become a father is a mixture of pride in his ability to procreate and concern about his readiness to assume the role of father and to provide for his family.

The initial shock of those involved is followed by confusion and preoccupation with the problems this disruptive event produces. During this period, various alternatives such as abortion or adoption may be weighed in light of their legal, moral, and economic consequences. Finally, decisions are reached, and a plan of action is formulated. Sometimes the action is, in fact, inaction, until the reality of the pregnancy can no longer be denied and is accepted. As the experience is mulled over and reviewed, learning takes place.

Perception of the event

Every woman brings to pregnancy her own idea of what a pregnant woman and mother is like. She forms this image from her own mother, her life experiences, and the culture in which she was reared. This perception affects how she responds to the stresses of pregnancy. Some women think of pregnancy as a means of securing nurturance, recognition, or emancipation from parental control. They may equate pregnancy with sickness, ugliness, or shame, or they may view it as a period of creativity and fulfillment.

The first pregnancy means the end of childhood and the beginning of adulthood. This maturational crisis may not be welcome. In many states a pregnant female is legally an adult, regardless of her age. She may give consent for care for herself and her child. In the United States, a pregnant woman is entitled to financial aid from the government and, if unwed, is the sole legal guardian of her child. As such, she has the right to care for the child herself, place the child in a foster home, or give the child up for adoption.

A man brings to pregnancy his own idea of what a father-to-be and father is like. He forms this image from his own father, his life experiences, and the culture in which he was reared. His perception affects how he cares for the mother of his child. Many men become extremely solicitous of the mother and take an active role in obtaining medical care for her. Some men develop the same symptoms as the woman, such as morning sickness, lassitude, or pain. This phenomenon is called *mitleiden*, or "suffering along," by some medical historians.

Pregnancy may represent a perpetuation of the family line. As such, the name and sex of the baby become highly significant. For many people, the ideal outcome of the pregnancy, especially the first one, is a male heir. To such parents, a girl represents failure to carry on the family name. Thus each member of the family associated with the pregnancy views the event from a different perspective. Those perceptions affect the resolution of the crisis.

Situational supports

The second factor that affects how those involved resolve a crisis is the situational supports they possess. These are the people and resources available to bolster, assist, and care. During pregnancy, the family or its substitute usually fills this important role. (See Chapter 2 for a discussion of family types and functions.)

Coping mechanisms

The third factor influencing the degree of success experienced in resolving a crisis is one's repertoire of coping skills. These are strengths and skills people learn to solve problems and to deal with stress. They may include such activities as "talking it out" with a friend, doing strenuous physical activity, listening to music, crying, writing prose or poetry, and seeking solitude. Defense mechanisms are somewhat self-deceptive (such as denial), but they may be helpful in providing temporary relief from anxiety. Such coping methods may be used by expectant parents and family members to adjust to the reality of the pregnancy and restore equilibrium to their disrupted lives.

Crisis intervention

The steps of crisis intervention are: (1) assess the situation, (2) plan intervention, (3) intervene and resolve crisis, and (4) give anticipatory guidance. When applied to pregnancy they are:

Assess the situation. Get the facts. Is the woman really pregnant? A physical examination and pregnancy test are in order. A missed menstrual period is not always caused by pregnancy. If the woman is not pregnant, intervention can move quickly to anticipatory guidance, and she can be given contraceptive information. If she is pregnant, focus on what she views as the problem. Is it fear of pregnancy, disappointment because of interrupted life goals, guilt for having been sexually active, fear of being ostracized by her family, concern for the needs of other children, conflict about the ethics of abortion? Will the prospective father assume responsibility for the child?

Does the mother want to establish paternity of the child?

Assess the coping skills of the persons in crisis: What are their perceptions of the pregnancy? Are there others who can give support, or is the woman or man alone? Whatever the problem, focus on the here and now, the present situation.

Plan intervention. Clearly define the problem before planning an intervention. Help clients sort out reasonable options. The nurse may need help from experienced or specially prepared counselors to adequately plan the intervention.

Intervene and resolve crisis. The intervener assists clients to carry out their decisions. This may involve asking pertinent questions that clarify conflict, giving information, making referrals, teaching, or arranging for direct care, financial assistance, shelter, or medical supervision.

With the facts of various alternative actions before them and an honest appraisal of how they feel about these alternatives, the expectant mother and father can resolve the crisis the pregnancy has created. The woman must decide whether to have an abortion or go on with the pregnancy. The man must decide whether to accept the woman's decision or to leave her. Other family members also must decide how supportive they will be. Ideally, each one will come to a mutually satisfactory solution. A return to emotional equilibrium is a sign of resolution of the crisis.

Give anticipatory guidance. Each life crisis produces lasting effects on those who have lived it. The coping skills learned will then be available in the future. In addition, practical means to control the future can be learned. In the case of unexpected pregnancy, the couple should be provided with family-planning information before another pregnancy occurs. In this way, they can control their future and avoid repeating this crisis if they so choose.

Abortion

Nurses who work with pregnant women need information about abortions. The definitions and legal-moral issues of abortion are discussed here. Operative procedures are described in Chapter 6.

Definitions

An abortion is any termination of a pregnancy before the fetus is viable or requires a fetal death certificate (before the twenty-fourth week of gestation). A *spontaneous* abortion is called a miscarriage in lay language and is an abortion that occurs of itself. An *induced* abortion is one that is deliberately caused. A *therapeutic* abortion is an abortion induced for medical reasons.

Legal considerations

Until 1803 there were no laws against abortion in the United States. During the next 50 years most of the states and other Western nations passed laws designed to protect women from the risk of unsanitary hospital abortions. The demand for abortions continued and led to a multimillion dollar business in butchery as desperate women sought abortions outside the law. This tragic situation generated pressure for legal reform. In 1962 the American Law Institute proposed a model code to be submitted to all states. Under it the patient's physician and a hospital committee were given power to grant or deny a woman's request for abortion using certain criteria. By 1970 many states had modified their abortion laws to include features of the model code.

In 1973 the Supreme Court of the United States wrote a landmark decision that overrode all state laws. It emphasized the constitutional guarantee of personal freedom of choice. The Wade and Bolton decision states that any woman is eligible for a legal abortion anywhere in the United States. During the first 12 weeks of pregnancy, the only legal requirement is that the abortion be performed by a licensed physician; from the thirteenth to the twenty-fourth week, a state may regulate the procedure only to the extent necessary to protect the mother's life.

The decision means that anyone may have an abortion for any reason through the first 6 months of pregnancy. After the sixth month a state may regulate or forbid abortion, except when it is necessary to preserve the life or health (including mental health) of the woman. The decision does not require a woman to have an abortion, and it excuses medical personnel morally opposed to abortion from participating in any such procedure. There have been numerous efforts to circumvent the Supreme Court decision, including attempted Constitutional amendments and laws that restrict funding or define the time life begins. To date the decision remains unchanged.

Moral considerations

Underlying the legal considerations of abortion is the moral consideration. There are two main points of view on this issue. Some consider the fetus to be a separate human being from the moment of conception; therefore they look on abortion as murder. Others view the fetus as a parasite in its biological host, the woman, until it can survive independently. Vital statistic regulations lend some support to this second view by requiring a fetal death certificate for any fetus that dies after 24 weeks and none for one that dies before that age.

Abortion counseling

Abortion counseling focuses on the specific issues that surround unwanted pregnancy and abortion. The counselor explores with the woman alternatives to abortion, their comparative risks and emotional consequences. Ideally, the woman is not pressured. The final decision is hers. If the woman decides to have the abortion, supportive care is provided during and after the procedure. Such counseling is not complete unless information about effective contraceptive methods is offered to the woman.

The single mother

The single mother cannot be stereotyped. She may be wealthy or poor or of any race. She may be dull or bright, innocent or sophisticated, a young teenager or a mature professional. The pregnancy may have been planned or accidental. Regardless of her background, a single mother has one need in common with all women in her situation: nonjudgmental counsel and care.

When a pregnancy is planned, the woman usually has considered her need for shelter, sustenance, and medical care before conception. When the pregnancy is accidental, realistic counseling and prenatal care may be needed.

Professional counseling is offered to the single mother by many agencies. If the mother is a student, counseling services may be available through her school. If not, mental health clinics and various charitable organizations offer these services.

The counselor's function is to help a woman cope with emotional stress, make realistic plans, and grow from the experience. Whether to relinquish the infant to adoptive parents or to parent the child is explored. Ultimately, the mother must decide. Ideally, regular counseling sessions go on for many months before delivery and continue afterward until the woman has made a satisfactory adjustment to postpartum life.

A single mother needs respect, genuine concern, and acceptance. The father of the baby may need help to resolve his feelings and to come to a decision about what his involvement with the mother and baby will be. Nurses also

may need to ventilate their feelings in confidence with other staff members or consultants so that they will be free to give nonjudgmental, supportive care.

Continued adjustment to pregnancy
First trimester (1 to 3 months)

Once the initial crisis brought about by the confirmation of pregnancy is resolved, most women experience a certain elation as they adjust their plans to the thrilling business of creating a new life. Since the body and emotions are an interconnected whole, the physical changes begin to affect the emotions. Soon after conception, progesterone and estrogen levels in the body start to rise. Morning sickness, weakness, fatigue, and a feeling of fullness result. The woman "doesn't feel good" and commonly experiences depression. Fathers may view the newly pregnant woman with awe and shun sexual intercourse because they fear it will harm the baby. Some men experience increased sexual excitement relative to the pregnant woman. Both groups of men need understanding and acceptance.

Second trimester (4 to 6 months)

The second trimester is usually the most pleasant. The woman's body has become accustomed to high hormone levels, her morning sickness has ceased, she has accepted her pregnancy, and she is using her mind and energies constructively. The fetus is still small and does not yet produce discomfort by its size. During this trimester, *quickening* occurs when the mother feels the baby move for the first time. The experience confirms the presence and growth of a new life, and it often gives the mother a great psychological boost.

Third trimester (7 to 9 months)

The third trimester is characterized by a crescendo of emotional elation climaxed by the birth of the baby. About the eighth month there may be a period of discouragement and depression, when the baby is large and discomforts increase. The woman is tired, and the waiting seems long. About 2 weeks before delivery, most women begin to experience a feeling of well-being. They may tell the nurse, "I feel better now than I have for months!" Unless an unusual physical problem develops, this elation carries the woman right through labor, a period of maximum stress.

A woman's emotional reaction to labor and delivery largely depends on her preparation for and her perception of this event. Her specific cooperation during these events will be discussed in connection with the nursing care given to her at that time. The high level of elation experienced by the mother in the weeks before delivery reaches a climax about 24 hours after delivery.

Postpartum "blues"

Sometimes the elation of delivery continues for 2 or 3 days, but it almost always passes by the fourth postpartum day. The mother may become depressed, tearful, and listless. A sudden drop in the progesterone and estrogen levels after delivery may account in part for the postpartum "blues," as these days of depression are called. There are other reasons why the mother may feel depressed and discouraged. The suspense is over, the baby has come, and the excitement has passed. The mother has a sore perineum, engorged breasts if she is breast-feeding, and after-pains. She may not really understand why, but she knows that her wonderful world of a week ago has soured.

Return to nonpregnant state

If the story ended at this point, there would probably be few families with more than one child. Fortunately, the period of depression is self-limiting. When the mother assumes her essential role in the family when she experiences the joy of nurturing a precious new infant, and when her body tissues heal and hormone levels return to normal, the depression lifts. It takes about 6 weeks for the effects of pregnancy to subside and for the woman to return to a nonpregnant state.

This characteristic picture of the emotional reaction of a woman to pregnancy is modified by individual personality differences. Some women have exaggerated mood swings, others seem to have none. In general, however, nurses can expect the characteristic pattern of behavior and can comfort mothers by explaining that their feelings are not unusual. Enthusiasm and zest for living return as surely as they departed.

PHYSIOLOGICAL CHANGES

While the reproductive system is the center of attention during pregnancy, the entire body is affected. All the body systems undergo change from the nonpregnant state to the pregnant state in what is generally called *maternal physiology.*

Reproductive system
Blood supply

Blood supply to the reproductive organs increases soon after conception because of the increased levels of steroid sex hormones. This vascularity provides a rich supply of blood for the growing fetus, typical signs in the organs, and various symptoms in the woman.

Cervix

Soon after the first missed menstrual period, the cervix begins to soften as a result of the increased blood supply (Goodell's sign). The cervical canal fills with a thick mucous plug called the *operculum.* During the pregnancy the operculum bars bacteria from entering the uterus. Its passage during labor, called the "bloody show," indicates that the canal is opening for the baby to pass through.

The cervix of a nullipara (a woman with no prior pregnancies) is round and smooth and protrudes into the vagina. The birth process stretches the cervix and almost always causes lacerations of the cervix. Thereafter, the cervix is oval. During the course of a pregnancy the consistency of the cervix changes. Before pregnancy it is likened to the tip of the nose; in early to midpregnancy to the earlobe; and at term to the lips.

Uterus

The most obvious change in maternal anatomy is the enlargement of the uterus to accommodate the growing fetus (Fig. 4-1). The uterus grows from a small, nearly solid organ into a thin-walled, muscular pouch that contains the fetus, placenta, and about 1,000 ml of amniotic fluid. Its weight increases 20 times, and its capacity increases 500 times.

This increase in size is caused by the growth of muscle fibers and related tissues, including new fibroelastic tissue, blood, and nerves.

The growth of uterine tissue in early pregnancy occurs because of estrogen stimulation of the muscle fibers and not because there is an embryo growing in the uterine cavity. Even when the ovum implants outside the uterus, as in ectopic pregnancy, the uterus enlarges to about the size of a 4-month intrauterine pregnancy.

The nonpregnant uterus feels like a firm green pear. Pregnancy produces noticeable softening, so that by the eighth week an examiner can bend it by palpation. This is called *Hegar's sign* of pregnancy.

As the uterus enlarges with the growth of the fetus, it is held in place by the ligaments, particularly the *uterosacral ligaments*, which connect the uterus to the sacral bones, and

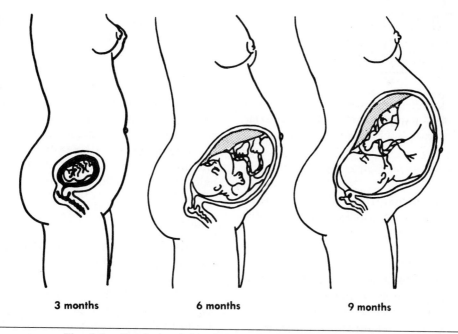

3 months   **6 months**   **9 months**

Fig. 4-1. Fetal growth in relation to the mother by trimesters.

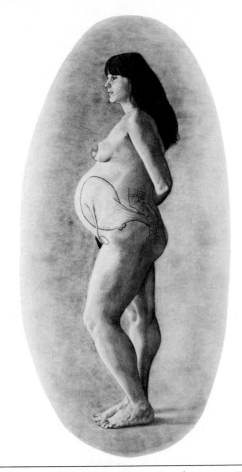

Fig. 4-2. Supporting ligaments of uterus. (From Davis, Elizabeth: A guide to midwifery: heart and hands, Sante Fe, 1981, John Muir Publications.)

the *round ligaments*, which extend from the uterus through the inguinal canal to the labia majora (Fig. 4-2).

Vagina

By the eighth week, increased vascularity of the vagina produces a typical sign of pregnancy called *Chadwick's sign*, a purplish hue that is visible to the examiner. In response to hormonal stimulation, the secretions of vagi-

nal cells increase noticeably. They are highly acidic in reaction and white in color, hence the term "whites" or *leukorrhea*. These secretions provide a rich medium in which Döderlein's bacilli flourish. These bacilli provide the body's first line of defense against *Candida albicans*, a pathogen that thrives on alkalinity.

As the pregnancy progresses, the increased vascular congestion of the vagina and pelvic organs results in a marked increase in sensitivity. This may lead to a high degree of sexual arousal, especially between the fourth and seventh months of pregnancy.

Integumentary system
Breasts

One of the first clues a woman may have that she is pregnant is a tingling tenderness of her breasts, which gradually enlarge as alveolar tissue grows and blood supply increases. The nipples become more prominent and erectile, and early in pregnancy a clear serous secretion, *colostrum*, oozes from them. The pigmented area around the nipple, the *areola*, grows darker, and the small Montgomery's glands stand out.

If breasts are not properly supported during pregnancy, their increased heaviness may cause discomfort. Fear that the figure will be "ruined" need not be true if a good supporting brassiere is worn during pregnancy. Frequent washing keeps dried colostrum from accumulating. Brisk drying with a rough towel may help toughen the nipples in preparation for breast-feeding.

Skin

Striae gravidarum. As the fetus grows, the uterus enlarges, pressing out from within. This causes the navel to flatten and later protrude. Elastic fibers of the deep layers of skin separate and are broken by stretching. The resulting stretch marks are called *striae gravidarum*. They appear on the abdomen and buttocks of about 50% of all pregnant women and fade to a lighter shade after delivery. The woman may experience considerable pruritus (itchiness) as a result of this stretching. Temporary relief may be gained by applying soothing lotions.

Pigmentation. Temporary deposits of pigment may appear on specific areas of the body, depending on the natural color of the skin. A *linea nigra* or "dark line," follows the midline of the abdomen. *Cholasma,* or the mask of pregnancy, looks like a blotchy suntan on the face. Areola around the nipple enlarges and deepens in color. All these areas of increased pigmentation fade after delivery.

Perspiration and oil secretion. Both the sweat and the sebaceous (oil) glands become more active during pregnancy. As a result, the woman may be troubled by body odor, embarrassing perspiration stains on her clothing, and oily, hard-to-manage hair. Frequent bathing, shampooing, and use of deodorants help control these unpleasant side effects.

Endocrine system

The glands of the endocrine system produce powerful chemicals that affect the entire body. During pregnancy, many changes occur in these glands.

Ovaries and placenta

The ovaries are the source of estrogen and progesterone in the nonpregnant woman. The ebb and flow of these hormones during the menstrual cycle is described in Chapter 1. At conception, dramatic changes occur. The corpus luteum from which the ovum came begins to produce estrogen and progesterone. As soon as the placenta develops sufficiently, it becomes the primary source of these hormones. The placenta also synthesizes steroids and three other hormones: human chorionic gonadotropin (hGC), human placental lactogen

(hPL), also called human chorionic somato-mammotropin (hCS), and human chorionic thyrotropin (hCT).

Thyroid gland

During pregnancy, basal metabolic rate (BMR) rises almost 20% and the thyroid gland enlarges, but the amount of hormone (thyroxin) it produces remains the same. Its increased size is caused by acinar cell growth, and the increased metabolic rate is caused by greater oxygen use.

Parathyroid glands

The parathyroid glands increase in size during pregnancy, particularly during the fifteenth to the thirty-fifth week when calcium needs of the fetus are greatest. Parathyroid hormone is necessary to maintain sufficient calcium in the blood, without which bone and muscle metabolism are hampered.

Pancreas

Insulin is produced by tiny cell groups called *islands of Langerhans,* which occur throughout the tissue of the pancreas. During pregnancy these islets grow and produce more insulin to meet the increasing needs. Even so, since glycogen storage is limited, the healthy pregnant woman is less able to handle large amounts of sugar, so some may spill into her urine. For a diabetic mother, pregnancy is especially precarious and requires continuous medical supervision. (See Chapter 6).

Pituitary gland

The anterior lobe of the pituitary gland enlarges slightly during pregnancy and continues to produce all of the tropic hormones, but in slightly different amounts. Follicle-stimulating hormone (FSH) is suppressed by the chorionic gonadotropin (hCG) produced in the placenta. Growth hormone is decreased and melanotropic hormone is increased, causing additional pigmentation of the nipples, face, and abdomen. Prolactin production increases and continues after delivery throughout lactation.

As the baby matures, the posterior lobe's production of oxytocin increases in preparation for its role in stimulating uterine muscle contractions during labor.

Adrenal glands

The adrenal glands increase in size during pregnancy, especially the cortical portion that produces *cortin*. The number of sodium and potassium ions in the bloodstream are regulated by cortin.

The medullary portion of the adrenal glands secretes *epinephrine*, the emergency hormone. Pregnancy does not change the size or function of the medullary portion.

Cardiovascular system

As the pregnancy advances, blood volume increases gradually until it is 30% to 50% above nonpregnant levels at term. Estrogen stimulates adrenal secretions of aldosterone, resulting in salt and water retention. This leads to increased blood volume and tissue edema. However, blood pressure normally remains relatively unchanged. A significant rise indicates preeclampsia.

The heavy uterus presses on the enlarged veins that drain the pelvis and lower extremities. Varicose veins may develop in the legs, thighs, vulva, and rectum (hemorrhoids). Varicose veins occur in 16% to 33% of all pregnant women.

Pressure of the uterus on the vena cava that occurs when the woman lies supine may produce a marked decrease in blood pressure, called *supine hypotensive syndrome*, causing temporary pallor, dizziness, and claminess.

Red blood cells increase by 33% and hemoglobin by 15%; but because of the increased plasma volume causing hemodilution, a *pseudoanemia* develops—the so-called physiological anemia of pregnancy.

Plasma fibrogen levels increase by 40% or more, and clotting time remains the same as prepregnant levels. As a result, blood clots more readily. This, coupled with venous stasis, causes the woman to be especially vulnerable to venous thrombosis.

Musculoskeletal system
Teeth, bones, and joints

During pregnancy the woman needs about one-third more calcium and phosphorus. With a well-balanced diet these needs are satisfied. Dental caries is not the result of decalcification, since the calcium in teeth is fixed. There is evidence that the acidic saliva of pregnancy encourages the activity of enamel-destroying bacteria that cause cavities.

The otherwise fixed joints of the pelvis soften during pregnancy and become slightly movable. The woman's posture gradually changes as the fetus enlarges in the abdomen. To compensate for the added weight, the woman throws back her shoulders and arches her spine. The resulting lumbar curve, combined with joint softening, may account for the backaches some women experience. Use of supporting girdles may be recommended in these special cases.

Muscles

Cramps of the leg muscles and feet are a common problem during pregnancy. The cause is not known but may be related to calcium and phosphorus metabolism, poor drainage of muscle wastes, or imbalanced posture. The cramps usually follow a long day of standing and occur in the evening when the body is relaxed. Movement or applications of heat may give some relief. A general moderation of activity and frequent rest periods with the legs elevated are probably the most successful ways to reduce this discomfort.

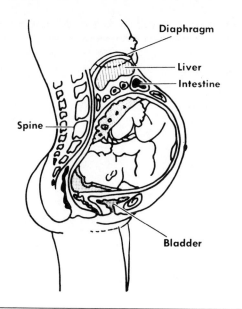

Fig. 4-3. Displacement of the mother's organs by the full-term fetus.

Respiratory system
Lungs and respiration

As the fetus grows and pushes the diaphragm upward, the shape and size of the woman's chest cavity are changed but not made smaller (Fig. 4-3). Lung capacity for inspired air remains the same as before pregnancy or may actually be increased. Respiratory rate and vital capacity are not changed. Tidal volume, minute ventilatory volume, and oxygen uptake increase. Because the shape of the chest cavity is changed and because the woman is breathing more rapidly, about 60% of pregnant women complain of a feeling of breathlessness.

Mucous membrane

Although the cause is not fully known, an allergic-like swelling of the mucous membrane is common in pregnancy. It produces symptoms of hoarseness, nasal stuffiness, dys-pnea, throat soreness, nosebleeding, and loss of smell and taste. Drugs that shrink the tissue both locally and systemically may be prescribed to relieve the symptoms, which disappear after delivery.

Gastrointestinal system

The gastrointestinal system is affected in a number of ways by pregnancy. High progesterone levels alter body fluid balance, increase blood cholesterol, and slow contractions of smooth muscles. Salivary secretions become acidic and increase, and stomach acid decreases. The enlarging uterus exerts pressure on the diaphragm, stomach, and intestine.

In the early months of pregnancy, one-third of all women experience nausea and vomiting. As the pregnancy proceeds, reduced stomach acid slows stomach emptying and causes bloating. Reduced peristaltic movement contributes not only to nausea but to constipation, because the longer fecal matter remains in the bowel, the more water is drawn from it and the harder it becomes. Constipation is also aggravated by the pressure of the uterus on the lower bowel early in pregnancy and again near term.

Teeth decay more readily in the acidic saliva of pregnancy and require conscientious care to prevent caries. In the later months, heartburn and esophageal regurgitation (acid indigestion) are common discomforts resulting from the upward pressure of the enlarging uterus. Engorged rectal vessels (hemorrhoids) may develop. At delivery, the rectum and supporting muscles are greatly stretched.

Urinary system

Under normal circumstances the increased work of filtering blood for the mother and growing fetus creates no unreasonable demands on the kidneys and ureters. They become dilated because the ureteral peristalsis is reduced. As a result, urine moves to the bladder more slowly. This urinary stasis increases the possibility of pyelonephritis.

Early in pregnancy, blood supply to the bladder lining increases, and the enlarging uterus presses against the bladder. These factors cause frequent urination. Near term the fetus drops low in the pelvis, again pressing against the bladder and increasing urinary frequency. Although this symptom is inconvenient, it does not cause medically significant problems.

Nervous system
Peripheral nerves

There are no "normal" nerve changes during pregnancy. Occasionally symptoms develop as a result of the softening of the joints, as was described in the discussion about bone and joint changes in pregnancy. Sometimes the altered posture of pregnancy may cause *acrodysesthesia*, or numbness, tingling, and stiffness of all or parts of the arms, hands, or fingers. This is purely a mechanical problem and is relieved by supporting the shoulders on a pillow at night and by assuming proper posture in the daytime.

Brain

Although brain tissue is probably not changed by pregnancy, the psychological effects may be profound. Mood swings are common. Occasionally a woman cannot accept pregnancy, and psychosis may result. This abnormal reaction to pregnancy is discussed in Chapter 12.

Weight gain

Although weight gain is highly individualized, pregnancy accounts for the averages found in Table 4-1. One should remember these are average, not absolute, amounts.

Women who are greatly underweight or carrying more than one baby should gain more weight during pregnancy. Those who are obese may gain less but should avoid starva-

Table 4-1 Components of maternal weight gain*

	Grams	Pounds
MOTHER		
Uterus	900	1.98
Breasts	450	.99
Blood	1,350	2.97
Tissue	1,350	2.97
Fat	4,050	8.91
Subtotal	8,100	17.82
FETUS	3,150	6.93
Placenta	675	1.49
Amniotic fluid	900	1.98
Subtotal	4,725	10.40
TOTAL	12,825	28.22

*From Guthrie, HA: Introductory nutrition, ed 6, St. Louis, 1986, The CV Mosby Co.

tion diets and drastic weight loss that may produce ketosis and endanger the fetus.

Normally, weight gain occurs as follows:

First trimester	2 to 4 pounds
Second trimester	12 to 15 pounds
Third trimester	8 to 10 pounds

In general, a liberal, well-balanced diet with adequate fluids is recommended. Strict weight control diets are no longer advised because mothers who gain less than 20 pounds (907 kg) have more low birth weight babies. Current recommendations for average women are that they should gain more than 25 pounds and less than 40 pounds during the pregnancy.

▶ *KEY CONCEPTS*

1. Pregnancy creates a crisis; a state of psychological disequilibrium that is affected by one's perception of the event, situational supports, and coping mechanisms. Crisis intervention: assess, plan, intervene and resolve, give anticipatory guidance.
2. Abortion: spontaneous and induced termination of pregnancy. Wade/Bolton decision: no restric-

tion to 12 weeks, 13 to 24 weeks, states may regulate. Moral issues: counseling indicated, should be nonjudgmental.

3. Single mothers: now common and universal, need medical care, shelter, acceptance, and counseling. Fathers: also need supportive, nonjudgmental counsel.

4. Adjustment to pregnancy during first trimester: crisis, response to hormones causes morning sickness and general malaise. Second trimester most pleasant: body has adjusted to hormone levels, fetus smaller, quickening occurs. Third trimester: more discomfort and depression, crescendo of elation occurs just prior to delivery. Postpartum period: postpartum "blues" common due to decreased hormones, physical fatigue, and discomfort.

5. Maternal physiology (changes due to pregnancy): reproductive system undergoes profound changes. *Goodell's sign:* soft cervix. *Hegar's sign:* soft uterus. *Chadwick's sign:* purplish hue of vagina. Vaginal secretions increase. Breasts enlarge and secrete colostrum; perspiration and oil secretions increase. *Skin pigmentation:* linea nigra on abdomen; chloasma on face. *Hormonal changes:* increased progesterone and estrogen, placenta produces hCG, hPL, hCT; islands of Langerhans produce more insulin, pituitary hormones significantly affected; adrenal cortex produces more cortin. *Cardiovascular system:* increased blood volume, body fluids, red cells, hemoglobin, and fibrin, with resultant pseudoanemia; supine hypotensive syndrome caused by pressure of uterus on vena cava; more vulnerable to venous thrombosis due to fibrin increase and venous stasis. *Skeletal changes:* calcium needs increase 33% but not taken from teeth, pelvic joints soften, lumbar curve develops due to fetal weight. *Lungs:* lung capacity not changed, in fact, tidal volume increases; mucous membrane swells in some women. *Gastrointestinal tract* greatly affected: stomach and oral acid increase, peristalsis decreases, constipation common, and engorged rectal vessels may cause hemorrhoids. *Other:* urinary frequency increases during first and third trimesters; stasis increases possibility of pyelonephritis; acrodysesthesia due to mechan-

ical pressure; mood swings common; weight gain should be 25 to 40 pounds.

■ ANNOTATED SUMMARY

I. Psychological changes—pregnancy is a time of crisis when life's equilibrium is disrupted
  A. Crisis theory—stages: shock and denial, confusion and preoccupation, action, and learning from experience; intervention helps facilitate return to a state of equilibrium
  B. Initial adjustment to pregnancy—both mother and father experience shock
    1. Perception of the event—varies with individual
    2. Situational supports—important to provide assistance and caring
    3. Coping mechanisms—the strengths and skills learned to deal with stress
    4. Crisis intervention
      a. Assess the situation
      b. Plan the intervention
      c. Intervene and resolve the crisis
      d. Give anticipatory guidance
  C. Abortion
    1. Definitions—termination of pregnancy before fetus is viable (24 weeks); may be spontaneous, induced, or therapeutic
    2. Legal considerations—from 1803 to 1973, induced abortions were illegal
    3. Moral considerations—revolve around issue of when life begins, at conception or when independent survival is possible
    4. Abortion counseling—focuses on issue of unwanted pregnancy; should be nonjudgmental
  D. The single mother—may be any age, race, or social status; pregnancy may be planned or unplanned; mother's needs for care and counsel are the same; professional counseling is helpful, aim is to help mother cope with stress, make plans, and grow from experience; father should not be forgotten
  E. Continued adjustment to pregnancy
    1. First trimester (1 to 3 months)—characterized by adjustment to idea of par-

enthood, high hormone levels, nausea and vomiting, and fatigue

2. Second trimester (4 to 6 months)—most pleasant time; increased sexual responsiveness; quickening gives psychic boost

3. Third trimester (7 to 9 months)—fatigue; body is big and awkward; crescendo of elation climaxed by birth

4. Postpartum "blues"—sudden decrease in hormones, tender perineum, and engorged breasts produce depression

5. Return to nonpregnant state—by sixth week body has healed, hormonal levels have stabilized, and lactation is regulated

II. Physiological changes—maternal physiology includes all the changes of pregnancy in the woman's body

A. Reproductive system

1. Blood supply—increase caused by hormones; produces typical signs and symptoms

2. Cervix—softens (Goodell's sign) and fills with mucous (operculum); changes to oval shape after first birth

3. Uterus—tremendous change in shape, size, and wall thickness; supported by ligaments that hold it in place; softens by eighth week (Hegar's sign)

4. Vagina—purple hue (Chadwick's sign) by eighth week caused by increased vascularity, as are leukorrhea of pregnancy and increased sexual arousal

B. Integumentary system

1. Breasts—tenderness, enlargement, colostrum, and areola darkening occur

2. Skin

a. Striae gravidarum—stretching of tissue that causes pruritus and marks

b. Pigmentation—temporary deposits occur on abdominal midline (linea nigra), on face (chloasma), and on areola

c. Perspiration and oil secretion—increase during pregnancy, requiring increased bathing

C. Endocrine system

1. Ovaries and placenta—corpus luteum produces estrogen and progesterone; placenta also produces hCG, hPL, and hCT

2. Thyroid gland—enlarges during pregnancy, but amount of thyroxin remains constant

3. Parathyroid glands—increase in size between fifteenth and thirty-fifth weeks, when calcium needs of fetus are greatest

4. Pancreas—insulin production increases during pregnancy, but glycogen storage is limited

5. Pituitary gland—FSH is suppressed by hCG of placenta; prolactin increases during pregnancy and lactation; oxytocin increases and stimulates uterine muscle contractions

6. Adrenal glands—cortin increases, but epinephrine remains constant

D. Cardiovascular system—blood volume increases 30% to 50%, but blood pressure remains unchanged; red blood cell production increases but because of hemodilution, pseudoanemia develops; pressure on vena cava produces supine hypotensive syndrome; venous stasis and fibrogen increase makes woman vulnerable to thrombosis.

E. Musculoskeletal system

1. Teeth, bones, and joints—calcium and potassium needs increase; dental caries is not the result of decalcification; joints soften

2. Muscles—cramps are a common problem

F. Respiratory system

1. Lungs and respiration—diaphragm is displaced by fetal growth; increased tidal volume, increased O_2 in blood

2. Mucous membrane—swelling common, causes stuffy nose, hoarseness, dyspnea, etc.

G. Gastrointestinal system—stomach acid decreases; nausea and vomiting are common in early pregnancy; slowed peristalsis causes bloating; constipation and esophageal regurgitation (heartburn) are common.

H. Urinary system
   1. Normal kidneys are able to handle added work without problems; pressure by growing fetus may cause urinary stasis
   2. Urinary frequency of early pregnancy caused by pressure of uterus on bladder

I. Nervous system
   1. Peripheral nerves—no normal changes
   2. Brain—no physical changes, but considerable psychic adjustment

J. Weight gain—25 to 40 pounds.

● STUDY QUESTIONS

1. What are the typical stages people pass through as they respond to crisis situations?
2. What factors affect how people react to crisis? Discuss the mother's and father's perceptions of pregnancy.
3. Describe the physical changes that take place in each of the body systems during pregnancy.
4. About how many additional pounds does pregnancy at term add to the woman's weight?

Discuss the mother's and father's perceptions of pregnancy.
3. Describe the physical changes that take place in each of the body systems during pregnancy.
4. About how many additional pounds does pregnancy at term add to the woman's weight?

REFERENCES

Danforth DN: Textbook of obstetrics and gynecology, ed 4, New York, 1980, Harper & Row Publishers, Inc.

Guthrie HA: Introductory nutrition, ed 6, St. Louis, 1986, The CV Mosby Co.

Hellman LM, and Pritchard J: Williams' obstetrics, ed 15, New York, 1975, Appleton-Century-Crofts.

Jensen MD, Benson RC, and Bobak IM: Maternity care: the nurse and the family, ed 3, St. Louis, 1985, The CV Mosby Co.

Marias V: Female sexual response during and after pregnancy, San Francisco, 1969, National Sex Forum.

Stave H, editor: Physiology of the prenatal period, ed 2, New York, 1970, Appleton-Century-Crofts.

CHAPTER 5

Prenatal Care

VOCABULARY

Ballottement
Braxton Hicks' contractions
Funic souffle
Leukorrhea
Presumptive sign
Pseudocyesis
Psychoprophylaxis
Quickening

LEARNING OBJECTIVES

- Describe the subjective, objective, and absolute signs of pregnancy.

- Discuss the TPAL system of identification and state its advantages over the GPA system.

- Discuss the usefulness of prenatal care.

- Describe the health history and physical assessment that take place at an initial prenatal visit.

- Calculate the EDC using the date of a woman's last menstrual period.

- Discuss the advantages and disadvantages of breast-feeding and bottle-feeding.

- Describe recommended prenatal breast care, exercise, bathing, elimination, intercourse, dental care, mental health, rest, and activity.

- Discuss effects of drugs, alcohol, and tobacco during pregnancy.

- List prenatal teaching needs of parents.

- List danger signs a mother should report during pregnancy.

- Describe natural childbirth methods of Lamaze and Bradley, hypnosis, and analgesic medications.

SIGNS AND SYMPTOMS OF PREGNANCY

Because of the tremendous effect of pregnancy on the life of the woman, it is important to her and her family to know if she is indeed pregnant. For this reason, the signs and symptoms of pregnancy have been classified according to their significance in establishing a positive diagnosis of pregnancy. These signs are divided into subjective, objective, and absolute evidence of pregnancy.

Definitions

symptoms Feelings that are experienced by a person but not necessarily observed by others.

signs Objective evidence that can be seen, heard, felt or measured by others.

presumptive evidence Early subjective signs and symptoms that make pregnancy a possibility.

probable evidence Objective signs and symptoms that provide valuable information, including laboratory tests.

positive signs Absolute evidence that a fetus is present; all appear late in pregnancy.

Subjective (presumptive) evidence

Amenorrhea

For healthy women who normally menstruate regularly, amenorrhea is one of the earliest evidences of pregnancy, especially if other early symptoms are also present. Other reasons for amenorrhea include anemia, central nervous system abnormalities, endocrine disturbances, altitude or climate change, infectious diseases, cervical obstruction, or emotional tension.

Breast changes

Tingling, tenderness, heaviness, and enlargement are early symptoms of breast change. Later, pigmentation, nipple change, colostrum secretion, and vein enlargement occur. These changes are especially significant in a woman who has never been pregnant before.

Nausea and vomiting

Beginning soon after the first menstrual period is missed, many women experience various degrees of nausea, dizziness, and vomiting. This is called *morning sickness* because the symptoms occur more often after periods of fasting. It is believed that morning sickness is the body's initial response to high progesterone levels. The sickness usually disappears by the third month although in rare cases vomiting may continue longer. This condition is then called *pernicious vomiting* and is treated as an abnormal complication of pregnancy.

Urinary frequency

Blood congestion in the pelvic organs increases the sensitivity of the tissues. The pressure of an enlarging uterus on the bladder stimulates nerves and triggers an urge to urinate during pregnancy. Urinary tract infection, trauma, and tumor growth may produce similar symptoms.

Leukorrhea ("whites")

Increased vaginal secretions caused by the stimulating effect of hormones on the glands and an increase in blood supply to the pelvis appear quite early in pregnancy. Any foul, yellow-green discharge or any bleeding during pregnancy is *not* normal and should be investigated immediately.

Chadwick's sign (purple vaginal hue)

An early change that can be seen on examination is the color of the vaginal mucosa, which becomes bluish purple because of an increased blood supply. However, any pelvic congestion can cause this symptom, not only pregnancy.

General symptoms

Some women say they "feel" pregnant. By this they may be describing the rather vague feeling of fatigue, dull-headedness, and even headache that are common during the first month of pregnancy. Some women find they need 12 hours or more of sleep per day. These symptoms may be caused by progesterone-induced water retention. Such signs also may be caused by mental depression. Although the dull headache of early pregnancy is relatively common, headaches that develop in later pregnancy may indicate hypertension. For this reason later headaches should be reported.

Quickening

Quickening is an archaic term that means "the first feeling of life." This thrilling sensation, like the fluttering of a butterfly, is first felt by the expectant mother about the twenty-second week of gestation. A woman who has been pregnant previously may feel movement at 20 weeks. Although an encouraging sign to the woman, quickening is not proof of pregnancy. This sign is subjective, not objective evidence that can be corroborated.

Objective (probable) evidence
Uterine growth and change

Hegar's sign is the softening of the lower segment of the uterus. *Goodell's sign* is the softening of the cervix. These signs are probable but not absolute evidence of pregnancy.

Uterine growth is not as significant a sign in the early weeks of pregnancy as change in the uterine muscle. By the end of the second month the uterus normally doubles in size. By the end of the third month the uterus is as large as an orange, and the fundus has begun to rise above the pubic bone. Thereafter, the size of the uterus is used to determine fetal growth.

By the end of the fifth month the fundus usually has risen to the navel; by the eighth month it has risen to the bottom of the sternum, or breast bone. At about the eighth month, *lightening* usually occurs. Lightening is the rather sudden drop of the fetus into the mother's pelvis in a position preparatory to birth.

Because cysts and tumors also can develop rapidly in the uterus, increasing uterine size is considered a useful sign, but not positive proof of pregnancy.

Ballottement is the rebound that occurs when an examiner's finger taps the floating fetus within the uterus, causing the fetus to float away and then to return to its original position. This rebound can only occur when the fetus is large enough to be felt and before it grows too large to move about freely, at approximately 4 to 5 months. Ballottement is not considered a positive sign of pregnancy because the same effect could conceivably be duplicated by a tumor within a fluid-filled abdomen.

The *uterine souffle* (pronounced soo-full) is a muffled, swishing pulse heard over the pregnant uterus. The pulse sounds in unison with the expectant mother's heartbeat and is caused by the rush of blood through the large uterine blood vessels. This sign is not a proof of pregnancy, since the same sound may be heard over large vascular tumors or an aneurysm (outpouching) of an artery.

Braxton Hicks' contractions are painless, intermittent contractions that may occur anytime throughout the pregnancy. Late in pregnancy they may be strong enough to be felt by the expectant mother and may even be mistaken for true labor.

Abdominal changes

As the uterus enlarges, it is quite natural that the abdominal walls should be pushed out to accommodate the increasing size of the uterus. A woman who is about 3 months pregnant begins to notice that her dress belts seem too small. This is caused by the rise of the uterus into the space of the abdominal cavity.

By the time she feels the fetus move, the woman's abdomen may have enlarged so that she can no longer wear her usual clothing. By the eighth month, when maximum distention occurs, the abdominal skin may be stretched tight.

Striae gravidarum occur as a result of stretching of the skin. They are irregular scar lines that may appear in the skin of the abdomen. Especially obvious in fair-skinned women, these striae occur whenever skin is stretched quickly and so by themselves striae are not diagnostic of pregnancy.

Pigmentation occurs as pigment is deposited in the skin of the breasts, face, and midline of the abdomen *(linea nigra)*. This sign is especially noticeable in dark-skinned women. Seen together with other evidence of pregnancy, this pigmentation is a significant sign of pregnancy, but not an absolute one.

Laboratory tests

All laboratory tests for pregnancy are based on the presence of human chorionic gonadotropin (hCG) in blood or urine. This hormone is produced first by the trophoblast when a fertilized ovum implants in the endometrium. The four types of pregnancy tests are bioassay, radioreceptor, immunoassay, and monoclonal antibody.

The *bioassay tests* were the first pregnancy tests and are done with rabbits, rats, mice, and frogs. Urine is injected into the animal; after various time periods the animals are killed and their ovaries examined for follicular changes. In the frog tests, production of sperm or a ripe ovum gives a positive test.

The *radioreceptor assay* uses radioiodine-labeled hCG. This sensitive test can be performed in 1 hour. By adjusting test sensitivity, luteinizing hormone (LH) cross reactions can be compensated for and false-positive test results reduced.

The *immunoassay types* are chemical tests that use the immunological principle causing clumping of animal red blood cells. These tests are 98% accurate and give results 10 to 14 days after the first missed menses. The most recently devised type is called a solid-phase

radioimmunoassay (RIA). It is especially desirable because it eliminates cross reaction with LH, thus giving fewer false-positive results.

The *monoclonal antibody test* is quick (20 minutes), accurate (100%), and uncomplicated (a dipstick read by direct visual observation). This test detects pregnancy by the time of the first missed menses. First approved in 1987, the monoclonal antibody test will probably replace other tests.

Positive (absolute) evidence

Presumptive and probable signs of pregnancy are based on changes observed or felt by the mother. Absolute proof, however, comes with evidence provided by the fetus itself. Positive proof of pregnancy is demonstrated when the examiner can do the following:

1. Hear the fetal heart tones and funic souffle (fetal blood rushing through the umbilical cord).
2. Feel the fetal parts.
3. See the products of conception on ultrasonograms or the fetal skeleton on x-ray films.
4. Feel the fetal movements.
5. Record a fetal electrocardiograph.

Fetal heart tone and funic souffle

The heartbeat of the fetus may be heard as early as the tenth week of gestation with ultrasound fetal pulse detectors (see Fig. 8-8) and by the seventeenth week with ordinary stethoscopes. The fetal heart tone (FHT) sounds like the rapid tick of a wristwatch, beating 120 to 160 times per minute. To obtain an accurate count, the mother's abdomen should be bared and room noises reduced to a minimum. If the woman is especially obese or there is excessive amniotic fluid, the sounds may be difficult to hear. Occasionally the uterine souffle is heard instead of the fetal heartbeat. Remember that the uterine souffle is the mother's pulse heard in an abdominal vessel.

To avoid error, her radial or apical pulse should be counted at the same time or immediately before or after the FHTs.

The *funic souffle* is the sound of fetal blood rushing through the umbilical vessels. This sound can be heard only in a small percentage of cases. Naturally it beats in time with the fetal heart but has a muffled, swooshing tone.

Fetal parts

Sometimes the fetal parts can be felt as early as the fifth month of gestation, but usually definite identification comes later (Fig. 5-1). If the woman is obese or a large amount of amniotic fluid is present, it may be difficult to identify the parts. Usually the head and back can be felt and sometimes the arms and legs.

Ultrasonography and x-ray examination

Ultrasonography is the use of high-frequency sound waves to produce an image of an organ or tissue (Fig. 5-2). The reflected sound waves are transmitted to a viewing screen as they strike tissues of different densities, producing a picture. Ultrasound is safe at any time during the pregnancy for both mother and fetus and can be used repeatedly, if necessary. Ultrasonography has successfully identified an embryo as early as the sixth week and has become a useful diagnostic tool in obstetrical practice, largely replacing x-ray films.

The fetal skeleton can be visualized by x-ray films as early as the twelfth week of gestation. Because of the possible harmful effects of radiation, x-ray examination rarely is used.

Fetal movement

Some time in the fourth month the woman feels the fetus move. To be a positive sign, these movements also must be felt and identified by an observer. The fetus may be so active that the movements can be seen through the mother's clothing.

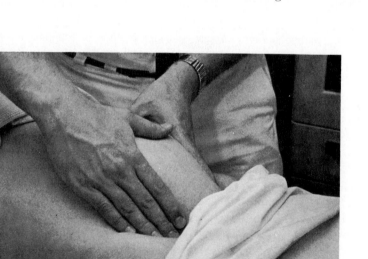

Fig. 5-1 Abdominal palpation.

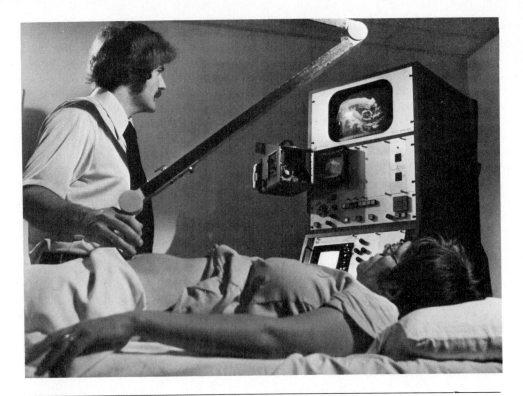

Fig. 5-2 Ultrasonography, a safe, painless method of scanning the mother's abdomen with high-frequency sound waves to follow fetal growth. *(Courtesy The National Foundation– March of Dimes.)*

Fetal electrocardiography

Fetal electrocardiography is a technique in which the electrical impulses coursing through the fetal heart are recorded by means of electrodes placed on the mother's abdomen. This is done in much the same way that electrodes are positioned for recording an adult's electrocardiograph. Fetal monitoring provides continuous information about the fetus. It is especially valuable during labor in high-risk pregnancies.

False pregnancy (pseudocyesis)

False pregnancy is a rather rare psychogenic condition in which the woman experiences subjective symptoms of pregnancy but is not pregnant. In this condition, sometimes called *hysterical pregnancy*, the signs of amenorrhea, morning sickness, weight gain, breast enlargment with colostrum secretion, and abdominal enlargement all may occur. The pituitary gland is affected by emotions sufficient to cause changes in the menstrual cycle and lactogenic hormone production, in turn causing breast changes.

Enlargement of the abdomen is caused by subconscious relaxation of abdominal muscles. When the patient sleeps, is anesthetized, or is hypnotized, abdominal distention disappears. The patient experiences fetal movement. After several months, often more than 9, symptoms of labor, complete with a bloody discharge may develop. Negative laboratory tests do not convince the patient that she is not pregnant. Psychotherapy is prescribed.

Terminology
Definitions

abortion Delivery that occurs before the end of 20 weeks' gestation.

ante Before.

fetal death Death of the fetus after 20 weeks' gestation; formerly called stillbirth.

gestation Growth of the fetus in the uterus.

gravida Any pregnancy, regardless of duration, including present pregnancy (memory aid: "grave condition").

multigravida A woman who is pregnant for a second or more times.

multipara A woman who has had two or more deliveries at more than 20 weeks' gestation.

nullipara A woman who has not had a delivery at more than 20 weeks' gestation.

para Delivery after 20 weeks' gestation, regardless of whether the infant is born alive or dead.

primipara A woman who has had one delivery at more than 20 weeks' gestation, regardless of whether the infant is born alive or dead.

primigravida A woman who is pregnant for the first time.

stillbirth Former term for death of fetus after 20 weeks' gestation.

weeks of gestation Number of weeks since the first day of the last menstrual period (LMP).

Usage

In maternal records women are identified by their gravid and parous history. The original system, called *gravida-para-abortion (GPA)*, focuses on the woman's deliveries. The newer system called *term-preterm-abortion-living (TPAL)*, focuses on the children that resulted from the pregnancies.

Gravida-para-abortion system. Examples of the GPA system include the following:

1. A woman enters the hospital with her first pregnancy and has not delivered yet: Gravida I, Para 0, Abortion 0.

2. The same woman leaving the hospital with her baby: Gravida I, Para I, Abortion 0.

3. The same woman pregnant for a second time: Gravida II, Para I, Abortion 0.

4. The same women after a spontaneous abortion of her second pregnancy at 8 weeks' gestation: Gravida II, Para I, Abortion I.

5. The same woman after delivery of twins: Gravid III, Para II, Abortion I. (Note that twins are considered as one pregnancy and one delivery.)

Term-preterm-abortion-living system. In the TPAL system the number of pregnancies is stated after the world *gravida,* just as in the GPA system. After the word *para,* however, the infants and abortions are listed in a four-digit sequence, as follows:

Digit one—**T:** *term* infants born; that is, the number of infants born at 37 weeks' gestation or after

Digit two—**P:** *preterm* infants born; that is, the number of infants born before 37 weeks' gestation

Digit three—**A:** *abortion;* that is, the number of pregnancies ending in either spontaneous or therapeutic abortion.

Digit four—**L:** *living;* that is, the number of currently living children.

Examples of the TPAL system include the following:

1. A woman, at term, enters the hosptial with her first pregnancy and has not delivered yet: Gravida 1, Para 0000.

2. The same woman leaving the hospital with her baby: Gravida 1, Para 1001.

3. The same woman pregnant for a second time: Gravida 2, Para 1001.

4. The same woman after a spontaneous abortion of her second pregnancy at 8 weeks' gestation: Gravida 2, Para 1011.

5. The same woman after her third pregnancy and delivery of twins at 40 weeks' gestation: Gravida 3, para 3013.
6. The same woman after her fourth pregnancy and delivery of a preterm infant at 36 weeks' gestation who survived: Gravida 4, Para 3114.

MEDICAL SUPERVISION
Importance of prenatal care

There is no question that one of the most important factors in reducing maternal and infant mortality is adequate medical supervision begun early in pregnancy. In 1915, of 10,000 live births, 60.8 mothers and 999 babies under 1 year old died. In 1987, of the same number of live births, 1.9 mothers and 140 babies died. Although the overall situation has vastly improved, not all groups have benefited equally. The maternal death rate for black women is 47% higher than for white women. Research show this to be largely because of more stress, poorer nutrition, and less medical supervision among black women. Nurses and nursing organizations must intensify their efforts to provide all women with early and continuous care throughout pregnancy.

Goal of prenatal care

The goal of all prenatal care is to provide maximum health for expectant mothers and their babies. This is accomplished by the following actions:

1. Determine that the woman is pregnant.
2. Evaluate and treat other medical conditions that may be present.
3. Diagnose and treat complications of pregnancy.
4. Provide support for the psychological needs of the woman to reduce stress-related complications.
5. Ensure a nutritious diet.
6. Prepare the woman for labor and child care by education and assistance.

7. Ensure and later provide postpartal care and medical supervision of newborn.

Preparation for pregnancy

Good prenatal care begins in childhood as the girl grows and develops emotional and physical health. When the young woman reaches puberty, she should have the benefits of medical supervision. Just before marriage she should arrange a premarital consultation. A prepregnancy examination is recommended and when the woman first suspects she is pregnant, she should seek medical supervision.

The first visit

The first visit to the midwife or physician is of great importance to the woman. The nurse plays a vital role in creating an atmosphere of cheerful confidence in which the apprehensive woman can relax. This visit sets the tone for a therapeutic relationship and establishes rapport between the nurse and the woman.

Usually the new patient has a brief interview with the midwife or physician during which she introduces herself and tells of her suspicion of pregnancy. A detailed medical history may be completed at this time or may be taken after a thorough physical examination, depending on the woman's needs. Before the woman leaves, the nurse should be sure that medical instructions are understood and that the woman knows when to return for her next appointment. Often the patient then proceeds to a laboratory for tests.

Medical history

A detailed medical history is important because it provides an accurate picture of the woman's past and present health status. Family diseases, childhood diseases, accidents, surgical operations, allergies, immunizations, and present disease conditions are all pertinent. Information about previous pregnancies is vital, including the number, whether they were full term or less, size of the babies at birth, length of the labors, and complications that may have occurred before, during, or after delivery. The menstrual history includes the age of menarche, the amount of flow, and the interval between and length of each menses. The date of the beginning of the last menstrual period (LMP) is used in determining the predicted date of delivery.

Determination of delivery date

The duration of pregnancy varies from 38 to 42 weeks or between 266 and 294 days. Any date that is set for the delivery can be only an approximation. The estimated date of confinement (EDC) usually is determined by a rule devised by Naegele, using a 268-day standard. To calculate a woman's EDC according to Naegele's rule, take the first day of her LMP, add 7 days to it, count back 3 months from the new date, and add 1 year. An error of 2 weeks either way may occur. For example, consider a woman who began her LMP March 1, 1988:

$$LMP = 3/1/88 + 7 \text{ days} = 3/8/88$$
$$3/8/88 - \underline{3 \text{ months}} = 1/8/88$$
$$1/8/88 + 1 \text{ year} = 1/8/89 = EDC$$

When a woman does not remember the date her LMP began or has irregular menses, other means of estimating the delivery date are used. These include palpating the fetus to estimate its growth rate and size and performing an ultrasonography examination (Fig. 5-2).

Physical examination

At the first visit the patient is examined from head to foot, including all body systems, general appearance, and psychological status. These initial findings are important for later comparison. If the patient has a known major

disorder such as diabetes, is younger than 18 or older than 35 years of age, or has a history of obstetric complications, she is classified as a *high-risk mother*. She then is given special attention throughout her pregnancy.

A physical examination list includes all of the following:

1. General appearance, including posture, nutritional status, and age
2. Height, weight, and body build
3. Eyes, ears, nose, mouth, and teeth (cavities may require immediate attention)
4. Blood pressure, heart, and lungs
5. Examination of breasts and nipples
6. Abdominal examination by palpation (feeling) for uterine enlargement, fetal heart tones (if the fetus is 10 weeks old or more), and any other abdominal finding
7. Examination of the extremities for edema or varicosities
8. Vaginal examination for signs of pregnancy such as Chadwick's sign
9. Cervical smear for cancer cytology test (Papanicolaou—usually taken from the cervix with an applicator, placed on glass slides, immediately immersed in 95% alcohol, and sent out for microscopic examination)
10. Vaginal secretion smear for gonorrhea
11. Manual examination of the pelvic organs for signs of pregnancy (Hegar's and other signs) and any abnormal condition
12. Pelvic measurements (pelvimetry) to determine the approximate size of the bony pelvic outlet through which the fetus must pass during birth
13. Urinalysis—sugar, acetone, and albumin, usually done by the nurse in the office or clinic using simple, rapid tests (sulfosalicylic acid drops added to urine coagulate albumin readily)
14. Blood tests—hemoglobin and blood

counts; standard tests for syphilis (fetal deformities possible from untreated maternal syphilis); determination of blood group, Rh status, and rubella antibody titer, which indicates whether the woman has immunity to German measles; and test for acquired immunodeficiency syndrome (AIDS)

Continuing medical supervision

Each return visit to the clinic becomes an important event in the life of the expectant mother. She should be encouraged to keep a note pad at home to write the questions she may have between visits.

The frequency of return visits depends on the patient's needs. For an uncomplicated pregnancy the usual pattern of office visits is every 4 weeks during the first 5 months, then more and more frequently until the last month, when visits are weekly.

Subsequent visits to the clinic usually include the following (Fig. 5-3):

1. Urinalysis: the woman brings a clean, midstream, early-morning voiding to be tested for sugar, acetone, and albumin.

2. Weight: weight gain of more than 2 pounds per week in the second trimester is usually caused by fluid retention. This condition is called *gestational edema* and is abnormal.

3. Blood pressure measurement: rise of 30 mm Hg systolic or 15 mm Hg diastolic is called *gestational hypertension* and is abnormal.

4. Interview midwife, physician, or nurse: at this time the mother discusses her problems or questions, thus building a trusting relationship.

5. Abdominal examination: height of the uterus, position of the fetus, and fetal heart tone are all measured.

6. Vaginal examination: performed as indicated to determine the presenting part and the status of the cervix as the EDC approaches.

7. Blood examination: performed to monitor such conditions as syphilis, anemia, and blood type incompatibility.

Nutritional needs

The diet of a pregnant woman must supply the needs of both the mother and the fetus. This does not mean doubling caloric intake. It means that nutrients required by the fetus will be supplied by either by the mother's diet or by her body tissues. Caloric needs of the fetus are small; protein, mineral, and vitamin needs of the fetus are considerably greater. For the fetus to develop properly, these needs must be met. Special diets for malnourished women or those with special problems must be adjusted during pregnancy to meet the added needs of the growing fetus.

A normal diet for a pregnant woman is described in Table 5-1.

Breast-feeding vs. bottle-feeding

Sometime during the prenatal period the mother needs to decide how she will feed her baby. Both bottle-fed and breast-fed infants grow into happy, healthy children, and most women can breast-feed their infants successfully if they so choose. Some women, however, have a definite aversion to the whole matter of breast-feeding. Others eagerly anticipate the experience. The factors to consider in making a decision include the following:

Breast	Formula
Less expensive and readily available	Expensive, requires some preparation
Sterile and warm at all times	Easily contaminated, must be refrigerated
Content uncontrolled and variable	Content known and easily controlled
Contains antibodies and more digestible fat with more cholesterol to stimulate enzyme production.	Antibodies and more digestible forms of fat not presently available in commercial preparations

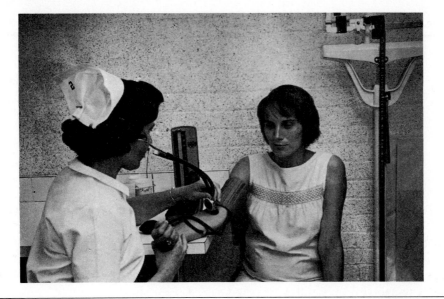

Fig. 5-3 Routine antepartum checkup includes urinalysis, weight, and blood pressure measurements, followed by an interview and examination by the physician or nurse-midwife.

Mother only person to feed baby	Father or substitute mother can feed baby
Quality affected by mother's physical and emotional state	Quantity or quality of milk not affected by emotions of mother
Baby always held during feeding	Baby may or may not be held
Increased possibility of breast abscess	Breast complications rare
Mother's life restricted to feeding schedule	No restriction on mother's life
Some mothers gain considerable psychosexual satisfaction	Infant feeding not associated with mother's psychosexual needs

Nurses should not shame mothers who decide to bottle-feed or discourage those who decide to breast-feed. Both groups need supportive care and information.

Breast care

During pregnancy breasts should be prepared for their unique function of producing milk for the newborn infant soon after birth. Because each breast may increase in weight more than 1 pound, a good uplift brassiere is essential for protection and support. If the mother does not plan to breast-feed, cleanliness is the only preparation needed. If she does plan to breast-feed, nipple toughening is recommended.

In cultures where breasts are exposed to the sun and air, a natural toughening of the nipple tissue occurs. In our society other methods, such as nipple rolling and twisting, have been advised. However, recent studies show that this practice does not help and may cause preterm uterine contractions. Daily washing without soap, careful drying, and application of lanolin-based ointment to the nipples are recommended.

Pelvic floor muscle (Kegel's) exercises

The pelvic floor muscles encircle the outlet through which the baby passes at birth. It is important for mothers to strengthen these muscles and gain conscious control over them

Table 5-1 Daily food guide

	One serving	Daily servings		
		Non-pregnant	Pregnant	Breast-feeding
Protein foods		4	4	4
Animal (meats)	60 gm or 2 oz			
Legumes (beans)	240 ml or 1 cup			
Nuts	120 ml or ½ cup			
Eggs	2 medium size			
Milk foods		2	4	5
Milk and yogurt	240 ml or 1 cup			
Cottage cheese	320 ml or 1½ cups			
Solid cheese	45 gm or 1½ oz			
Bread and cereals		4	4	4
Bread	24 to 28 gm or 1 slice			
Rice and cereal	120 ml or ½ cup			
Ready-to-eat cereal	180 ml or ¾ cup			
Dark green vegetables (chard, romaine, spinach, cabbage, etc.)		1	1	1
Cooked	180 ml or ¾ cup			
Raw	240 ml or 1 cup			
Vitamin C–rich fruits and vegetables (tomatoes, greens, brussels sprouts, broccoli, cauliflower, peppers, cantaloupe, citrus fruit, guava, strawberries, mango, papaya, etc.)	180 ml or ¾ cup 120 ml or ½ cup 30 ml or 2 tbsp 240 ml or 1 cup	1	1	1
Any other fruits and vegetables	To taste (unless physician prescribes otherwise)	1	1	1
Fats and oils		1	1	1
Liquids (water, tea, coffee, juices, soups)		6	6	8
Salt		1	1	1
Supplementary minerals and vitamins				
Iron	Per physician's order		1 to 3	1 to 3
Folic acid (folacin)	Per physician's order		1 to 3	
Avoid all alcohol, unprescribed drugs, and cigarettes.				

Modified from Daily food guide. In Maternal-child health, Sacramento, Calif, 1977, California Department of Health.

so that they can contract or relax these muscles at will.

To begin Kegel's exercises, the woman first must learn to control the muscles. To teach her, the examiner places two fingers in the vagina and asks the woman to squeeze them as if stopping the flow of urine. Once the woman has learned this control, she can carry out the exercises at any time or place. The exercises are as follows:

1. Contract the pelvic floor muscles and hold for 10 seconds.
2. Relax for 10 seconds. Repeat eight to ten times.

3. Repeat this exercise five to ten times each day.

Dental care

Losing a "tooth per child" is not necessary. Women should go to their dentist early in pregnancy to have cavities filled and infected teeth treated. These procedures can be done safely at any time during the pregnancy, although it is better to have them taken care of early. To prevent additional caries, the mother is encouraged to:

1. Brush her teeth regularly.
2. Floss between teeth.
3. Rinse the mouth with water after eating or drinking anything.
4. Use an *alkaline* mouthwash to counteract the acidic saliva of pregnancy, which provides a favorable medium for the growth of enamel-destroying bacteria.

Clothing

A great deal of imagination has been displayed by designers of maternity fashions. The criteria for these garments are that they should be adjustable to the expanding contour; washable because of increased perspiration; loose fitting, so that they will not bind; and reasonably priced because they are to be used for only a few months. A wide variety of costumes have been added to the traditional smock, including attractive garments for sports, formal wear, and dressy occasions so that expectant mothers can continue to look and feel pretty—an important factor in maintaining morale.

High-heeled shoes are no longer taboo if the woman is used to them and is careful to avoid falls. Round garters are not recommended; they cut off circulation in the legs and increase the likelihood of varicose veins. Stretch-front pantyhose are comfortable, safe, and recommended. Abdominal supports and maternity corsets are seldom ordered except for severe backache or prior skeletal disability. Some physicians believe these supports and corsets contribute to muscular weakness. Other physicians leave the use of supports up to the woman's preference.

Bathing

Daily bathing stimulates circulation, refreshes, and removes body wastes. With caution to avoid falls, both showers and tub baths are acceptable for pregnant women.

Intercourse

Many women experience heightened sexual tension during pregnancy. This is caused in part by increased blood congestion of the vulva and a heightened awareness of their sexual role. Unless there is a history of repeated spontaneous abortions, no medical reason exists to restrict intercourse. The frequency, intensity, and positions for sexual activity need to be adjusted to the woman's changing body contour.

Elimination

Constipation is common during pregnancy because of hormonal action that reduces the peristalsis of the bowel and the enlarging uterus that crowds it. A regular "time," together with extra fluids and laxative fruits, is the best nonmedicinal remedy. Stool softeners and mild laxatives may be prescribed if necessary.

Urinary frequency is a common occurrence during the first and last months of pregnancy because of the space taken by the uterus and the increased sensitivity of the blood-congested tissue. If, however, this frequency is accompanied by burning or by blood and pus-streaked urine, the physician should be notified at once.

Albuminuria is a danger signal of abnormal kidney function. Since this condition cannot be seen by the naked eye, an albumin test is performed at each prenatal visit to determine if albumin is present in the urine.

Drugs, alcohol, and tobacco

Studies done in 1964 on babies deformed by thalidomide have revealed that during the extremely critical time when the baby is first being formed, even single doses of otherwise harmless drugs taken by the mother may cause serious deformities of the embryo. For this reason, pregnant woman should avoid *all* drugs except those specifically ordered by their physician. This precaution is especially important when the body organs are forming during the first trimester.

Addictive drugs such as heroin taken by the mother pass into the fetal blood and cause the fetus to become dependent on the drug as well. When these babies are born, their source of the drug is withdrawn, and they exhibit typical life-threatening withdrawal symptoms. At birth such infants may be admitted to the noenatal intensive care unit for observation. (See Chapter 14.)

All alcoholic beverages should be avoided during pregnancy. Recent studies reveal that a pregnant woman who drinks as little as 3 ounces of liquor a day runs a significant risk of bearing a child with congenital defects. Fetal alcohol syndrome (FAS) deformities include retarded physical and mental growth and defects of the heart, eye, ear, face, and brain. The risk is greatest among babies of chronic alcohol abusers.

Recent studies show that cigarette smoking or even continual exposure to a smoke-filled environment is harmful to both the fetus and the mother, causing retarded fetal growth and a higher incidence of neonatal and infant mortality. Besides aggravating acute and chronic respiratory conditions, smoke also interferes with the body's ability to use vitamin C, a vitamin needed for synthesis of connective tissue in the growing fetus.

Rest and activity

Fatigue is an early symptom of pregnancy. As the body becomes accustomed to pregnancy and the woman learns to space her work and rest, this symptom lessens. During the first trimester most women find an afternoon nap most helpful. Blood congestion in the pelvis and legs is lessened, the work of the heart is reduced and mental stress is relieved.

Walking is considered an ideal exercise for pregnant women. Other forms of exercise depend on the degree of fatigue and muscular cramping that follow. Standing too long without moving the legs may cause fainting. Climbing chairs and ladders is dangerous because of possible falls. Moderation is the key to health.

Travel in itself does not cause abortion or premature labor, but the excessive fatigue often produced by travel should be avoided. The chief objection to travel is that it may take the mother away from competent care in case of an emergency. If long distances are involved, air travel is recommended, since it is rapid and usually between populated areas where medical care is available.

Mental health

Recent studies indicate that pregnant women who are subjected to continuous severe interpersonal tension have a 50% greater risk of bearing a child with physical handicaps. When there is evidence that a pregnant woman is living in a highly stressful environment, appropriate intervention should be made. Community resources may be called on to help, including mental health, public health, and social welfare services. During each prenatal visit the expectant mother needs an opportunity to speak in confidence with someone who will listen empathically to her concerns.

Father's role

Fathers were once forgotten, but today they are included in the entire maternity cycle. They are encouraged to participate in preparation-for-childbirth classes, where they learn to work with their wives during labor and go with them to the delivery room. Fathers learn how to feed, diaper, and bathe the newborn infant. Such full participation in parenthood strengthens child-father and husband-wife relationships.

Preparation for the baby

One of the joys of motherhood that can be shared with family and friends is planning and buying a layette. Some families spend large sums of money on elaborate equipment and supplies, but this is not necessary. A modest layette will meet the infant's needs as well as an expensive one if it is well planned. Some factors to consider follow:

1. Babies grow rapidly. A few items in each size are more practical than many in one size.
2. Safety and cleanliness are vital. Every item should be judged by these criteria.
3. Disposable diapers are expensive, and they must be changed as often as cloth ones.
4. Babies need to be warm, but not too hot. Weather and the environment affect the type of clothes.
5. Bottle-feeding requires nursing units. Disposable units are expensive; reusable ones must be clean.
6. Babies move and stretch. Heavy clothing or covers and tight bindings restrict movement.

Prenatal teaching

Prenatal teaching is the responsibility of health care providers. Table 5-2 presents a guide for such teaching.

Some physicians' offices and clinics give each mother a packet of information at her first visit. The information answers the most common questions women ask concerning such factors as weight gain, diet, bathing, and intercourse. Nurses should be prepared to discuss these concerns. Their instructions should be consistent with the other members of the obstetrical team, however, because minor differences in practice do exist among authorities.

Danger signals

Often mothers are given a list of danger signals so that they may recognize a possible emergency. Nurses may need to explain the significance of these signals. A typical danger list may read as follows:

Notify your physician *at once* if any of the following symptoms occur:

1. Any bleeding from the vagina or leakage of water
2. Severe or continuous headaches
3. Disturbance of vision
4. Chills and fever
5. Swelling of face, hands, feet, or ankles
6. Pain in the abdomen or chest
7. Scant or bloody urine
8. Persistent vomiting

Preparation for childbirth

Modern expectant couples prepare for the birth of their child. Such preparation, especially by men, is relatively recent.

Dick-Read method

Grantly Dick-Read, an English obstetrician, was a pioneer in the childbirth preparation movement. He is reported to have been asked, "Must childbirth be painful?" He began to explore the problem of pain in childbirth and in 1933 published his first work, *Natural Childbirth*. Eleven years later, he published his now-famous *Childbirth Without Fear*, a work that was destined to change the accepted ideas of centuries.

Dick-Read taught that pain resulted from fear and that when a woman knows what is happening in and to her body during childbirth, she will not be terrified. He also believed that weak muscles contribute to fatigue and

Table 5-2   Prenatal teaching guides

1st-12th weeks **Woman is more concerned with herself, physical changes with pregnancy, and her feelings about the pregnancy.**	**12th-24th weeks** **Woman usually has resolved the issue of the pregnancy and becomes more aware of the fetus as a person.**	**24th-32nd weeks** **Woman becomes more interested in baby's needs as a corollary to her own needs now and after birth.**

Changes that are normal for pregnancy
  Breast fullness
  Urinary frequency
  Nausea and vomiting
  Fatigue
EDC—calculate and explain
  Compare with uterine size
Expectation for care
  Initial visit
  Subsequent visits
Clinic appointments
Need for iron and vitamins
Resources available
  Education
  Dental evaluation
  Medical service
  Social service
  Emergency room
Danger signs
  Drugs, self-medication
  Spotting, bleeding
  Cramping, pain
	Growth of fetus
	  Movement
	  FHT
	Personal hygiene
	  Comfortable clothing
	  Breast care and supportive bra
	  Recreation, travel
	  Vaginal discharge
	Employment or school plans
	Method of feeding baby
	  Breast or bottle
	  Give literature on methods
	Avoidance or alleviation of
	  Backache
	  Constipation
	  Hemorrhoids
	  Leg ache, varicosities, edema, cramping
	  Round ligament pain
	Nutritional guidance
	  Weight gain
	  Balanced diet
	  Special nutritional needs
		Fetal growth and status
		  Presentation and position
		  Well-being—FHT
		Personal hygiene
		  Comfortable clothing
		  Body mechanics and posture
		  Positions of comfort
		Physical and emotional changes
		Sexual needs/changes; intercourse
		Alleviation of
		  Backache
		  Braxton Hicks' contractions
		  Dyspnea
		  Round ligament pain
		  Leg ache or edema
		Confirm infant's feeding plans
		Prepare for breast- or bottle-feeding
		  Nipple preparation
		  Massage and expression of colostrum
		Preparation for baby
		  Supplies
		  Household assistance
		Danger signs
		  Preeclampsia
		  Headache, excessive swelling, blurred vision
		Tubal ligation (papers prepared ahead)

From Roberts, J: JOGN Nurs 5:17-20, 1976.

32nd-36th weeks **Woman anticipates approaching labor caring for baby after birth.**	**36th week to term** **Woman should feel "ready" for labor and for the assumption of care-taking responsibilities for baby, even though she may feel anxious about both of these as well.**
Fetal growth and status	Review signs of labor (or teach)
Personal hygiene	Review or continue instruction about relaxation
Positions of comfort	and breathing techniques
Rest and activity	Finalize home preparations
Vaginal discharge	Anticipation of hospitalization
Alleviation of discomfort	Admission (ER and labor admitting room)
Backache	Examination, IV, mini-shave, possible enema
Round ligament pain	Care in labor
Constipation or hemorrhoids	Medication and anesthesia available
Leg ache or edema	Postpartum care
Dyspnea	Supplies needed: bra, personal items, money
Recognition of "false labor"—Braxton Hicks' contractions	May have visitors
How to cope and "practice" with these signs	Tour of maternity unit
Nature of "true labor"—signs; difference between "bloody show" and bleeding	Confirm plans to get to hospital; care of other children
What happens during labor	When to go and where
Labor contractions and progress	Consider family planning needs
What woman will experience	Emergency arrangements
Relaxation techniques	Precipitate delivery
Breathing techniques	Premature rupture of membranes with or without contractions
Abdominal	Care away from home
Accelerated pattern	Vaginal bleeding
Panting and pushing	
Involvement of husband or significant other	
Provision for needs of other children	
Anticipation of baby	
Care for children at home while mother is in hospital	

pain and that the ability to relax completely would contribute to a painless labor. The *Dick-Read method* includes (1) education about the physiology of labor, (2) exercises for the abdominal and perineal muscles, and (3) practice in relaxation. The Dick-Read positions and exercise are pictured in Fig. 5-4.

Dick-Read's ideas were widely read and argued both in Europe and the United States. Some authorities accepted his theories; others scoffed at them; still others attempted to improve and extend his pioneer ideas.

Russian psychoprophylaxis

Scientists in Russia had been doing extensive work in the field of nervous reflexes and behavioral patterns. Pavlov's famous experiments with salivating dogs had opened the way for others to apply these theories of conditioned reflexes to obstetrics. By 1949 Nicolaiev declared that the pain of childbirth depended on the nervous system and the relationship between the cortex and the subcortex. A system was devised whereby pregnant women were conditioned to respond to the spoken word in specific ways, thus preparing them for childbirth and removing their fear and pain. He called the system *psychoprophylaxis*, meaning prevention, and presented it to the world at the Karkov conference of 1949. By 1950 the system had been perfected, and by 1951 the Russian government ordered the method used throughout the whole country.

Lamaze method

During these same years a French obstetrician, Fernand Lamaze, became committed to the idea of painless childbirth. He attended the Karkov conference when the Russian system was presented and was so impressed that he went to Russia to observe and study their method. He returned to France convinced that psychoprophylaxis was indeed a valid means

by which women could have their babies without pain.

Lamaze developed a well-defined, step-by-step system of education and instruction, which has proved itself so effective that it is now used worldwide. In the United States, increasing numbers of mothers are turning to this system. At first glance the system sounds quite similar to Dick-Read's, and both include education and exercises. The Lamaze method, however, is based on the use of conditioned reflexes and focuses on particular objectives, whereas the Dick-Read method is quite general. The Lamaze system includes the husband or support person as a necessary assistant in the process of childbirth and makes the woman an active participant in her delivery rather than a victim of uncontrolled forces.

The Lamaze method has been modified over time. An important change has been in regard to use of analgesics. Originally, "successful" Lamaze mothers used *no* anesthesia. Today the Lamaze method is taught as a *tool*. The couple set their own goal, using the method as needed according to their situation.

Classes. The Lamaze psychoprophylactic method is usually taught through group instruction of five to ten women. Beginning at about their thirtieth week of pregnancy, these women attend one class a week for 8 weeks, preferably with a support person (Fig. 5-5). During eight carefully planned lectures and practice sessions, the mothers-to-be and their husbands learn the following:

1. Physiology of labor and delivery
2. The importance and method of proper breathing
3. How to relax certain muscle groups
4. How to use the painless Braxton Hicks' contractions to practice correct breathing
5. How to behave during the first, second, and third stages of labor.

Then the participants see a film of an actual

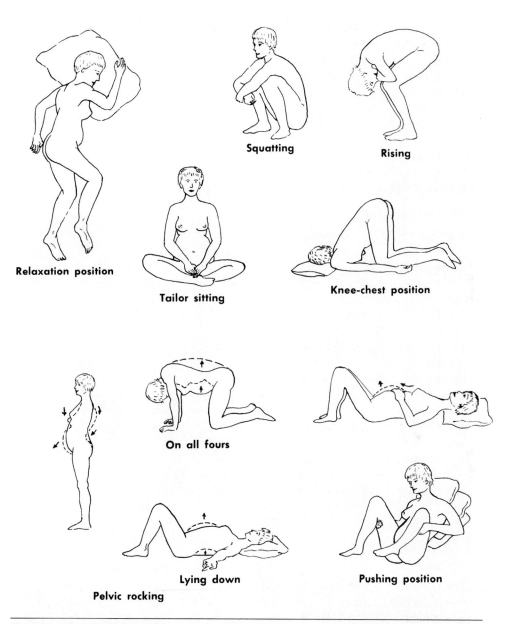

Squatting

Rising

Relaxation position

Tailor sitting

Knee-chest position

On all fours

Pelvic rocking

Lying down

Pushing position

Fig. 5-4 Dick-Read positions and exercises. Relaxation position requires that all parts of the body are supported by mattress. Tailor sitting and squatting positions stretch perineal muscles. Knee-chest position relieves pelvic pressure. Pelvic rocking helps relieve low backache and abdominal pressure. Pushing position is used during second stage of labor.

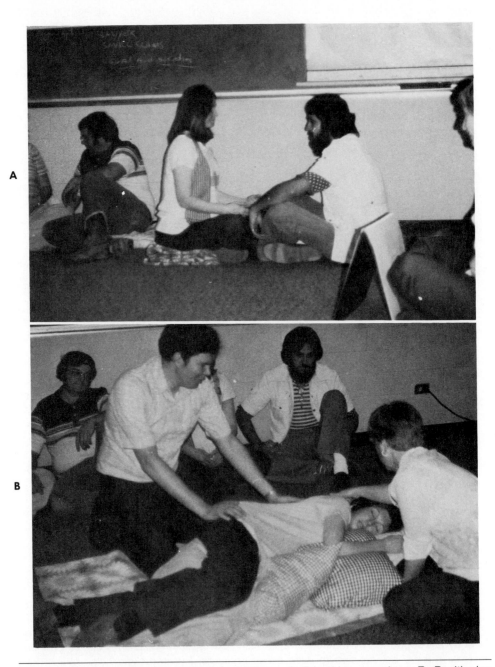

Fig. 5-5 Prenatal class for mothers and fathers. **A,** Breathing exercises. **B,** Positioning practice by husband and mother; it will be used during the preliminary phase of labor.

labor and delivery without pain in which the mother and support person take an active and vital role in the entire process. As a result of this training, many American women are experiencing what they feel is the fulfillment of the goal of childbirth without pain.

EXERCISES*
Body-building

Objective: To strengthen and stretch muscles.

Instructions: Do these exercises on the floor. Do not use pillows. Repeat pelvic rock exercises 10 times daily and other exercises three to five times daily.

Exercises:

1. PELVIC ROCK. Lie on back with legs bent, feet firmly on floor. Press back and shoulders against floor, contracting abdominal muscles. Release. Do exercise with breathing, as follows: flatten back while exhaling, release back while inhaling.
2. PELVIC FLOOR (KEGEL'S). Any body position. Contract anal sphincter, vagina, and urethra. Hold for count of six. Release.
3. CROSS-LEG SITTING. Sit cross-legged on floor to stretch thigh and pelvic muscles.
4. THIGH STRETCH. Sit on floor. Pull feet as near body as comfortable. Press knees gently to floor.
5. LEG STRENGTHENING. Lie down, arms at sides, inhale through nose, raise right leg slowly, point toes. Exhale through lips; flex foot and lower right leg slowly. Repeat with left leg.
6. RISE FROM LYING POSITION. Bend knees, turn from back to side. Push up with both arms.

Neuromuscular

Objective: To learn to control muscle groups.

Instructions: Contract the particular part strongly while completely relaxing the rest of the body. Practice three times daily.

Exercise: Contract right arm. Release. Contract left arm. Release. Contract right leg. Release. Contract left leg. Release. Contract right arm and left

---

* Compiled from various teachers of Lamaze techniques.

leg. Release. Contract left leg and right arm. Release.

Breathing, relaxation, and muscle control

Objective: To learn to control breathing and muscles.

Instructions: Practice for 1 minute three times daily.

Position and exercise:

1. Preliminary labor. Lie on side as coach massages back. Inhale–exhale deeply. Inhale through nose and exhale through lips with slow rhythmic chest breathing (six to nine breaths per minute). Inhale–exhale deeply.
2. Accelerated labor. Lie on side. Coach or mother uses effleurage (gentle stroking of abdomen with both hands in circular movement). Inhale–exhale deeply. Pant faster and faster as contraction builds and slower and slower as it subsides. Inhale–exhale deeply.
3. Transition labor. Lie on side as coach uses counterpressure on sacrococcygeal area and effleurage. Inhale–exhale deeply. Take four to eight fast, shallow breaths and blow. Repeat six times. Inhale–exhale deeply.
4. Expulsion labor. Lie on back at 45-degree angle. Inhale–exhale, inhale–exhale. Inhale, hold breath, hold legs under the knees, bringing legs as close to the shoulders as possible, elbows out, head bent forward; leaning on diaphragm, push out through vagina. Exhale, relax head. Inhale and repeat until contraction is over. Take two or three deep breaths. (During delivery, when asked not to push, use transition breathing. If urge to push is strong, blow through mouth.)

Bradley method

The Bradley method was proposed by Dr. Robert Bradley, a Colorado obstetrician. In 1965 he published *Husband-Coached Childbirth.* This method is essentially the Dick-Read method with the addition of a support person. Bradley advocates that what he proposes is truly natural childbirth, without any form of analgesia or anesthesia, using breathing techniques and a "husband-coach." The American Academy of Husband-Coached Childbirth (AAHCC) was founded to prepare teachers and make the method available to the general public.

Hypnosis

Before the age of modern medicine hypnosis was an effective, but often unrecognized, aid to healing. In recent years, hypnotism has come into its own as a recognized tool in the art of healing. It is being used in psychiatry, anesthesiology, obstetrics, medicine, and dentistry.

Hypnosis is an altered state of consciousness, in which subjects are suggestible to whatever the hypnotists tell them. It involves physical relaxation and focusing the mind so that outside influences are disregarded. There are four levels, or depths, of hypnosis described by various authorities: (1) light, (2) cataleptic, (3) medium, and (4) somnambulistic, or deep. Some people are highly suggestible and therefore are easily hypnotized. About 10% of the population cannot be hypnotized, perhaps because they resist losing control.

The use of hypnosis in obstetrics is not new. What is new in current practice is the way in which it is used and the fact that it is no longer a rare and secretive matter. Hypnotists begin instructing patients in small group sessions about the sixth month of pregnancy. Instruction in self-hypnosis is included so that the woman can practice between classes. The goal of the classes is to have each woman reach the fourth, or deepest, level of hypnosis with ease. This is the level at which she will be free from painful sensations and will respond to directions readily. The degree of suggestibility varies with each woman. Some can arrive at the fourth level in but a few sessions (five to ten), while others take considerably longer. Posthypnotic suggestion is used successfully

to facilitate elimination, breast-feeding, and control of afterpains.

Some physicians who successfully use hypnosis believe that whether Dick-Read, Lamaze, and others recognize it or not, their patients have in fact experienced a degree of hypnosis. Except for those few women who are not suggestible, hypnosis has proved itself effective in attaining childbirth without pain.

Acupuncture and acupressure

In recent years ancient Chinese medicine has gained popularity in some Western countries. The tradition is based on principles of Yin and Yang, the five humors, and the meridians of the body. One of the modes of treatment is acupuncture, in which long needles are inserted into identified points of the body to relieve pain in other areas. The exact physiological explanation has not been determined, but it has proved effective in blocking pain, including pain in childbirth. Acupressure is similar to acupuncture except that pressure is exerted on identified points instead of the insertion of a needle. Acupuncture may be used more frequently as more Western midwives and physicians learn its use.

Commonalities of childbirth preparation

It should be emphasized that no two women are alike and no two pregnancies are alike. The method that works for one may not work for another. The box provides a list of exercises common to all methods. The important thing is that women need not suffer any longer from medieval myths. They can take advantage of any or all the means available to them to experience a joyful birth.

▶ KEY CONCEPTS

1. Signs and symptoms of pregnancy are classified into three groups according to accuracy of diagnosis: subjective (presumptive), objective

---

CHILDBIRTH EXERCISES COMMON TO ALL METHODS

RELAXATION

Find a quiet environment.
Assume a comfortable position.
Concentrate on an object or a visual image.
Release tension from muscles.
The aim is to bring your body under control using your mind and to develop a harmony between your body and mind. For example, you may think of a cool stream or a color that soothes you. Let yourself go; be limp like a rag doll. Try tension and release—tighten muscles, then release.

Early labor

Do deep chest or abdominal breathing.
Breathe in through the nose and out through the mouth. You are taking in oxygen to provide a fresh supply of oxygen for you and your baby.

Transitional or later labor

Take a deep breath as the contraction begins.
Do shallow chest breathing. If you wish, you may increase the rate as the intensity of the contraction increases.
As the contraction ends, take another deep breath.
Relax between contractions to conserve energy.

PREPARATION FOR PUSHING

Take two deep breaths, then a breath and hold (if you wish, count to 10).
Round your back, chin on chest, hands on knees.
Practice for *not* pushing by panting (mouth-centered breathing).

EXHALE BREATHING

Assume the fetal position with the spine totally flexed.
Take several deep breaths.
When ready, hold your breath for 5 or 6 seconds to fix your thorax and abdominal muscle. Keep your rib cage as still as possible.
Begin slow, light exhalation through slightly pursed lips.
As you feel the urge to push, use the abdominal muscles to push with the uterine contraction.
Keep the pelvic floor muscles relaxed.
When ready for your next breath, straighten your neck and inhale slowly.
Repeat as before. Take as many breaths as needed during the contraction.
When the contraction is over, take a deep breath and release the muscle tension.

(probable), and positive (absolute) evidence.

2. Subjective evidence includes breast amenorrhea, breast changes, morning sickness, leukorrhea, Chadwick's sign, and quickening.

3. Objective evidence includes uterine change and growth, abdominal changes, and laboratory tests (bioassay, radioreceptor, and immunoassay types).

4. Positive evidence includes fetal heart tone (FHT), funic souffle, fetal parts, fetal movement, and electrocardiographic readings.

5. Pseudocyesis (false pregnancy) is a psychiatric disorder that produces subjective and some objective evidence of pregnancy.

6. Gravida-para-abortion (GPA), which focuses on deliveries, and term-preterm-abortion-living (TPAL), which focuses on the children produced, are two systems for designating an obstetrical history.

7. Medical supervision helps reduce maternal and infant mortality; it consists of regular prenatal care with early treatment of complications.

8. The first prenatal visit involves a medical and obstetrical history, determination of estimated date of confinement (EDC) using Naegle's method, and physical examination.

9. Continuing prenatal care involves selected physical assessment, teaching, and supervision regarding nutrition, breast care, exercises, dental care, clothing, bathing, intercourse, elimination, substance abuse, rest and activity, mental health, participation of significant other, preparation for baby, and danger signals.

10. Preparation for childbirth to reduce pain was pioneered by Dick-Read. Russian psychoprophylaxis, Lamaze, Bradley, hypnosis, acupuncture, and acupressure are all used to facilitate the birth process and reduce labor pain.

■ *ANNOTATED SUMMARY*

I. Signs and symptoms of pregnancy
   A. Definitions
   B. Subjective (presumptive) evidence—early symptoms, not conclusive
      1. Amenorrhea
      2. Breast changes
      3. Nausea and vomiting
      4. Urinary frequency
      5. Leukorrhea ("whites")
      6. Chadwick's sign (purple vaginal hue)
      7. General symptoms
      8. Quickening
   C. Objective (probable) evidence
      1. Uterine growth and change
      2. Abdominal changes
      3. Laboratory tests
   D. Positive (absolute) evidence
      1. Fetal heart tone (FHT) and funic souffle
      2. Fetal parts
      3. Ultrasonography and x-ray examination
      4. Fetal movement
      5. Fetal electrocardiography
   E. False pregnancy (pseudocyesis)—rare psychogenic condition
   F. Terminology
      1. Definitions
      2. Usage
         a. Gravida-para-abortion (GPA) system
         b. Term-preterm-abortion living (TPAL) system

II. Medical supervision
   A. Importance of prenatal care—to reduce infant and maternal deaths
   B. Goal of prenatal care—maximum health for mothers and babies
   C. Preparation for pregnancy—begins in childhood with emotional and physical health; continues with premarital and prepregnancy examinations
   D. The first visit—rapport established
      1. Medical history—taken in detail
      2. Determination of delivery date— Naegele's rule: LMP + 7 days − 3 months + 1 year = EDC
      3. Physical examination
   E. Continuing medical supervision
      1. Nutritional needs—balance with added milk and supplementary minerals and vitamins
      2. Breast-feeding vs. bottle-feeding— mother needs to make decision during prenatal period; nurse should support her decision

CHAPTER 6

Complications of Pregnancy

VOCABULARY

Eclampsia
Ectopic pregnancy
Estriol
Hyperemesis gravidarum
Hyperglycemia
Leiomyoma
Sensitization
TORCH diseases

LEARNING OBJECTIVES

- List six categories of factors that carry unusual risk for the fetus and cause a pregnancy to be identified as high risk.

- Discuss pregnancy-induced hypertension, stating its cause, symptoms, prognosis, treatment, and nursing care.

- Describe various categories of spontaneous abortion, their causes, treatment, and nursing care.

- Discuss ectopic pregnancy and its locations, management, prognosis, and nursing care.

- Discuss hydatidiform mole, myomas, and cervical polyps and their prognoses, treatment, and nursing care.

- Describe the causes, effects on the mother and fetus, and treatment of the TORCH diseases.

- Discuss diabetes in the pregnant woman and its classifications and effects on the fetus.

- Discuss heart disease during pregnancy, its classifications, prognosis, nursing care, and complications.

- Explain the process of maternal sensitization, Rh factor and ABO incompatibility, and how RhoGAM works.

• Describe the following diagnostic procedures and their purposes and implications for care: ultrasound, estriol determination, nonstress test, contraction stress test, and amniocentesis.

Pregnancy is a normal function of the body, not a disease. Several factors can complicate pregnancy, however, including preexisting conditions and those that develop during pregnancy. Pregnancies that threaten the health of the fetus or mother are termed *high risk* and are listed in the box. Women with any of these complications need special care before, during, and after delivery.

PREEXISTING MEDICAL CONDITIONS
Diabetes mellitus
Description

Diabetes is an endocrine disorder characterized by high blood levels of glucose (hyperglycemia) and glucose in the urine (glycosuria). Diabetes results from inadequate production or use of insulin, an essential hormone, normally produced by the beta cells of the islets of Langerhans in the pancreas. Insulin lowers blood glucose levels by enabling glucose to move from blood into tissue cells. Without adequate insulin, glucose cannot enter the cells to be used as a source of energy. Instead, the body uses fat and protein for energy, causing tissue wasting, negative nitrogen balance, and ketosis caused by fat metabolism. High blood sugar pulls water from the cells into the blood, causing cellular dehydration. Glucose spills over into the urine, which increases osmotic pressure and prevents reabsorption of water by kidney tubules, causing extracellular dehydration. As a result, the four cardinal signs and symptoms of diabetes mellitus occur: *polyuria* (excessive urine excretion), *polydipsia* (extreme thirst), *weight loss*, and *polyphagia* (excessive eating).

HIGH-RISK PREGNANCIES

COMPLICATIONS OF PREVIOUS PREGNANCIES

Prolonged labor
Cesarean birth
Abnormal fetal position
Pregnancy-induced hypertension
Bleeding

ANATOMICAL ABNORMALITIES

Small pelvis
Incompetent cervix

METABOLIC AND ENDOCRINOLOGICAL DISORDERS

Diabetes
Thyroid disorder

CARDIOVASCULAR DISORDERS

Hypertension
Congenital heart disease

KIDNEY DISORDERS

Acute pyelonephritis
Acute cystitis

HEMATOLOGICAL DISORDERS

Anemia (hemoglobin <10 gm)
Sickle cell anemia

OTHER FACTORS

Age—under 16 or over 35
Weight—<100 pounds (45 kg) or >200 pounds (90 kg)
Syphilis
Tuberculosis
Smoking
Drug addiction

Adapted from Korones, SB: High-risk newborn infants: the basis for intensive nursing care, ed 4, St. Louis, 1986, The C.V. Mosby Co.

Classifications

Altered carbohydrate (glucose) metabolism has been classified in several ways. A special committee of the National Institute of Health (1979) suggested three main categories:

1. Diabetes mellitus
   a. Type I, insulin dependent
   b. Type II, non–insulin dependent
   c. Secondary diabetes
2. Impaired glucose tolerance
3. Gestational diabetes (onset or first diagnosis during pregnancy)

Another classification of diabetic mothers made by White is especially useful to those planning nursing care (Table 6-1).

Complications

Diabetes complicates 1 in 300 pregnancies. Before the discovery of insulin in 1921, maternal mortality was 30% and fetal mortality 65%. Even today, with intensive treatment, the incidence of hyperemesis gravidarum, pregnancy-induced hypertension, hydramnios, and cesarean births resulting from large fetal size is great. Fetal mortality is about 20%, and major fetal defects occur much more often than in normal pregnancies. Fetal respiratory distress syndrome, hyperbilirubinemia, and hypoglycemia also occur.

Pregnancy effects diabetes as follows:

1. Changing insulin requirements: decrease during first trimester, then an increase as human placental lactogen (hLP), an insulin antagonist, increases; an increase during labor; and a sudden decrease after delivery
2. Decreased renal threshold for spilling glucose and nephropathy
3. Dietary fluctuations resulting from nausea, vomiting, and cravings
4. Increased risk of ketoacidosis, insulin shock, and coma
5. Hypertension (increased systolic pres-

Table 6-1 White's classification of diabetic mothers

Class	Description
A	Chemical (subclinical) diabetes only, with a normal fasting blood glucose level but elevated 1- or 2-hour levels after a glucose load. Most likely complications: large baby, intrapartum fetal loss
B	Diabetes for less than 10 years, with onset after age 19; no vascular disease. Most likely complications: hydramnios, excessive maternal weight gain, pre-eclampsia, large placenta, large baby, intrapartum fetal loss, intensified diabetes
C	Diabetes for 10 to 19 years or onset between ages 10 and 19; no vascular disease. Most likely complications: all those in class B, but with slightly less risk
D	Diabetes for more than 20 years or with vascular disease, including retinitis and arteriosclerotic retinal and leg-vessel changes
F	Diabetes with nephropathy, including intercapillary glomerulosclerosis (Kimmelstiel-Wilson syndrome), pyelonephritis, and papillary necrosis. Most likely complications: spontaneous abortion, intrauterine fetal loss, neonatal loss
R	Diabetes with malignant retinopathy, including vitreous hemorrhage and neovascularization of scars. Most likely complications: spontaneous abortion, superimposed pre-eclampsia, intrauterine fetal loss, neonatal loss

sure of 30 mm Hg and diastolic of 15 mm Hg)

6. Retinopathy

Goals of nursing care

The goals of nursing care of the diabetic woman during pregnancy are to maintain the physiological equilibrium of insulin production and glucose use and to deliver a healthy mother and neonate. To achieve these goals, prenatal care based on the following principles is essential:

1. Assessment of disease and client information
2. Instruction and support
3. Dietary regulation
4. Urine and blood testing for glucose levels
5. Establishment of insulin needs
6. Evaluation of fetoplacental functioning
7. Assessment of fetal maturity

Assessment

All pregnant women should be tested for glycosuria, although during pregnancy some glycosuria may occur. If urine tests are positive, blood tests may be prescribed, including fasting plasma glucose (FPG), also called fasting blood sugar (FBS); oral glucose tolerance (OGT); and the preferred test, intravenous glucose tolerance (IGT). Prescription of insulin and dietary glucose are based on the findings of these tests.

Women who have been insulin dependent for many years may be quite knowledgable about their disease. Those who develop gestational diabetes may know nothing about the disease and its treatment and may be extremely frightened. Information and support are based on need.

Interventions

Diabetic women need continuous medical and nursing supervision during pregnancy. Therefore, prenatal visits are scheduled every 1 to 2 weeks for the first 32 weeks, then weekly until delivery.

Interventions are based on identified problems, as follows:

Dietary regulation need. The recommended diet is 30 to 35 calories per kg body weight, 150 to 200 gm carbohydrate, 125 gm protein, 60 to 80 gm fat, and possible sodium restriction. Mothers should not gain more than 3 to 3½ pounds (1.3 to 1.6 kg) per month and may need instruction and encouragement to maintain the diet.

Insulin need. Insulin dosage is based on blood and urine glucose levels. Oral hypoglycemics are not used because they are fetotoxic and do not provide adequate control. Mothers need to learn how to test for glucose and administer correct amounts of insulin. They need to know the symptoms of hypoglycemia and hyperglycemia and appropriate emergency treatment for each.

Preeclampsia potential. Because diabetic mothers are prone to pregnancy-induced hypertension (PIH), their blood pressure is monitored frequently. If signs and symptoms of PIH appear, treatment is begun at once.

Infections potential. Vaginitis and urinary tract infections are common. If symptoms appear, diagnosis and medical treatment are begun at once.

Inadequate rest. Mothers need to lie down and rest frequently during the day.

Fear and inadequate knowledge. Mothers are encouraged to ask questions and involve their partner as much as possible. Prenatal classes and support groups are encouraged.

Excessive fetal size and condition. Periodic tests are done to determine estriol and creatinine levels, the lecithin/sphingomyelin (L/S) ratio to determine fetal lung maturity, and ultrasonographs to evaluate fetal size. The mother is kept informed of test results and their meaning.

Hydramnios. Size of the mother's uterus and signs of respiratory distress are evaluated.

Sometimes amniotomy may be performed to remove excessive fluid.

Labor induction. At about 37 weeks, if fetal lungs have matured enough, labor may be induced. Blood glucose levels and fetal conditions are monitored closely.

Postpartum considerations. After delivery, the mother's insulin need is monitored closely. She is watched carefully for hemorrhage caused by uterine relaxation, which often follows hydramnios. If the infant was placed in a special care unit, efforts are made to assist the parents with infant bonding. If the fetus dies, grief counseling is indicated.

Heart disease

Every pregnancy places extra demands on the cardiovascular system, especially on the heart. Blood volume and cardiac output are increased 40%, and the rate is accelerated. The normal heart is well able to compensate for the added work, but the damaged or diseased one may not, and decompensation may develop. The symptoms of *cardiac decompensation* are increasing fatigue and breathlessness with usual exertion, a smothering feeling, episodes of palpitation and tachycardia, murmurs and rales in the lungs, and hemoptysis. There is progressive generalized edema and irregular pulse, and fluid collects in the base of the lungs.

Incidence

Heart disease affects 0.5% to 2% of pregnant women. Of these, rheumatic heart disease, which causes valve damage, is responsible for 95%; congenital defects of the conductive system, septa, and valves account for 3%. Of women with severe heart disease, pregnancy precipitates death in 1% to 3%. Perinatal mortality (infant death) is 50%, and fetal growth is retarded. Spontaneous abortions in early pregnancy and premature labor are common.

Classifications and interventions

Women with heart disease are classified in four groups from I to IV, according to the level of activity tolerated without symptoms. Medical and nursing care is adjusted accordingly.

Class I patients are women who have no limitation of activity. They need extra rest at night and must be monitored closely during the perinatal period. During the second stage of labor bearing down should be limited. Pudendal block anesthesia with low forceps delivery may be used to shorten the stage and reduce strain on the mother's heart.

Class II patients are women with slight limitations of activity. They must have a daily rest period and regular prenatal supervision. They are admitted to the hospital near term and given prophylactic antibiotics against bacterial endocarditis and mask oxygen to increase the available supply for the baby during delivery. Second-stage labor is shortened to reduce stress on the mother's heart as much as possible. Reliable contraception or tubal ligation is recommended.

Class III patients are women with considerable limitation who develop symptoms just doing the activities of daily living. They must spend 1 day in bed each week during pregnancy. If they go into cardiac decompensation (30% do), they are admitted to the hospital until delivery. Breast-feeding is too strenuous and not recommended. Therapeutic abortion may be necessary. Sterilization surgery may be recommended.

Class IV patients are women who cannot engage in any activity without symptoms. Their hearts barely maintain them. If pregnancy is not interrupted, more than 50% die. Fetal death rate is even greater. Therapeutic abortion is indicated. For those who attempt pregnancy, absolute bed rest, hospitalization, and intensive care are necessary.

The immediate postpartum period is especially dangerous for all categories of women with heart disease because of the increased blood flow to the heart produced by the sudden change in abdominal pressure at delivery. Some physicians favor alternating tourniquets or the use of an abdominal binder to counteract this effect and reduce the work of the heart.

Postpartum hospitalization is usually prolonged. Ergonovine maleate (Ergotrate) and estrogen are contraindicated, since they foster fluid retention and blood clotting. Dilute oxytocin may be administered cautiously to shorten the second stage of labor and control postpartum bleeding.

Nursing care includes bed rest with gradual resumption of activity, frequent opportunities to hold but not care for the baby, stool softeners to prevent straining, and constant supervision of vital signs. Preparation for discharge requires careful planning. The mother needs help to care for the new baby.

MEDICAL CONDITIONS ASSOCIATED WITH PREGNANCY
Hyperemesis gravidarum

About 75% of all women experience a mild form of nausea in early pregnancy. This so-called morning sickness usually disappears by about the twelfth week as the woman's body becomes accustomed to the tremendous changes within it. In about 3.5 in 1,000 pregnancies, however, vomiting persists, causing serious dehydration and starvation. Such a condition is called *hyperemesis gravidarum* (excessive vomiting of pregnancy).

Cause

A single cause for this reaction has not been found, but there is evidence that nausea is common to most women when gonadotropic hormone levels are elevated and when the endocrine glands undergo drastic change. In some people vomiting is a habitual response to stress. It is thought that when women with this habit experience the normally mild nausea of early pregnancy, they react in an exaggerated manner and begin to vomit. Once they have begun the pattern of vomiting, they cannot stop.

Course

Hyperemesis gravidarum usually begins with morning sickness and becomes increasingly severe until the woman cannot retain food or fluids. She loses weight and becomes dehydrated. Signs of vitamin deficiency such as polyneuritis may also develop. Other serious signs include jaundice caused by liver damage and blindness caused by retinal hemorrhages. Convulsions and death have been known to occur.

If the fetus dies and is expelled, nausea usually stops immediately, but damage to major organs of the mother may be permanent.

Interventions

Treatment for hyperemesis gravidarum should begin long before damage occurs. If signs of dehydration develop, the woman is usually hospitalized. Intravenous fluids are started immediately, with glucose, electrolytes, and vitamin B complex added to combat vitamin deficiency and nausea. All food and fluid by mouth are withheld for a time and then introduced with great caution and in small amounts. Sedative, tranquilizing, and antiemetic drugs and psychotherapy may be ordered. Visitors, especially family, may be restricted because of their psychic effect.

The nurse can play an important role in the woman's treatment by showing a sincere concern for the patient's welfare and a cheerful expectancy for rapid improvement. It may be helpful for the same nurse to care for the patient each day so that a relationship of mutual respect and trust can be developed.

If treatment is begun before irreversible damage to the mother has occurred, the pregnancy usually can be carried to term. Only in rare situations is pregnancy terminated because of hyperemesis gravidarum.

Bleeding disorders

Any bleeding during pregnancy is abnormal. When bleeding occurs early in pregnancy, the most common causes are abortion, ectopic pregnancy, and hydatidiform mole. When hemorrhage occurs late in pregnancy, the most common causes are placenta previa and abruptio placentae; these will be discussed as complications of labor and birth. Bleeding disorders that follow pregnancy are discussed as complications of the postpartum period.

Abortion

Abortion is the termination of pregnancy before the fetus is viable (28 weeks' gestation or a weight of 600 gm). Spontaneous abortions (miscarriages) occur without planning. Induced abortions are performed deliberately for medical (therapeutic) or social (elective) reasons.

Causes. The immediate cause of a spontaneous abortion is death of the embryo or fetus early in pregnancy or disruption of the implantation site. Some of the reasons are:

Defective germ plasm
Defective implantation
Maternal disease or nutritional deficiency
Abnormal reproductive organs
Psychic or physical trauma
Endocrine deficiencies
Blood group dyscrasias such as Rh factor

Assessment and classification. The most common symptoms of a spontaneous abortion are bleeding and cramplike pain. Since delayed menses may produce similar symptoms, further assessment is necessary. Such assessment includes a history of menses, intercourse, and past pregnancies; a pregnancy test; vaginal examination; and other tests as indicated.

Abortions are classified according to various criteria, as follows:

Threatened—small to moderate amount of bleeding with a closed cervix

Imminent—large amount of bleeding with uterine cramping and a partially open cervix

Complete—passage of all products of conception after which bleeding stops and no other symptoms appear

Incomplete—continued bleeding, discharge of pieces of tissue, cramping, and soft or open cervix

Septic—Infected conceptus with a soft tender uterus, odorous discharge, persistent bleeding, fever, and pain

Missed—no knowledge of an abortion, irregular bleeding, anemia; condition may persist for many years

Habitual—occurs in a woman who has had more than three abortions, often caused by an "incompetent cervix"

Interventions. The goal of interventions is to prevent damage to the mother and save the pregnancy. To that end, interventions for threatened or imminent abortions include bed rest with close observation of all vaginal discharge, emotional support, measures to promote relaxation, and a quiet comforting environment.

When a spontaneous abortion is incomplete, preparations are made to evacuate all the products of conception from the uterus. The surgical procedure of dilation and curettage (D and C) usually is performed. With the woman anesthetized, the cervix is opened with blunt-ended sounds, or dilators, of increasing size. The uterine cavity is scraped with a curette to dislodge tissue that keeps blood sinuses open. Postoperatively the woman is monitored closely for signs of hemorrhage, infection, pain, urinary retention, appetite, and grief. Fluids, analgesic medications, light foods, moderate activity, and emotional support are provided.

Women who have habitual abortions because of an incompetent cervix may elect the Shirodkar-Barter operation. This surgery is performed at about 15 to 18 weeks' gestation, when a purse-string suture is placed around the cervix. The suture may be removed to permit a vaginal birth or left in place, in which case a cesarean birth is performed.

When an invasion of pathogenic organisms causes a septic abortion, the woman is placed on bed rest with intravenous fluids and antibiotic therapy. When her condition stabilizes, a D and C is performed to remove the infected tissues. Postoperatively she is monitored closely for signs of hemorrhage, infection, pain, and urinary retention. Much emotional support is needed, with gradual return to normal activities.

Ectopic pregnancy

Incidence and types. When a fertilized ovum implants any place other than the endometrium of the uterus, the pregnancy is called ectopic, or *extrauterine*. This unfortunate event occurs in 0.5% to 12.5% of pregnancies. Most (90%) occur in the uterine tubes; other sites include the ovaries, abdominal cavity, cervix, fimbrae, and supporting ligaments (Fig. 6-1). Even though the pregnancy is outside the uterus, it responds to the action of hormones, softening and enlarging to about the size of a 4-month pregnancy. Obviously none of these sites is constructed to maintain a developing embryo or to provide an outlet for the fetus if it did grow to term. As a result, fetal mortality is 100%. Maternal mortality is 0.125% in the United States, probably because of delayed diagnosis.

Description of tubal pregnancy. In a tubal pregnancy the woman experiences the usual early symptoms of pregnancy, with some irregular vaginal bleeding. As the pressure within the tube increases, she may have intermittent pelvic side pain. Gradually the ovum erodes and weakens the tissue, bulging

out into the tubal lumen. Eventually a rupture occurs, causing hemorrhage, severe pelvic pain, and referred pain up into the shoulder. If internal hemorrhage is massive, signs of shock develop.

Assessment. Signs and symptoms include a weak rapid pulse, cold sweat, pallor, prostration, air hunger, and extreme anxiety. Diagnosis is difficult because the symptoms are similar to many other conditions, such as appendicitis, salpingitis, pelvic inflammatory disease, and ruptured ovarian cyst. Assessment includes a medical history, physical examination (including the pelvis), pregnancy test, and blood analysis. Laparoscopy, culdotomy, or laparotomy may be performed.

Interventions. Nursing interventions include close observations for signs of shock or a sudden change in the woman's condition and preoperative preparation as prescribed by the surgeon. Emotional support is especially important because the diagnosis is not known before surgery. Postoperative care may include blood transfusions and fluid replacement. Supportive interventions of appropriate empathy, genuineness, and warmth to help the woman cope with the initial stage of grief for her lost pregnancy should be provided.

Hydatidiform mole

Description and incidence. Hydatidiform mole is an abnormal change of the chorionic villi into numerous grapelike cysts filled with viscid material. The embryo dies and the mole grows rapidly, enlarging the uterus and producing large amounts of human chorionic gonadotropin (hCG). The cause is unknown. Incidence in the United States is 1 in 1,500 pregnancies but is much higher in some other countries, such as Mexico where the incidence is 1 in 200. This condition occurs more often in women over 45 years of age, who have a 35% chance of developing the extremely malignant *choriocarcinoma*.

Initially the pregnancy appears normal;

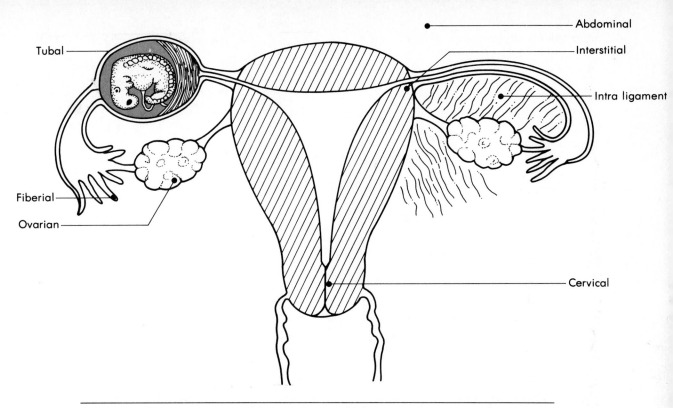

Fig. 6-1 Ectopic pregnancy. Various sites at which extrauterine pregnancies occur.

Labels in figure: Tubal, Fiberial, Ovarian, Abdominal, Interstitial, Intra ligament, Cervical

however, severe nausea and vomiting soon develop as hCG increases to higher than normal levels. Toward the end of the third month vaginal bleeding appears, which may be bright red or "prune juice" brown. If grapelike clusters pass, they are of great diagnostic significance. The uterus enlarges rapidly, but there is no fetal movement or heart sound, and no fetal skeleton can be seen on sonography.

Assessment and treatment. Women over 45 years of age with typical symptoms are tested for hCG levels, and sonographs are made every 1 to 2 weeks. Vaginal discharge is observed closely. If diagnosis is confirmed, uterine content is removed by suction and curettage. Because the incidence of choriocarcinoma in older women following hydatidiform mole is so high, hysterectomy may be performed. If not, follow-up monitoring of hCG levels is es-sential. If these remain normal for 1 year, another pregnancy can be safely attempted.

Leiomyomas (smooth muscle tumors)

Description and incidence. Uterine leiomyomas are benign growths that develop from immature smooth muscle cells in the uterine wall. The muscle bundles grow in whorllike fashion and often degenerate into fibers, thus the name *fibromyomas* or simply *fibroids*. Multiple myomas are common. They are named according to their location in the uterine wall: *submucous, interstitial, subserous, cervical,* and *ligamentous* (Fig. 6-2). Some grow out into the abdominal cavity or into the uterine cavity on stems or pedicles. *Pedunculated myomas* may become twisted or completely detached, adhering to abdominal tissue, in which case they are called *parasitic*.

115

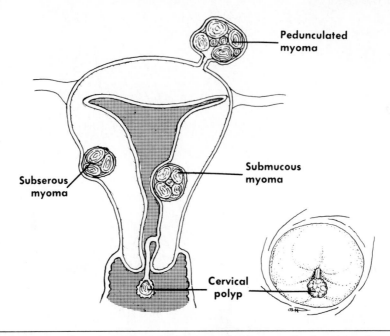

Fig. 6-2 Myomas and cervical polyps. Myomas are benign growths from immature smooth muscle cells named for their location in the uterus. Cervical polyps are growths from epithelial tissue of the cervix.

Malignant changes are rare, and the presence of myomas does not increase the likelihood that cancer of the cervix or endometrium will develop. Small myomas usually produce no symptoms and cause no problems. However, submucous myomas may double the abortion rate.

Assessment and interventions. During pregnancy myomas grow rapidly because of the increased blood supply and estrogen level. There may be spotting, pain, and a feeling of pressure as the baby grows. During labor myomas may impede or stop contractions, causing uterine inertia; obstruct the birth canal; cause malposition of the baby for delivery; and interfere with complete separation of the placenta, causing hemorrhage.

When myomas are diagnosed during pregnancy, surgical excision (myomectomy) is postponed until after delivery. If the birth canal is obstructed or hemorrhage develops, cesarean birth is necessary. Hysterectomy may be performed at the time of birth or afterward, depending on the number and size of myomas and the woman's wishes.

Prenatal teaching regarding potential hemorrhage and preparation for birth are important. The mother needs to understand her medical condition, including the possibility of cesarean birth or hysterectomy, so that she can make informed decisions. During labor and after birth she needs emotional support and encouragement.

Cervical polyps

Description. Cervical polyps are small outgrowths from the epithelial tissue of the cervix (Fig. 6-2). They occur often, bleed easily, and only rarely undergo carcinomatous change. Polyps tend to increase in size during pregnancy and occasionally twist on their pedicle and become necrotic.

Interventions. Polyps may be removed safely during pregnancy by various surgical means. The procedure is carried out in the clinic or office, and the tissue is sent to the laboratory to rule out cervical cancer. The mother needs to understand the procedure, give her consent, and be supported during their painless removal. Postoperatively she should undertake only moderate activity and report any bleeding.

Hypertensive disorders
Pregnancy-induced hypertension

Description and incidence. Pregnancy-induced hypertension (PIH), once called toxemia, has two stages: preeclampsia and eclampsia. In *preeclampsia,* hypertension, proteinuria, and excessive fluid retention develop with resultant edema and weight gain. Symptoms may be mild or severe. In *eclampsia,* convulsive seizures and coma develop. When preeclampsia is treated intensively, however, eclampsia may be prevented. The only cure for PIH is termination of the pregnancy.

The cause of PIH is unknown; however, recent studies implicate an organism named *Hydatoxi lualba.* PIH develops in the last 10 weeks of gestation, during labor, or in the first 12 to 48 hours after delivery. It occurs in 5% to 7% of all pregnancies. Adolescents, young primiparas, and low-income women have a 10% to 30% risk. Women who have had PIH before or those who have chronic hypertensive disease have a 25% to 35% chance of developing PIH. Of those who develop preeclampsia, 5% go on to develop eclampsia. Fetal death with preeclampsia is about 10% and with eclampsia 20%. Although the incidence of eclampsia is rare, PIH remains the third leading cause of maternal death in the United States.

Mild preeclampsia is characterized by a blood pressure rise of 30 mm Hg systolic or 15 mm Hg diastolic, proteinuria of +2, and weight gain during the second trimester of more than 3 pound (1.3 kg) per week and during the third trimester of more than 1 pound (0.45 kg) per week.

Severe preeclampsia is characterized by blood pressure of 160/100 or higher, albuminuria of +3 or +4, generalized edema, weight gain of 2 pounds (0.9 kg) in less than a week, headaches, blurred vision, oliguria, and elevated blood urea nitrogen, uric acid, and serum creatinine.

Eclampsia may be preceded by epigastric pain and an elevated temperature followed by a grand mal seizure. Such seizures are characterized by a *tonic phase,* during which the muscles contract, the back arches, arms and legs stiffen, the jaw snaps shut, respirations cease, and the woman becomes cyanotic. The tonic phase lasts 15 to 20 seconds. This phase is followed by the *clonic phase,* which begins with alternating contraction and relaxation of all muscles, during which incontinence of urine and feces may occur. Apnea may continue, or the woman may inhale and exhale irregularly. The clonic phase lasts about 60 seconds. The *coma phase* follows and may last for hours; it may be interrupted by other seizures, or the woman may awaken. Only one seizure or many may occur.

Mild preeclampsia

Assessment. An essential part of prenatal assessment of all women is to establish a baseline blood pressure in early pregnancy against which later readings are compared. At each prenatal visit blood pressure is measured and other signs of PIH assessed. Assessment includes testing a clean-catch urine specimen for proteinuria, weighing on the same scale at about the same time of day, observing for edema, and asking about headaches, dizziness, or gastric disturbances. Blood tests are prescribed as indicated.

Assessment of the fetus is essential to achieve a safe outcome. This includes assessment of fetal movement, nonstress test, serial ultrasonography to determine growth, contraction stress test, estriol and creatinine levels, and amniocentesis to determine fetal lung maturity.

Interventions. Nursing interventions for women with mild preeclampsia focus on support and teaching as follows:

DIET. High-protein diet with moderate sodium intake of 2.5 to 7.0 gm per day and 6 to 8 glasses of water per day. No longer are fluids and salt restricted or diuretics prescribed.

REST AND ACTIVITY. Resting in the left lateral recumbent position is beneficial by increasing renal plasma flow, glomerular filtration rate, and placental perfusion. Lying in a supine position is harmful because it compresses the inferior vena cava and aorta and diminishes blood supply to the uterus. The supine position also compresses renal arteries and decreases blood flow to the kidneys. Although complete bed rest may not be necessary, reduced activity is beneficial.

MENTAL HEALTH. Family members are helped by sharing areas of concern about the unborn fetus, sexual relations, finances, social relations, boredom and isolation, and ability to care for other family members. When these problems are identified, solutions may be found, such as referral to community agencies such as homemaker services.

MEDICAL SUPERVISION. Office visits are scheduled every 2 weeks or less, depending on the symptoms. Assessment of blood pressure, albuminuria, weight gain, edema, mental health, and fetal development are made at these times.

DANGER SIGNS. Mothers are instructed to report any sudden change in their condition,

such as generalized edema, headaches, fever, muscle tremor, or seizure. If they are testing their urine for protein and keeping a weight chart, they are asked to report sudden increases in these measures.

Severe preeclampsia

Assessment. If preeclampsia becomes severe, hospitalization is necessary. The goal of care is to prevent seizures, decrease blood pressure, establish adequate renal function, and continue the pregnancy until the fetus matures. If the pregnancy is at 36 weeks or more and fetal lung maturity confirmed, labor is induced or cesarean birth performed. If the L/S ratio indicates immaturity (see Tables 3-1 and 6-4) or the pregnancy is less than 36 weeks, interventions are aimed at reducing maternal symptoms to allow time for fetal maturation.

Assessment of hospitalized preeclamptic women includes:

1. *Blood pressure, pulse, respirations* at least every 2 to 4 hours
2. *Temperature* every 4 hours, or less if elevated
3. *Fetal heart rate* every 2 to 4 hours or monitored continuously
4. *Urinary output* measured at each voiding or hourly if indwelling catheter is in place (Output should be greater than 700 ml per 24 hours or 30 ml per hour.)
5. *Urinary protein* determined hourly if indwelling catheter (Readings of +3 indicate loss of 5 gm protein in 24 hours.)
6. *Specific gravity of urine* determined hourly if indwelling catheter in place (Readings of 1.040 correlate with oliguria and proteinuria.)
7. *Edema* evaluated of face, extremities, and sacrum every 4 hours; pitting determined by pressing over bony areas
8. *Weight* determined daily at same time unless strict bed rest

9. *Deep tendon reflexes* evaluated every 4 hours for hyperactivity of such tendons as the biceps, triceps, or Achilles

10. *Pulmonary edema* determined every 4 hours by auscultation

11. *Placental separation* assessed hourly by checking vaginal bleeding or uterine rigidity

12. *Headache* assessed every 2 to 4 hours by questioning woman

13. *Visual disturbances* assessed every 4 hours by questioning or daily by funduscopic examination

14. *Level of consciousness* assessed continuously for changes in alertness, mood, understanding, and signs of seizure or coma

15. *Laboratory blood tests* determined daily for hematocrit, blood urea nitrogen, creatinine, uric acid serum, estriol, clotting, and electrolytes.

Interventions. During the time the woman is hospitalized with severe preeclamptic symptoms, interventions include the following:

1. *Bed rest, quiet private room, no phone, and few visitors* to reduce stimuli that might precipitate seizures

2. *High-protein, moderate-sodium diet* as tolerated if no nausea or indications of impending seizure activity

3. *Fluid balance and electrolyte replacement* to correct hypovolemia, prevent circulatory overload, and replace electrolytes as indicated by daily serum tests (Fluid intake should be 1,000 ml plus urine output for prior 24 hours.)

4. *Sedatives* such as diazepam or phenobarbital to promote rest

5. *Antihypertensives* such as hydralazine to promote vasodilation without adversely effecting the fetus (Given when diastolic pressure is higher than 110 mm Hg, IV drip or push.)

6. *Anticonvulsants* to reduce risk of seizures, such as magnesium sulfate ($MgSO_4$) administered IM or IV to maintain blood levels between 4.0 and 7.5 mg/dl (At 10 mg/dl deep tendon reflexes fade, and at 15 mg/dl respiratory paralysis and/or cardiac arrest occurs.)

7. *Support and teaching* to decrease anxiety and promote understanding and cooperation by keeping the couple informed of fetal status, listening attentively, maintaining eye contact, and communicating with genuineness, warmth, and appropriate empathy

Eclampsia

A seizure is frightening to family members and nurses as well, although the woman will not remember it when she recovers. Therefore preparation for such an event is essential. Nurses need to know their duties, remain calm, reassure family members, and explain to them and to the woman later what happened and why certain interventions are taken.

During the tonic phase of the convulsion, turn the woman to her side to allow saliva to drain from her mouth. Inserting a padded tongue blade may prevent injury to the mouth if it can be done without force. Side rails should be padded or a pillow placed between them and the woman. Call for assistance.

When the clonic phase begins, remain nearby and assist as an oral airway is inserted, oxygen administered, fetal heart tones and maternal vital signs monitored, and magnesium sulfate administered. Diazepam, furosemide, and other drugs may be given as determined by the physician. The woman remains in the left lateral recumbent position to relieve pressure on the aorta and inferior vena cava.

A decision about delivery is made based on maternal and fetal signs and maturity of the fetus. If induction of labor for a vaginal delivery is chosen, the mother remains on her side and delivers in Sims' or semisitting position.

If delivery is by cesarean birth because of fetal distress, a wedge is placed under the woman's right buttocks during the procedure. An anesthesiologist or pediatrician should be available for care of the baby at birth.

Postpartum recovery of the woman with PIH usually is rapid, although seizures still may occur during the first 48 hours. Because the woman is hypovolemic, even normal blood loss can be serious. Rapid pulse rate and falling urine output are indications of excessive blood loss. The uterus should be palpated frequently and massaged to keep it contracted.

Blood pressure and pulse are checked frequently and intake and output records maintained. Ergot products are not given because of their hypertensive effect.

Postpartum depression typically follows such difficult pregnancies. Support by family members and infant-mother contact is encouraged as much as possible. It is recommended that at least 2 years elapse before another pregnancy and that prenatal supervision begin immediately.

Chronic hypertensive disease

When women have a blood pressure of 140/90 or higher before the twentieth week of gestation and/or blood pressure of 140/90 that persists indefinitely after delivery, they are said to have chronic hypertensive disease (CHD). These women need careful medical supervision during pregnancy. The antihypertensive medications and diuretics that they have been taking usually are continued during pregnancy at the lowest effective dose. These women are watched carefully for development of edema or proteinuria.

When vascular changes such as arteriosclerosis, retinal hemorrhage, and renal disease have occurred as a result of longstanding hypertension, the condition is called *chronic hypertensive vascular disease.*

When women with CHD develop systolic blood pressure 30 mm Hg or diastolic 15 to 20 mm Hg *above baseline* on two occasions at least 6 hours apart, show proteinuria, or develop edema in the upper half of the body, they need close monitoring. Often they progress quickly to eclampsia, sometimes before 30 weeks of gestation.

Infectious diseases

Pregnancy does not protect women from infectious diseases. In fact, their heavily taxed bodies may be even more susceptible to infection. These diseases are classified in various ways, by affected body area such as the urinary tract, by their method of transmission such as sexually transmitted diseases, and by causative agent (Fig. 6-3) such as bacterial. They also are classified as common diseases affecting mothers and infants.

Sexually transmitted diseases

Sexually transmitted diseases (STDs, venereal diseases) are infectious disorders contracted primarily by intimate oral and genital sexual contact. The most common ones are syphilis, gonorrhea, herpes simplex, *Chlamydia* infection, cytomegalovirus, *Trichonomas vaginalis* infection, candidal (monilial) vulvovaginitis, and condyloma acuminatum. When mothers are infected with these conditions, their infants may contract them during intrauterine life or at birth and may suffer serious consequences. For this reason, some sexually transmitted diseases are included among the common TORCH diseases described next.

TORCH diseases

Common diseases that cause adverse maternal, fetal, or neonatal effects are described by the acronym TORCH, for the initial letter of the diseases. Table 6-2 describes the effects, diagnostic procedures, prevention, and management of the following diseases:

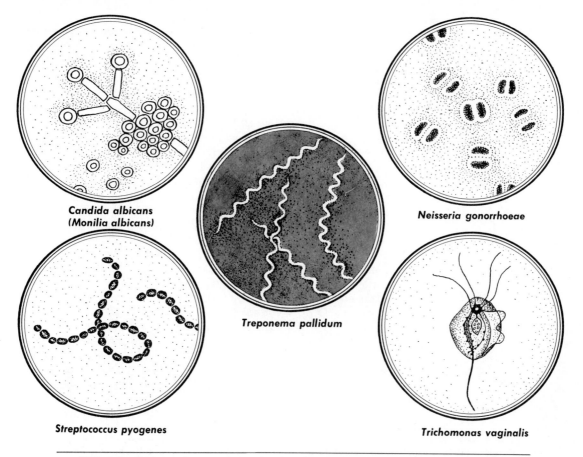

Fig. 6-3 Pathogenic organisms that frequently invade the reproductive organs.

T Toxoplasmosis
O Other diseases: hepatitis A and B, syphilis, gonorrhea, acquired immunodeficiency syndrome (AIDS), *Chlamydia* infections, candidal vulvovaginitis, *Trichomonas* and *Listeria* infections, various urinary tract infections
R Rubella
C Cytomegalovirus (CMV)
H Herpes genitalis (genital herpes)

Substance use and abuse

Once it was believed that the placenta acted as a protective barrier, keeping dangerous substances from reaching the fetus. This is not true. Substances that can harm the fetus (teratogens) do pass through the placenta and can adversely affect the developing fetus. The seriousness of these effects depends on:

1. Developmental stage of the fetus
2. Chemical properties of the substance
3. Whether the substance was taken alone or with other chemicals that enhance its effects

It also has been found that many commonly used substances such as caffeine, nicotine, and alcohol are harmful to the fetus.

Table 6-2 TORCH diseases

Infection	Maternal effects	Neonatal effects	Prevention, diagnosis, and management
Toxoplasmosis (protozoa)	Acute infection similar to influenza: swollen lymph glands, malaise, or may be asymptomatic	Transmitted to 50% of fetuses; high spontaneous abortion rate and congenital defects; if born, 15% die, 85% severe defects, 50% visual problems	Avoidance of infected raw meat or cat feces; diagnosis by serology test; some drugs control progression of damage; therapeutic abortion counseling
Other Hepatitis A (virus)	Spontaneous abortion; liver failure during pregnancy	Fetal defects, premature birth or death, neonatal hepatitis	Spread by fecal contamination; Y globulin for prophylaxis if exposed
Hepatitis B, serum hepititis (virus)	Fever, malaise, arthralgia, abdominal pain, jaundice, enlarged liver	25%-40% infected at birth; high risk for chronic hepatitis, cirrhosis & liver cancer	Spread by amniotic fluid, blood, urine, and other secretions Clean baby of all secretions; give immune globulin or HBIG vaccine IM within 12 hours, second dose at 1 month, third dose at 6 months

Adapted from Bobak, IM, and Jensen, MD: Essentials of maternity nursing: the nurse and the childbearing family, ed 2, St. Louis, 1987, The C.V. Mosby Co.

Maternal effects

Women who are addicted to street drugs such as heroin, cocaine, and psychotropics usually are malnourished, receive little or no prenatal care, and are more susceptible to all types of infection, including AIDS and hepatitis. As a result, they have a much higher risk of PIH, third-trimester bleeding, and puerperal sepsis. In addition, the risk of drug toxicity is present, and their ability to handle the stress of pregnancy is severely reduced.

Women who are addicted to alcohol often are malnourished and have folic acid and thiamine deficiencies, bone marrow suppression, liver disease, and reduced resistance to infection. If alcohol is abruptly stopped, they may experience withdrawal seizures, hallucinations, and delirium tremens.

Women taking prescription drugs and those who drink coffee and alcohol or smoke in moderation may not know they are pregnant. They may not know about the effects of such drugs or common substances on their infants. When they find out, they may become extremely anxious and guilt-ridden, fearful that their infants have been damaged.

The psychosocial effects of substance abuse are enormous. Street drugs are expensive and

Table 6-2 TORCH diseases—cont'd

Infection	Maternal effects	Neonatal effects	Prevention, diagnosis, and management
Syphilis (*Treponema pallidum*—spirocyte)	Incubation: asymptomatic for many weeks Primary stage: painless chancre; in 4-6 weeks clears without treatment Secondary stage: malaise; fever; nontender rash causes hair loss; condylomata on moist skin surface; clears in 2-6 weeks without treatment Early latent stage: lesions reappear up to 4 years later Late latent: lifetime—50%-70% have no symptoms Tertiary stage: damages described by acronym *paresis* for *p*ersonality, *a*ffect, *r*eflexes, *e*yes, *s*ensorium, *i*ntellect, *s*peech	Primary and secondary stages lead to fetal death Latent and tertiary stages lead to congenital infection Congenital: spirocytes cross placenta after 16-18 weeks' gestation Signs: snuffles, rhagades, hydrocephaly, corneal opacity, saddle nose, saber shin, Hutchinson's teeth, and diabetes If mother treated adequately before fifth month, no fetal-neonatal effects	Spread by blood, lesion exudate, and semen through intact mucosa and breaks in skin Begin penicillin before fifth month of gestation to avoid congenital syphilis; if not done, begin intensive treatment of both mother and infant as soon as possible; treat birth defects
Gonorrhea (*Neisseria gonorrhoeae*—diplococcus)	Lower urogenital (early stage): purulent vaginal discharge, dysuria Upper urogenital (later stage): abscesses, chronic pain, ectopic pregnancy Anorectal, systemic, and oropharyngeal infections	Gonococcal ophthalmia neonatorum and neonatal sepsis	Spread by direct contact and by fomites; all infected persons must be treated until two cultures negative Incubation: 2-5 days; females may have no symptoms in early stage No vaccine available; penicillin treatment of choice

Table 6-2   TORCH diseases—cont'd

Infection	Maternal effects	Neonatal effects	Prevention, diagnosis, and management
Acquired immunodeficiency syndrome (AIDS); human immunodeficiency virus	Incubation: 4+ years; normal immune defenses reduced; pregnant women more vulnerable to opportunistic diseases; 100% fatal when these conditions overwhelm body	Early symptoms: failure to thrive, lymphadenopathy, respiratory distress, fever, progressive weakness, sepsis	At-risk women: those with infected partners, IV drug users
Test women and infants
Use blood and secretion precautions and supportive care; no vaccine available; various drugs for specific symptoms
Chlamydia trachomatis (intracellular bacterium)	Mucopurulent discharge from infected cervix; urethritis; sore throat; conjunctivitis; can lead to pelvic inflammatory disease and salpingitis	Fetal death and preterm birth 10 times more common
Inclusion conjunctivitis occurs in one third of infected infants; pneumonia life threatening	Spread by direct contact through mucous membrane
Tetracycline drug of choice; in men linked to nongonococcal urethritis
Candida (Monilia) albicans infection (yeast)	Present in 20% of pregnant women; thrives when Döderlein's bacilli reduced or in carbohydrate-rich environment
Thick vaginal discharge, dysuria, itching	Thrush: infected at birth or from unclean practices of mother; swallowing difficulty	Vaginal creams or suppositories of miconazole, nystatin, or clotrimazole; bathing vulva with weak soda; treat sexual partner; teach clean practices
Trichomonas vaginalis (protozoa)	Thrives in alkaline environment; 20%-30% of pregnant women harbor organism; profuse white, frothy, irritating discharge; strawberry-colored cervix and vagina with dysuria	Metronidazole may cause fetal defects so contraindicated during first trimester; found in breast milk	Sexual partner may harbor organism without symptoms and reinfect woman
Metronidazole only effective drug; treat locally with weak acid douche, then both partners with drug

Table 6-2   TORCH diseases—cont'd

Infection	Maternal effects	Neonatal effects	Prevention, diagnosis, and management
Listeria mono-cytogenes (bacteria)	No vaginal inflammation; systemic influenza-like symptoms: fever, malaise, back pain May account for habitual abortions in some women	If contracted in early pregnancy, spontaneous abortion; if contracted between 17th and 28th week, may cause premature birth, fetal or neonatal death If infant infected up to 4 weeks, meningitis develops	Spread by contact with birds and animals; teach woman to wash hands well Diagnosed by microscopic examination or antibody studies With antibiotic treatment of mothers: 71% of neonates survive; when mothers untreated, only 29% of neonates survive
Urinary tract infection, usually *Escherichia coli* (bacteria)	Affects 2%-10% of women; caused by urinary stasis, decreased bactericidal leukocyte capacities, and pressure on right ureter from larger bowel mass on left Cystitis, fever, urgency, dysuria Acute pyelonephritis, chills, high fever, flank pain, nausea, dehydration, ileus	Amniotic fluid infection and placental growth retardation; risk of premature labor if infection occurs near term Sulfonamides during last 6 weeks interferes with protein binding of bilirubin	Diagnosis by symptoms: culture and sensitivity of urine Treatment: sulfonamides before last month; later with nitrofurantoin and antibiotics; tetracycline retards fetal bone growth; force fluids Pyelonephritis: IV fluids; bed rest; keep woman on left side to enhance kidney emptying
Rubella (German measles) (virus)	Rash, mild symptoms, some photophobia, occasionally encephalitis or arthritis	Incidence of congenital defects: 90% of infected infants show signs by 5 years; mental retardation and motor impairment; more severe if mother infected in 1st trimester	Vaccination of all nonpregnant females; prevent pregnancy for 2 months Diagnosis: viral cultures of amniotic fluid, placenta, or infant's blood Isolation: use gown and gloves; breastfeeding allowed

Table 6-2 TORCH diseases—cont'd

Infection	Maternal effects	Neonatal effects	Prevention, diagnosis, and management
Cytomegalovirus (CMV) (a herpesvirus)	Asymptomatic illness; may have cervical discharge; transmitted to 50% of fetuses	Most common cause of perinatal infection; 10%-12% will be born with CMV inclusion disease: microcephaly, encephalitis, bone lesions, heart disease, cataracts	Fetal infection may occur during birth; subsequent pregnancies may be infected Viral cultures, anti-CMV IgM antibodies in cord or baby's serum; treat infant with antimetabolite or antiviral agents to reduce CNS destruction; use gown and glove isolation
Herpes genitalis (herpes simplex virus, HSV I and II)	Symptoms more severe at first infection; painful blisters that rupture; shallow ulcers heal in 2-6 weeks; vaginal discharge, fever, malaise, painful inguinal lymphadenopathy Cervical lesions may lead to invasive carcinoma in middle age	Spontaneous abortion, premature birth Transplacental infection: microcephaly, mental retardation, heart defects Symptoms appear at 4-7 days: lethargy, convulsions, jaundice, bleeding, skin and mouth lesions	Spread by sexual contact and by fomites Incubation: 2-4 weeks; remains in cells for life, so infections recur; lies dormant in sensory nerve ganglia; triggered by emotional upsets, menses, and pregnancy Diagnosis: cultures; herpes IgM antibodies in cord and blood Treat infant: gamma globulin, systemic antimetabolites; gown and glove isolation Treat woman: acyclovir; no vaccine, no cure

often lead to prostitution and crime to support the addiction. As a result, these women may feel fearful, angry, sad, guilty, hopeless, worthless, and helpless.

Fetal-neonatal effects

The effects of various substances on the fetus and neonate are described in Table 6-3.

Interventions

Antepartum nursing care of pregnant women relative to substance use and abuse includes the following:

Goal of interventions. To provide maximum health for the mother and infant.

Assessment

1. General health status, with particular attention to infections and nutrition
2. Obstetrical condition of mother and fetus
3. Substances being used by mother

Diagnosis. Diagnosis is made according to specific teratogenic (fetal-damaging) substance (e.g., woman: addicted to alcohol; fetus: possible fetal alcohol syndrome).

Planning. A plan for care is devised in cooperation with mother, physician or midwife, social worker, and other health professionals.

Implementation

1. Prenatal health teaching:

   Alcohol use—stop drinking altogether.

   Nicotine—stop smoking altogether.

   Prescription drugs: use with caution after consultation with physician or pharmacist.

   Caffeine—drink less than 600 mg per day (coffee: about 100 mg per cup).

2. Management of heroin addicts: metha-

Table 6-3 Effects of various substances on fetus and neonate

Drug	Effect on fetus and neonate
Alcohol	Intrauterine growth retardation (IUGR), cardiac defects, fetal alcohol syndrome (FAS)
Heroin	Withdrawal symptoms, convulsions, death, respiratory acidosis, hyperbilirubinemia, IUGR
Methadone	Fetal distress, meconium aspiration, withdrawal symptoms, neonatal death
Barbiturates	Increased incidence of defects, neonatal depression, withdrawal symptoms, convulsions, hyperactivity, hyperreflexia, vasomotor instability
Pentazocine (Talwin)	Safe for use in pregnancy (depresses respirations if taken near birth)
Diazepam (Valium)	Hypotonia, hypothermia, low Apgar score, respiratory depression, poor sucking reflex, possible cleft lip
Phenothiazine derivatives	Withdrawal symptoms, extrapyramidal dysfunction, delayed respiratory onset, hyperbilirubinemia, decreased platelet count, hypotonia, hyperactivity
Lithium	Congenital defects, lethargy, cyanosis in neonate
Racemic amphetamine (Benzedrine)	Cleft palate, transposition of great vessels, learning disabilities, poor motor coordination, generalized arthritis
Dextroamphetamine (Dexedrine)	Congenital heart defects, hyperbilirubinemia
Cocaine	Learning disabilities
Caffeine (more than 600 mg/day, about 6 cups)	Spontaneous abortion, IUGR, cleft palate, congenital defects
Nicotine (10-20 cigarettes/day)	Spontaneous abortion, placental separation, decreased length, small head circumference, small for gestational age (SGA)
PCP (angel dust)	Flaccid appearance, poor head control, impaired neurological development
LSD	Possible chromosomal breakage
Marijuana	Potential impaired immunological mechanisms, IUGR

done treatment preferred to "cold turkey" because of potential risk to fetus; discharge planning for long-term rehabilitation; give particular attention to intercurrent infections.

3. Management of neonates of heroin addicts: provide immediate intensive care and discharge planning with possible placement in foster care.

4. Management of alcoholics: sedate as needed; provide seizure precautions, IV fluids, and discharge planning for long-term rehabilitation.

5. Management of fetal alcohol syndrome (FAS) infants: provide immediate intensive care and discharge planning with possible foster care placement.

Blood dyscrasias

Of special significance in obstetrics is the typing of blood according to the inherited presence or absence of certain antigens. The two most important types are the Rh and A and B antigens.

Rh factors

Several forms of Rh antigens exist. Those factors responsible for problems are D, C, E, c, e, and d. The D antigen produces the strongest stimulus for antibody production in Rh-negative people. Those whose genotype is DD are Rh positive; those with dd are Rh negative. About 85% of white, 95% of black, and 99% of Oriental populations are Rh positive.

Fetal-neonatal implications. In the United States each year 10,000 infants die of Rh hemolytic disease. If treatment is not begun, the anemia resulting from this disorder can cause severe fetal edema called *hydrops fetalis.* Congestive heart failure may result, as well as profound jaundice called *icterus gravis,* leading to neurological damage called *kernicterus.* This severe hemolytic syndrome is known as *erythroblastosis fetalis.*

Rh hemolytic disease occurs when Rh antigens pass through the placenta into the woman's blood. The woman produces antibodies against the antigens *(sensitization).* The antibodies then pass back into the fetus and destroy the erythrocytes. The fetus attempts to make up for this destruction by producing increased numbers of immature red cells called *erythroblasts,* thus the name *erythroblastosis.* Sensitization also can occur whenever a Rh-negative person receives a Rh-positive blood transfusion.

Prenatal screening and assessment. At the first prenatal visit a history is taken concerning prior blood transfusions, abortions, children born with jaundice, and the presence of medical diseases. Blood typing (ABO), Rh factor, and Rh antibody screening are done. If the woman is Rh negative (dd), the father of the unborn child is assessed for Rh factor and blood type. If the father is DD, all his children will be Rh positive. If he is Dd, half will be heterozygous (Dd). If he is Rh negative, all the children will be Rh negative, and no incompatibility with the mother will exist.

When tests identify a Rh-negative woman who may be pregnant with a Rh-positive fetus, an indirect Coombs' test is performed to determine if she is sensitized to the Rh antigen. This test measures antibody amounts in the blood. Results are expressed as a *titer,* or proportion of antibodies to serum. A titer of 1 : 16 or less indicates that the fetus is *not* at risk. When titers are higher than 1 : 16, a *delta optical density (ΔOD) test* of amniotic fluid is performed at 26 weeks' gestation to plan treatment. ΔOD test results are indicated as zones. Zone I indicates a normal neonate who can be delivered at term with good prognosis anticipated. Zone II indicates an infant possibly at risk. Zone III indicates a severely affected fetus who many require intrauterine transfusions every 1 to 2 weeks until viability at about 32 weeks. Then a cesarean birth is performed, when an exchange transfusion will be anticipated.

Interventions. Prenatally, if tests indicate a severely affected fetus, plans will be made for an early delivery. In addition, intrauterine transfusions of the fetus may be considered. Mortality of nonhydropic fetuses who receive transfusions is 50% to 60%; 6% die from the procedure. Fresh packed cells are introduced through a catheter that passes through the woman's abdomen into her intrauterine space, then into the fetal peritoneal cavity. In this cavity diaphragmatic lymphatics absorb the red blood cells into the fetal circulation within a week after the transfusion. Few maternal complications occur.

In the postpartum period the Rh-negative woman whose indirect Coombs' titer is negative and who has delivered an Rh-positive fetus is given an intramuscular injection of anti-RhO(D) gamma globulin such as RhoGAM within 72 hours. This is done so that she does not have time to produce antibodies to fetal cells than entered her bloodstream when the placenta separated. The anti-RhO(D) gamma globulin works to destroy fetal cells before sensitization occurs, thereby blocking maternal antibody production and protecting future babies if she should become pregnant again (Fig. 6-4). Sometimes RhoGAM is given to Rh-negative nonimmunized women at 28 to 32 weeks' gestation as well as after delivery. Protocol for administration of RhoGAM is similar to that for other blood products.

ABO blood types

In the ABO system there are two kinds of antigens: A and B. People who have neither are said to be type 0 (zero). The rest of the population has type A, B, or AB (both). When a fetus inherits a blood type from the father that is different from that of the mother, fetal blood may cross the placenta and sensitize the mother to antigens of the foreign blood type. During a subsequent pregnancy, another baby with the same type as the first infant might be affected by hostile antibodies in the blood of the mother. This baby might develop ABO hemolytic disease.

ABO incompatibility is less predictable than is Rh incompatibility. To date no immune globulin such as RhoGAM has been developed to counter the antibody buildup in the sensitized mother.

DIAGNOSTIC PROCEDURES

A variety of procedures are used to determine the status of the fetus, especially when complications of pregnancy are present. Such procedures include ultrasound, maternal assessment, nonstress testing, contraction stress testing, estriol determinations, analysis of amniotic fluid, and fetoscopy.

Ultrasound
Description and purpose

Ultrasound examination makes possible the study of the inner organs of the body by means of sound waves. In an ultrasound scan high-frequency sound waves are directed into the abdomen. In the abdomen the waves rebound from structures and surfaces, producing "echoes," which are then measured and recorded on a video display screen. Ultrasound uses nonionizing energy, in contrast to the ionizing energy of x-ray films. The major types of diagnostic equipment are the static B scan, real-time imaging, and Doppler ultrasound.

Ultrasound is noninvasive, painless, and nonradiating and gives immediate information to the physician. Ultrasonography is a valuable tool to monitor pregnancy whenever problems

WITHOUT RH₀ (D) IMMUNE GLOBULIN

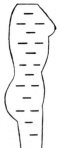 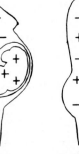 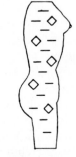 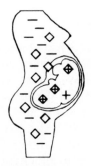

Before pregnancy

Rh- woman
Rh+ man

Pregnancy
Rh+ baby
Some Rh+ blood passes into the mother's blood

At delivery
Some Rh+ blood remains in mother

After delivery
Mother becomes sensitized to Rh+ blood

Later pregnancy
Rh+ sensitized mother actively produces Rh+ antibodies that destroy baby's blood

WITH RH₀ (D) IMMUNE GLOBULIN

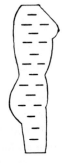 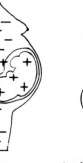 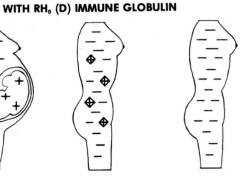 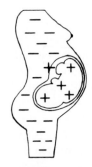

Before pregnancy

Rh- woman
Rh+ man

Pregnancy
Rh+ baby
Some Rh+ blood passes into the mother's blood

At delivery
Rh₀ (D) immune globulin given to mother within 72 hours of delivery destroys remaining Rh+ blood and then is eliminated from mother

After delivery
No Rh+ blood within mother to cause her to become sensitized to produce Rh+ antibodies

Later pregnancy
Same as first pregnancy; Rh+ baby is protected

Fig. 6-4 How Rh₀(D) immune globulin prevents disease.

are suspected, such as placental malposition, multiple fetuses, and fetal abnormalities, or to detect fetal presentation, position, and breathing movements.

Procedure

Usually the woman is scanned with a full bladder to enable the sonographer to assess other structures in relation to the bladder. She is asked to drink a quart of water about 2 hours before the examination and to refrain from emptying her bladder.

The procedure takes 20 to 30 minutes. Ultrasound is uncomfortable because the pregnant woman must lie flat on her back with a distended bladder. Some women develop supine hypotension because of compression of the abdominal aorta and inferior vena cava by the heavy uterus. This hypotension can be relieved by elevating the feet or turning to the side. Mineral oil or transmission gel is spread over the abdomen. The sonographer slowly scans with a transducer longitudinally and transversely in sections across the abdomen to gain an entire picture of the contents of the uterus.

Maternal assessment of fetal activity

A screening test used by some clinicians involves asking women to count fetal movement during the third trimester. These women keep a fetal movement record (FMR) or fetal activity diary (FAD). Two movements or more per hour is reassuring. Fewer than two per hour is an indication for a nonstress test. Although fetal movement is a sign of well-being, mothers should be assured that fetal rest-sleep states of up to 75 minutes occur in perfectly healthy infants.

Nonstress test

Nonstress testing (NST) has become a widely accepted method of evaluating fetal status. The test involves observing how the fetal heart rate (FHR) varies in relation to fetal movement. This variation is absent or decreases when the fetus is premature, asleep, affected by sedatives administered to the mother, and not receiving enough oxygen. Increased variability indicates that the central and autonomic nervous systems are normal and that the fetus is not suffering from hypoxia.

The mother is placed in a semi-Fowler's position, and an electronic fetal monitor disc is strapped to her abdomen over the area of best reception. Recordings of the FHR are obtained for about 30 minutes. The nurse or mother are asked to depress a "mark button" whenever fetal movement is observed. If no fetal movement occurs during the time, the woman is asked to eat a light meal and return for retesting. Fetal movement often occurs in response to an increase in blood sugar and to distention of the maternal stomach.

Contraction stress test
Description and purpose

The contraction stress test (CST) is an external means of monitoring the circulatory-respiratory reserve of the utero-placental-fetal unit before labor. CST enables the health care team to evaluate the ability of a high-risk fetus to withstand the stress of labor by recording the effect of oxytocin-induced contractions on the FHR.

With an increase in intrauterine pressure during contractions, blood flow is temporarily reduced in the intervillous space of the placenta. Therefore there is a decrease of oxygen to the fetus. In most instances this brief oxygen reduction is tolerated well by a healthy fetus. If placental reserves of blood are insufficient, however, fetal hypoxia, myocardial depression, and late deceleration of the FHR occur. These symptoms are associated with fetal metabolic acidosis, newborns with low Apgar scores, and fetal intrapartal death.

Procedure

To perform the CST, uterine contractions must occur at least three times in 10 minutes. Contractions may occur spontaneously or more often are induced either by IV ocytocin or breast stimulation. When IV ocytocin is used, the test is called an *oxytocin challenge test (OCT)*. When contractions are stimulated by manually rolling a nipple, the test is called a *breast self-stimulation test (BSST)*.

During the test the woman is placed in a semi-Fowler's position to avoid supine hypotension. An ultrasonic transducer is placed on her abdomen where the FHR most accurately can be recorded on the monitor strip. The tachodynamometer (pressure transducer) is placed on the uterine fundus to record uterine contractions. Baseline measures are recorded for 15 minutes. These measures include blood pressure, fetal activity, fetal movement, spontaneous contractions, and medical and obstetrical information. If three spontaneous contractions of good quality lasting 40 to 60 seconds occur during the 15-minute period, the test is concluded and the results evaluated. If no contractions occur or if they are insufficient for interpretation, IV oxytocin solution is administered or breast stimulation is begun.

A *negative* CST implies that placental support is adequate and the fetus could likely tolerate the stress of labor should it occur within a week. A *positive* CST does not give specific prognostic answers. Many other factors must be taken into consideration regarding ability of the fetus to tolerate labor. The test is repeated as indicated.

Estriol determination

Estriol is a by-product of estrogen metabolism. As the fetus grows and matures, estriol production increases. When growth is retarded, estriol production levels off. When there is fetal distress and the placenta reaches its limits, estriol production decreases. To maintain optimum estrogen metabolism, there must be a healthy fetus, a functioning intact placenta, and a healthy mother. The amount of estriol found in plasma or excreted in urine is an indicator of fetal well-being. Thus, by serially measuring estriol levels of high-risk women, fetal status can be assessed. Estriol is measured by testing blood plasma or a sample of urine collected for 24 hours.

Amniotic fluid analysis
Description and purpose

Analysis of amniotic fluid yields valuable information for those who provide health care to pregnant women (Table 6-4). Amniotic fluid is obtained by a technique called *amniocentesis*.

Procedure

Amniocentesis is performed on an outpatient basis but should be done near a delivery suite in case acute fetal distress occurs. The woman empties her bladder just before amniocentesis. To avoid inserting the needle into the bladder, placenta, fetus, uterine arteries, or umbilical cord, the abdomen is scanned to locate a pocket of fluid. The site is cleansed, may be anesthetized, and a 3- to 6-inch spinal needle is inserted into the uterine cavity. A specimen of 20 ml of amniotic fluid is withdrawn, placed in a test tube, shielded from light to prevent bilirubin breakdown, and sent to the laboratory for analysis. The needle is withdrawn and the FHR and vital signs of the woman are assessed for 15 minutes. She is allowed to leave if these signs stabilize.

The procedure may be a frightening experience, not only because a long needle is inserted into the abdomen, but because the findings of fluid analysis may be unfavorable. Dur-

Table 6-4 Amniotic fluid analysis

Test	Purpose	Interpretation
Bilirubin concentration test	To determine degree of Rh sensitization of mother	Three zones of optical density indicate degree that fetus is affected: I—none to mild, II—moderate, III—severe.
Lecithin/sphingomyelin (L/S) ratio test	To determine degree of lung maturity by measuring proportion of lecithin to sphingomyelin	Surfactant consists of phospholipids secreted by epithelial cells of the lungs, including lecithin and sphingomyelin. Lecithin is more active but is not manufactured in significant amounts until 34-35 weeks' gestation. When L/S ratio is 2:1, respiratory distress syndrome is less likely.
Foam stability (shake) test	To determine degree of lung maturity by observing ability of surfactant to make foam	Inexpensive, quick test with low false-positive rate; when test is positive, L/S ratio test is usually not done (see above).
Cytological examination of fat cells	To determine degree of fetal maturity by percentage of fat cells	When 20% of cells are fat cells, fetus will weigh at least 2500 gm.
Meconium staining	To determine presence of fetal hypoxia by clarity of amniotic fluid	Hypoxia in a fetus causes increased peristalsis, relaxation of the anal sphincter, and passage of meconium.
Genetic screening	To determine abnormal chromosomal forms	Fetal cells are examined for chromosomal defects, such as trisomy 21.

ing the procedure the woman needs to be attended continuously and kept informed of each step. Before she goes home, an appointment to review test results is made.

Fetoscopy

Fetoscopy is a technique for directly observing the fetus and obtaining a sample of fetal blood or skin. Ultrasound is used to locate an area in which to insert a cannula and trocar through the mother's abdomen and uterus. The endoscope is inserted through the opening, and ultrasound is used to direct it to the desired part of the fetus for viewing and sampling. Skin biopsies may be obtained and blood samples drawn from the umbilical cord under direct visualization. The procedure is done only in a few perinatal centers because fetal

mortality is 7.5% from the procedure and 2% from fetal death from the premature labor that fetoscopy initiates.

▶ *KEY CONCEPTS*

1. Diabetes seriouusly complicates pregnancy by changing insulin requirements, decreasing renal threshold for spilling glucose, causing dietary fluctuations, increasing risk of ketoacidosis, producing hypertension, causing retinopathy, and jeopardizing the fetus. Interventions for diabetic mothers include dietary regulation, insulin adjustment, monitoring of hypertension and infections, frequent rest periods, patient teaching, and monitoring of hydramnios and the fetus.

2. Heart disease is classified into four groups according to level of activity the woman can sustain without symptoms. These women require

constant monitoring during and after delivery.

3. Hyperemesis gravidarum occurs in 3.5 of 1,000 pregnancies and may cause maternal and fetal death. Interventions include hospitalization, IV fluids, vitamins and nutrients, rest, and psychotherapy.

4. Abortion is termination of pregnancy before 28 weeks' gestation; its multiple causes are classified by various criteria. Except for therapeutic abortion, goal is to save the pregnancy and prevent damage to mother.

5. Ectopic pregnancy is extrauterine; tubal pregnancy is the most common type. Tubal pregnancy causes rupture of uterine tube with hemorrhage, pain, and shock. The diagnosis is difficult, and surgical intervention and supportive nursing care are required.

6. Hydatidiform mole is an abnormal change of chorionic villi into grapelike cysts. The embryo dies and the mole grows, producing large amounts of hCG. High incidence of malignant cancer occurs in women over age 45 years. Symptoms include bleeding, high hCG, and passing of cysts. Surgical intervention and follow-up hCG studies for 1 year are done. A hysterectomy is performed for women over 45 years.

7. Leiomyomas are benign growths of smooth muscle cells. These tumors may cause abortions, impede labor, obstruct the birth canal, and cause hemorrhages. Intervention involves excision or hysterectomy.

8. Cervical polyps are benign growths of epithelial cells that may cause bleeding. They can be removed during pregnancy.

9. Pregnancy-induced hypertension (PIH) has two stages: preeclampsia and eclampsia. Hypertension, proteinuria, and fluid retention are primary symptoms. The only cure is to end the pregnancy. The cause of PIH is unknown; a high incidence occurs in young primiparas, low-income women, and those with chronic hypertensive disease. Mild preeclampsia is managed at home with diet, rest, and close medical supervision. Severe preeclamptic women are hospitalized with bed rest and a quiet environment. They are monitored continuously. If a seizure occurs, the woman is protected from injury; the infant is delivered immediately by induced labor or cesarean birth. Ergot is not given in the postpartum period, and emotional support is needed.

10. Common infectious diseases that cause adverse maternal, fetal, or neonatal effects include the TORCH conditions: toxoplasmosis, other (hepatitis; syphilis; gonorrhea; AIDS; *Chlamydia, Candida, Trichomonas,* and *Listeria* infections; urinary tract infections), rubella, cytomegalovirus, and herpes genitalis.

11. Many substances taken by the mother can harm the fetus. Some are found in common foods such as caffeine, frequently prescribed drugs such as diazepam (Valium), and street drugs such as heroin. Health education and supervision are needed.

12. Hemolytic disease of fetus may be caused by sensitivity of mother to Rh or A and B antigens. Prenatal screening and monitoring of antibody titer are performed with possible intrauterine transfusions or early delivery to save baby.

13. Diagnostic tests used to monitor the fetus include ultrasound, maternal assessment, nonstress testing, contraction stress testing, estriol determination, analysis of amniotic fluid, and fetoscopy.

■ ANNOTATED SUMMARY

I. Preexisting medical conditions
   A. Diabetes mellitus
      1. Description—endocrine disorder characterized by hyperglycemia and glycosuria
      2. Classification—diabetes mellitus, impaired glucose tolerance, gestational
      3. Complications—numerous and severe
      4. Goals of nursing care—physiological equilibrium and delivery of a healthy mother and neonate
      5. Assessment—FPG (FBS), OGT, IGT
      6. Interventions—based on problems: diet, insulin, pregnancy-induced hypertension, infections, rest, knowledge, fetal size and condition, hydramnios, labor, postpartum care
   B. Heart disease—pregnancy places great demands on heart; if disease present, decompensation results
      1. Incidence

2. Classification and interventions—I to IV; all care aimed at reducing workload of heart

II. Medical conditions associated with pregnancy
  A. Hyperemesis gravidarum—excessive vomiting
    1. Cause—not firmly established
    2. Course—morning sickness continues, becomes severe with dehydration and even death
    3. Interventions—hospitalization, IV fluids, sedatives, psychotherapy
  B. Bleeding disorders—any bleeding is abnormal
    1. Abortion—termination of pregnancy before 28 weeks' gestation or fetal weight of 600 gm
      a. Causes—multiple
      b. Assessment and classification: threatened, imminent, complete, incomplete, habitual, missed, septic
      c. Interventions—depend on status
    2. Ectopic pregnancy—extrauterine
      a. Incidence and types—90% in uterine tubes
      b. Description of tubal pregnancy
      c. Assessment—shock, similar to many other conditions such as appendicitis, salpingitis, pelvic inflammatory disease
      d. Interventions—support, observations
    3. Hydatidiform mole—abnormal change of villi
      a. Description and incidence—high hCG levels
      b. Assessment and treatment—hCG levels
    4. Leiomyomas (smooth muscle tumors)
      a. Description and incidence—benign growths
      b. Assessment and interventions—surgical excision or hysterectomy
    5. Cervical polyps: description and interventions—small outgrowths; may be surgically removed
  C. Hypertensive disorders
    1. Pregnancy-induced hypertension (PIH)
      a. Description and incidence—hypertension, proteinuria, and excessive fluid retention with edema
        (1) Mild preeclampsia
          (a) Assessment—blood pressure (BP), proteinuria test
          (b) Interventions—diet, rest, mental health, knowledge of danger signs
        (2) Severe preeclampsia
          (a) Assessment—BP, temperature, pulse, respirations, fetal heart rate (FHR), output, edema, tendon reflexes, level of consciousness, laboratory tests
          (b) Interventions—bed rest, quiet, fluid balance, sedative, antihypertensives, anticonvulsants
        (3) Eclampsia—convulsions
    2. Chronic hypertensive disease—BP 140/90
  D. Infectious diseases
    1. Sexually transmitted diseases (STDs)
    2. TORCH diseases—*t*oxoplasmosis, *o*ther, *r*ubella, *c*ytomegalovirus, *h*erpes genitalis (Table 6-2)
  E. Substance use and abuse—effects depend on fetal development, chemical, single or multiple substances
    1. Maternal effects—high risk for PIH, bleeding, infection; reduced ability to handle stress
    2. Fetal neonatal effects—Table 6-3
    3. Interventions—antepartum care
  F. Blood dyscrasias
    1. Rh factors
      a. Fetal-neonatal implications—congestive heart failure, icterus gravis, erythroblastosis fetalis, hydrops fetalis
      b. Prenatal screening and assessment—indirect Coombs' test, delta optical density
      c. Interventions—intrauterine transfusions, early delivery, RhoGAM injection of mother
    2. ABO blood types
III. Diagnostic procedures

A. Ultrasound
   1. Description and purpose—fetus visualized
   2. Procedure—full bladder, abdomen scanned
B. Maternal assessment of fetal activity—two movements per hour
C. Nonstress test (NST)—relation of FHR to movement
D. Contraction stress test (CST)—effect of contraction on FHR
   1. Description and purpose—three contractions in 10 minutes
   2. Procedure—baseline for 15 minutes, then stimulate with oxytocin IV or breast self-stimulation test; monitor FHR
E. Estriol determination—fetal growth parallels estriol levels in plasma and urine
F. Amniotic fluid analysis—Table 6-4
   1. Description and purpose—provides information about fetal status
   2. Procedure—amniocentesis using ultrasound
G. Fetoscopy—direct observation of fetus or obtaining of sample through endoscopy using ultrasound to locate insertion site

● STUDY QUESTIONS AND LEARNING ACTIVITIES

1. What is diabetes mellitus? Describe its adverse effects in pregnancy. How is prenatal care altered to reduce these effects?
2. Describe the care of a pregnant woman with Class III heart disease. What is the immediate concern after delivery? Why give mask oxygen to the mother with heart disease during delivery?
3. Describe the nursing care and treatment for a woman admitted with hyperemesis gravidarum.
4. Define abortion. What are the causes of spontaneous abortion?
5. What is an ectopic pregnancy? What is the most common site?
6. Describe mild and severe preeclampsia and discuss its treatment. What should the nurse do if a seizure occurs?
7. Name the TORCH diseases and describe their neonatal effects and management.
8. What are the effects of alcohol and heroin on the fetus and neonate?
9. Explain what happens to cause Rh hemolytic disease. How does RhoGAM work?
10. What are the purposes of ultrasonography, NST, CST, and estriol determination?

REFERENCES

Bobak IM, and Jensen HD: Essentials of maternity nursing: The nurse and the childbearing family, ed 2, St. Louis, 1987, The CV Mosby Co.

Diabetes in pregnancy, Nursing '80 10:44, 1980.

Hare JW, and White P: Pregnancy in diabetes complicated by vascular disease, Diabetes 26:953, 1977.

Olds SB, London ML, and Ladewig PA: Maternal-newborn nursing: a family-centered approach, ed 3, Reading, Mass, 1988, Addison-Wesley.

Pardue SF: Hydatidiform mole: a pathological pregnancy, Am J Nurs 77:836, 1977.

Sonstegard L: Pregnancy-induced hypertension: prenatal nursing concerns, Maternal-Child Nurs J 4:90, 1979.

White P: Classification of obstetric diabetes, Am J Obstet Gynecol 130:228, 1978.

Zuspan FP: Treatment of severe preeclampsia and eclampsia, Clin Obstet Gynecol 9:954, 1986.

UNIT THREE
LABOR AND BIRTH

CHAPTER 7

Mechanism of Labor

VOCABULARY

Attitude
Breech
Engagement
Fetal position
Lie
Lightening
Station
Vertex

LEARNING OBJECTIVES

- Describe the relationships of the mother's pelvis, fetal skull, and fetal shoulders.

- Define lie, presentation, presenting part, attitude, positions, and stations.

- Discuss lightening, false labor, vaginal discharge, show, and rupture of the amniotic membrane in relation to the process of labor.

- Discuss causes of the onset of labor and list the signs of true labor.

- Describe the three phases of a uterine contraction.

- List the stages of labor and describe the phases within them and their average time spans.

- Describe the mechanism of labor, including descent, flexion, internal rotation, extension, restitution, and external rotation.

- Describe Schultze's mechanism and Duncan's mechanism of placental expulsion.

The mechanism of labor is the process by which the baby passes from the uterus to the outside world at birth. To understand this process, one first must know the anatomy of the mother's pelvis in relation to the baby's head, that is, the passageway, the passenger, and the positions.

ANATOMICAL RELATIONSHIPS
The passageway—the mother's pelvis

The pelvis is a funnel-shaped canal of irregular form and size. It is composed of the sacrum, the coccyx, and two innominate bones. The innominate bones are joined together at the symphysis pubis in front and at the sacroiliac synchondroses in back. These joints soften somewhat in the months before labor, but they are still fixed joints. From an obstetric point of view, the "true" pelvis begins at the level of the sacral prominence in an internal ridge running around to the symphysis pubis in front. This is called the *brim,* or *inlet,* to the pelvis. The middle portion of the funnel is larger than the inlet or the outlet and is called the *pelvic cavity*. The *outlet* is the smallest part of the funnel. It is bordered by the two ischial spines, the lowest part of the symphysis pubis, and the tip of the sacrum. (The coccyx bone bends back during delivery of the head.)

The passenger—the baby
Fetal skull

The fetal skull is the widest part of the baby. Labor is primarily the process of pushing the skull through the mother's pelvis. The bones of the skull are two frontal, two parietal, two temporal, the occipital, and the wings of the sphenoid (Fig. 7-1). These are separated by sutures, or membranous spaces. Where these sutures come together, there are irregular spaces that are closed by membranes, called *fontanels,* or soft spots. The largest one is the *anterior fontanel* on the top of the baby's head. A smaller one, the *posterior fontanel,* is lo-

cated on the back of the head just above the occipital bone. Two other fontanels, *mastoid* and *sphenoid,* are found on each side of the head. These large spaces between the bones enable the head to be compressed enough during labor to squeeze through the narrow birth canal. This compression, called *molding,* produces a temporary elongated shaping of the baby's head (Fig. 13-11).

Fetal shoulders

The shoulders are almost as wide as the head. They may need to turn or move up or down to pass through the birth canal.

Fetal body

Compared to the head and shoulders of the fetus, the body is relatively small. It normally slips through the birth canal after the larger head and shoulders without difficulty.

Positions of the baby within the mother
Lie and presentation

While the fetus is small, it may turn about freely within its watery sac; but as it grows larger and larger, it tends to remain in the same general position in relation to the mother. *Lie* refers to the relationship of the spinal column of the baby to the spinal column of the mother. A *transverse lie* means the baby is lying crosswise in the mother's abdomen. A *longitudinal lie* means the baby is lying lengthwise, with either its head down or its buttocks down (Fig. 7-2). *Presentation* refers to the general area of the baby's body that is toward the outlet. There are three presentations: cephalic (head down), breech (buttocks down), and shoulder (arm and shoulder down).

Presenting part

The presenting part is that part of the baby lowest in the mother's pelvis and the part that would come out first if nothing altered its passage (Fig. 7-3).

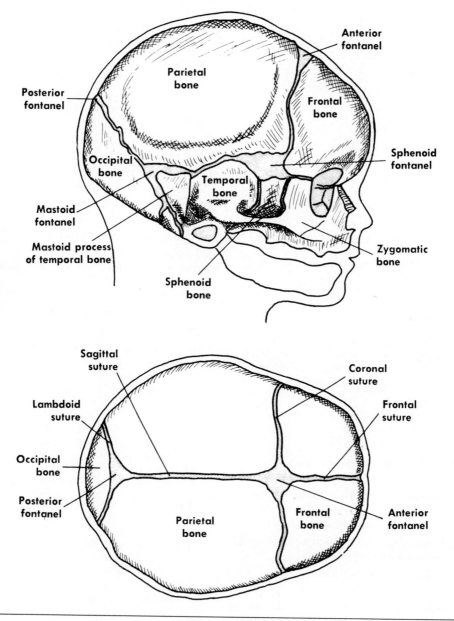

Fig. 7-1 Fetal skull.

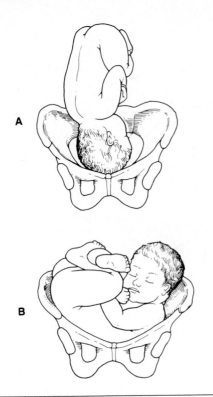

Fig. 7-2 Lie. The relationship of the fetal and maternal spinal columns: **A,** Longitudinal lie. **B,** Transverse lie.

Attitude

Attitude is the relation of various fetal parts to one another. The most common attitude of the fetus in the uterus is with the head flexed on the chest, arms folded, legs drawn up on the abdomen, and spine gently curved in flexion. This flexed attitude is called *the fetal position*. Other attitudes include the military attitude, deflection, and extension (Fig. 7-4).

Positions

The position of the fetus refers to the relation of some designated point on the presenting part to the mother's pelvis. If the vertex, or head, presents, the location of the occiput (abbreviated O) is the designated point. In any breech presentation, the sacrum (S) is the point; if the face presents, the chin or mentum (M) is the point; if the brow presents, the brow (B) or bregma (Br) is the point; and if the baby lies transversely, the scapula (Sc) is the designated point.

Viewed from below, the mother's pelvis also provides certain fixed points of reference. The symphysis pubis at the top is anterior (abbreviated A), and the coccyx is directly posterior (P). Exactly halfway between and on each side is the transverse point (T). The mother's left (L) and her right (R) tell the side.

A description of the fetal position can be made by combining the two sets of designated points. For example, LOA (left occiput anterior) means that the occipital bone of the fetus will present first in the left anterior quadrant of the mother's birth canal (Fig. 7-5).

Correlation of positions

Table 7-1 may help clarify the terms used in describing the positions of the baby.

In order of frequency, the vertex positions are as follows:

Left occiput anterior	LOA
Right occiput posterior	ROP
Right occiput anterior	ROA
Left occiput posterior	LOP
Right occiput transverse	ROT
Left occiput transverse	LOT
Occiput anterior (directly up)	OA
Occiput posterior (directly down)	OP

The breech positions are as follows:

Left sacrum anterior	LSA
Right sacrum posterior	RSP
Right sacrum anterior	RSA
Left sacrum posterior	LSP
Sacrum anterior (directly up)	SA
Sacrum posterior (directly down)	SP
Left sacrum transverse	LST
Right sacrum transverse	RST

Brow (B), bregma (Br), face (M), and scapula (Sc) are designated in the same manner

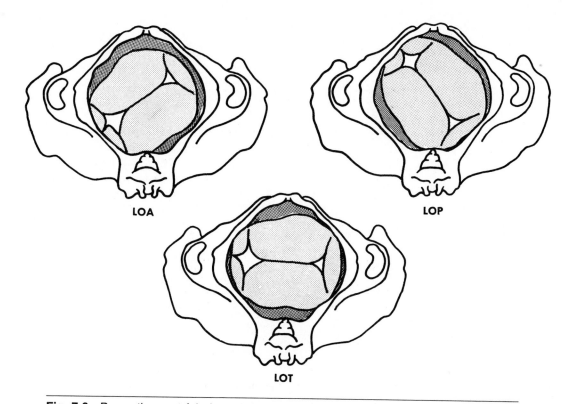

LOA

LOP

LOT

Fig. 7-3 Presenting part felt through the vagina in relation to the mother's pelvis. **LOA,** Left occiput anterior; **LOP,** left occiput posterior; **LOT,** left occiput transverse.

in relation to the mother's pelvis, but these are very rare.

Stations

The relationship of the presenting part to the level of the ischial spines of the pelvic bones is called the *station* (Fig. 7-6). When the presenting part is at the level of the spines, it is said to be at Station 0. If it is above the spines, the distance is designated in minus figures, such as − 1 cm or − 2 cm. If the presenting part is below the spines, the distance is designated in plus figures, such as + 1 cm or + 2 cm. In a vertex position, when the presenting part can move freely above the brim of the pelvis, it is said to be *floating*. As the part moves lower into the brim, it becomes

fixed and is no longer movable, but the largest diameters have not yet entered the inlet. When they do, the presenting part is usually at the level of the ischial spines and is said to be *engaged*. As the presenting part descends, it enters the midpelvis at about + 2 cm and finally reaches the pelvic floor at station + 4, where it causes the perineum to *bulge*. *Crowning* occurs as the presenting part is forced against the vaginal orifice, opening it larger and larger with each contraction until it passes through to the outside.

PROCESS OF LABOR
Before labor begins

Near the end of pregnancy the woman may notice certain changes or character-

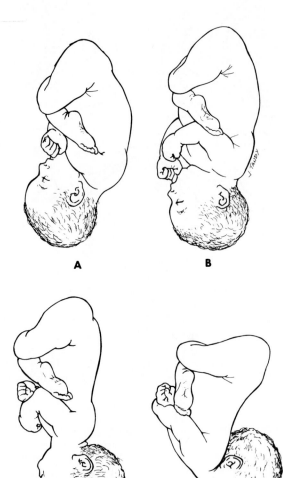

Fig. 7-4   Differences in attitude (flexion) cause different presentations. **A,** Complete flexion: vertex presentation. **B,** Moderate flexion (military attitude): upper head presentation. **C,** Marked extension (deflection): brow presentation. **D,** Excessive extension (deflection): face presentation. *(From Bobak, IM: Essentials of maternity nursing, ed. 2, St. Louis, 1987, The CV Mosby Co.)*

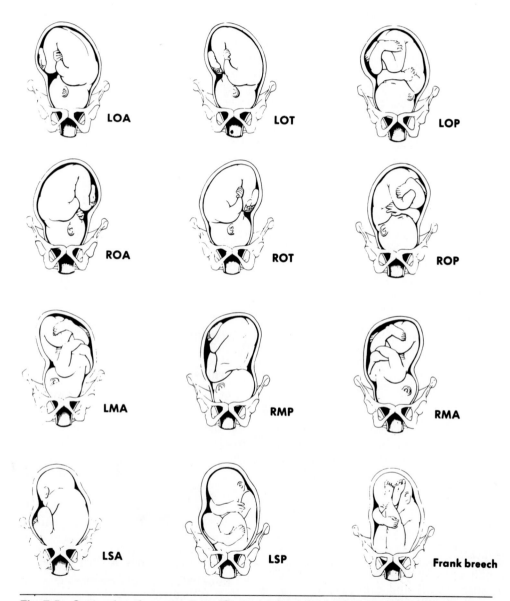

Fig. 7-5 Categories of presentations (Occiput: LOA, LOT, LOP, ROA, ROT, ROP. Mentum: LMA, RMP, RMA. Sacrum: LSA, LSP, Frank breech). *From Obstetrical presentation and position, Ross Laboratories, Nursing Education Service. Reprinted with permission of Ross Laboratories, Columbus, OH 43216.)*

Table 7-1 Correlated positions of the baby

Lie	Presentation	Presenting part	Description	Abbr.
Longitudinal (baby lengthwise in relation to mother)	Cephalic (head down): normal, occurs in 96% of all deliveries	Vertex (occiput)	Chin flexed on chest	O
		Bregma (anterior fontanel)	Head somewhat flexed	Br
		Brow (forehead)	Head upright	F
		Face (mentum)	Head bent back onto spine	M
	Breech (buttocks down): infrequent, occurs in 3% to 4% of all deliveries	Complete (full)	Squatting with feet tucked against thighs	S
		Frank (buttocks)	Legs straight up with feet near chin	S
		Footling (foot or feet)		S
		Knee	One or both feet preceding buttocks	S
			Flexed knee or knees present	
Transverse (baby crosswise in relation to mother)	Shoulder: rare, occurs in less than 1% of all deliveries	Scapula (shoulder bone)	Difficult; baby must be turned to another position	Sc

istic signals indicating that labor is not far off. An alert nurse will be aware of their significance.

Lightening (dropping)

About 2 to 4 weeks before the onset of labor, the fetal head begins to settle deeper into the pelvis. This reduces the pressure on the diaphragm, seems to lighten the load of the baby's weight, and allows the mother to breathe more freely. She also may notice urinary frequency and more pelvic pressure because the baby is lower in her pelvis.

False labor

Throughout pregnancy the uterine muscle contracts irregularly and painlessly in an action known as Braxton Hicks' contractions. In the weeks just before delivery these may become strong and regular enough to make the mother believe that labor has begun. If the cervix does not dilate, if walking has no effect or if it lessens contractions, or if contractions stop after a while, the incident is called *false labor.*

Vaginal discharge and show

As pressure from within thins the cervix, the woman may notice an increase in vaginal discharge. Labor often begins soon after this discharge occurs. Another important sign is the passage of the *operculum,* or mucous plug, that has filled the cervical canal during pregnancy. When the cervix thins sufficiently, the blood-tinged plug dislodges and passes. This is called the *show,* since it may introduce or "show" labor. Frank hemorrhage, however, is not normal and should be reported at once.

Rupture of amniotic membrane

During the 9 months of gestation the baby safely floats in an ever-increasing amount of amniotic fluid. By the fortieth week the volume normally reaches 1,000 ml. Before the baby can be born, the strong amniotic membrane must break and allow the fluid and baby

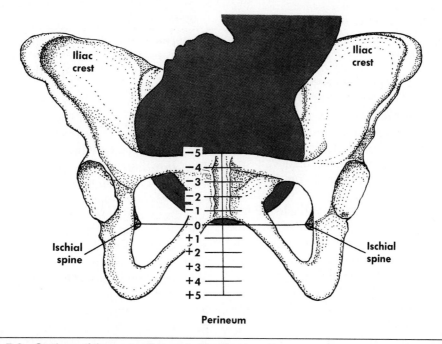

Fig. 7-6 Stations of the presenting part. *(Modified from Mechanism of normal labor, Ross Clinical Educational Aid No. 13. With permission of Ross Laboratories, Columbus, OH 43216.)*

to escape. Occasionally the membrane breaks before the baby is ready to be born. If this happens, there is danger of infection to the baby. The mother is hospitalized until the break heals and no more fluid escapes or until the baby is born, whichever comes first.

A simple tape test using phenaphthazine (Nitrazine paper) has been devised to determine whether the membranes are intact. The test is based on the fact that amniotic fluid is neutral to slightly alkaline (pH 7 to 7.5), while vaginal secretions are normally slightly acidic (pH 5 to 6.5). Test tape changes color from yellow (acid) to blue (alkaline) in the presence of amniotic fluid.

The enclosed amniotic fluid serves two important functions during labor: that of a battering ram and of a dilator. The bulging membrane in front of the presenting part focuses the force of contractions on the cervix, thinning and dilating it. When the membrane ruptures suddenly, the lower uterine segment and cervix are distended and contractions stimulated. For this reason, if the progress of labor slows, the physician may rupture the membrane artificially to stimulate the process.

Spontaneous rupture of the membranes frequently initiates labor. For this reason, women are instructed to immediately report any sudden gush of water. The nonmedical but descriptive term for this important sign of approaching labor is "the bag of waters breaking."

Onset of labor
Causes

Although it has been the subject of many studies, the exact cause of the onset of labor is still a mystery. However, a number of factors seem to work together to initiate and maintain the rhythmic uterine muscle contractions of labor.

Muscle fibers of the uterus become more irritable as they are stretched by the growing baby. Near the end of pregnancy, complex hormonal changes occur that are associated with the aging placenta and the failing corpus luteum. Estrogen and prostaglandin levels increase just before labor begins. The pituitary gland produces oxytocin, which stimulates contraction of the sensitized muscle fibers. Nervous pathways are stimulated by distention of the lower uterine segment, prolonged jolting movements, or the sudden pressure produced when the membranes rupture. Other factors, such as strong emotions or unconscious controls, may trigger the complex mechanism to begin.

True labor

Regardless of the exact cause of the onset of labor, the signs of true labor are:
1. Contractions are at regular intervals.
2. Intervals between contractions gradually shorten.
3. Duration and intensity of contractions increase.
4. Discomfort begins in the back and radiates around to abdomen.
5. Walking usually causes intensity of contractions to increase.
6. Cervical dilation and effacement progress.

Power of labor

The delivery of the baby is made possible by the combined powers of the uterine and abdominal muscles as they open the cervix and push the fetus through the birth canal. The uterine muscle is the primary force, and the abdominal muscles are secondary forces.

Uterine contractions

Uterine contractions during labor resemble the waves of the sea. They are rhythmic, regular, and involuntary, and they follow a repeating pattern.

Each uterine contraction has three phases:
1. Increment—when intensity builds
2. Acme—peak or maximum
3. Decrement—when muscle relaxes

The *duration* of a contraction is measured from the beginning of the increment to the end of the decrement. The *frequency* is the time from the beginning of the increment of one contraction to the beginning of the increment of the next.

At the beginning of labor, contractions may come intermittently from 10 to 30 minutes apart and last for only a few seconds. As labor progresses, they come closer together, last longer, and have greater force. When labor is well established, contractions may recur every 2 to 3 minutes and may last 90 seconds.

When the uterine muscle is relaxed between contractions, it feels soft and compressible. As it contracts, the muscle becomes harder and harder, and the whole uterus seems to rise up in the abdomen to a climactic height. Then it gradually relaxes and becomes soft again.

Each time the muscle contracts, the uterine cavity becomes smaller and the presenting part or the amniotic sac is pushed down into the cervix. The cervix is first thinned out, effaced, and then opened; and the muscle at the fundus becomes thicker (Fig. 7-7).

In multiparas, effacement and dilation tend to occur together. The lower uterine segment is actually pulled up or retracted, which makes dilation of the cervix possible even when the presenting part is not pushed with direct force against it, as in a shoulder presentation. A

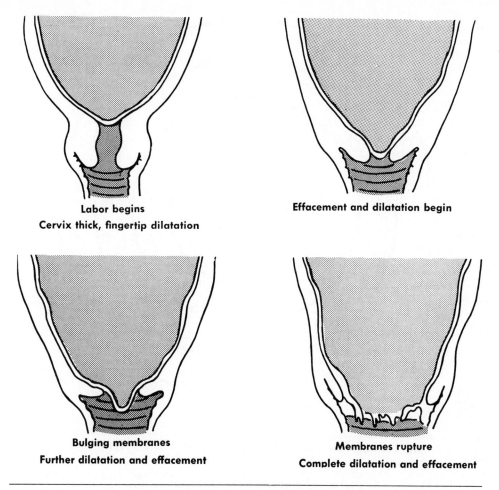

Labor begins
Cervix thick, fingertip dilatation

Effacement and dilatation begin

Bulging membranes
Further dilatation and effacement

Membranes rupture
Complete dilatation and effacement

Fig. 7-7 Cervical dilation (dilatation) and effacement.

completely dilated cervix is about 10 cm in diameter (Fig. 7-8).

Abdominal muscle contractions

The uterus is an upside-down pouch within a compressible cavity. By its own independent action the cervix gradually opens. Only after it opens can its contents be forced out. The abdominal muscles, which are under conscious control, then can tighten and compress the abdominal cavity, put added pressure on the open pouch, and push the baby out. Until the cervix is fully dilated, abdominal pressure only serves to tear it. After it is dilated, bearing-down efforts can greatly assist the final expulsion of the baby. In fact, when the presenting part presses on the rectum and perineum, there is an involuntary need to bear down. Paralysis of the woman's lower body by nerve damage or anesthesia removes this secondary force and thus prolongs the expulsive stage of labor.

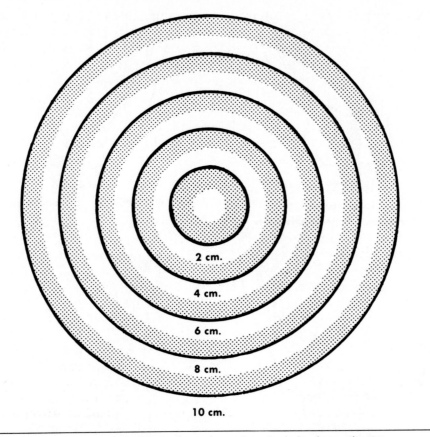

Fig. 7-8 Cervical dilation chart, drawn to actual size in centimeters.

Stages and duration

Labor has been divided into three stages or steps. Some authorities enlarge and divide the third stage, adding a fourth, or uterine, stage.

First stage

The first stage lasts from the onset of labor until the cervix is completely dilated (10 cm). It includes a beginning *latent phase* (0-4 cm), in which contractions are irregular or very weak; an *active phase* (4-10 cm), in which contractions come more frequently, last longer, and are of greater force; and a brief, intense *transition phase* (8-10 cm), which occurs as dilation is completed. The entire first stage averages 6 to 18 hours in primiparas and 2 to 10 hours in multiparas, with great individual variation.

Second stage

The second stage begins with complete cervical dilation and ends with the birth of the baby. Contractions are usually very strong during this stage. The mother's ability to use her abdominal muscles and the position of the presenting part influence its duration. In multiparas the second stage lasts about 20 minutes. In primiparas it takes up to 2 hours for the baby to pass through the dilated cervix and the birth canal.

Third stage

The third stage begins with the baby's leaving the uterus and ends with the expulsion of the placenta. This process usually lasts only a few minutes in both multiparas and primiparas.

Fourth stage

The so-called fourth stage begins with the expulsion of the placenta and ends when the uterus no longer tends to relax, that is, when the danger of postpartum hemorrhage has passed. The fourth stage may continue much longer in multiparas than in primiparas, but it usually averages from 4 to 12 hours.

Generally speaking, labor for primiparas is about twice as long as for multiparas. (Labor in a woman who has not delivered for 10 years is more like that of a primipara.) Of course, the length of labor for any woman depends on the size of the birth canal in relation to the baby, the number of prior pregnancies, the baby's position, and the quality of uterine contractions.

Mechanism of labor

Because of the irregular shape of the birth canal, the full-term baby cannot just slip out. Beginning with its attitude, or posture, in the uterus as labor commences, the fetus must be turned and twisted to find the path of least resistance as it is pushed out. The fetus is entirely passive. The mother's muscles must do the work. This series of movements is called the *mechanism of labor* (Fig. 7-9).

Descent

About 96% of all labors begin with the fetus in a flexed attitude with its head down and its body turned slightly to the left or right side in the uterus. As contractions begin the head is moved deeper into the pelvis in a sideways position, with the face to the right and the occiput to the left, or vice versa.

Flexion

As the head descends, the chin is flexed more and more on the chest, which causes the occipital bone at the back of the head to lead the way.

Internal rotation

As the head reaches the level of the ischial spines, which is called station 0, the structure of the pelvis causes the head to turn, or rotate, so that it will be able to pass through this extremely narrow place in the pelvis. It is then face down, moving under the pubic bone.

Extension

At this point in the canal the angle changes. The head, which has been pressed down on the chest in flexion, slips out from under the pubic bone and through the introitus, or vaginal opening, to the outside. The chin lifts up, or extends, and the head is born.

Restitution

Now the head is free to turn back to its normal position in relation to the shoulders.

External rotation

The shoulders and body of the infant usually slip out with relatively little difficulty because the head has opened the path for the smaller body. As this happens, the head turns, or rotates, in its normal relation to the shoulders.

If the occiput is to the posterior, the infant's head and body do not fit the normal curvature of the mother's pelvis. The infant will be born face up instead of face down, and the mother may experience greater back pain and a longer labor.

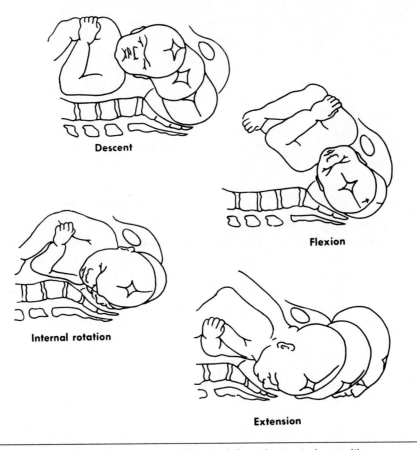

Descent

Flexion

Internal rotation

Extension

Fig. 7-9 Mechanism of labor in left occiput anterior position.

Placental expulsion

As soon as the baby is born, the uterus contracts, reducing its inner surface by 400%, while the placenta remains the same size. This causes the placental "roots," or villi, to be dislodged from the endometrium, separating the placenta from the uterus. If the edges remain attached, blood collects behind the placenta. Then when the placenta is dislodged, there is a gush of blood, and the amniotic surface leads the way out like an inverted umbrella. This is called *Schultze's mechanism,* named for the man who first described it (Fig. 7-10, *A*). (A memory aid

is to think of the shiny side as Schultze). It occurs in 80% of deliveries.

If the whole placenta separates at about the same time, there is no pooling of blood, and the placenta simply slides out with the decidual (dull) side exposed. This was first described by Duncan, so it is named *Duncan's mechanism* (Fig. 7-10, *B*). (A memory aid is to think of the dull side as Duncan.) It occurs in 20% of deliveries.

After the placenta has separated and before the uterus contracts again, the uterine muscle tends to relax. This allows blood to flow from the large exposed sinuses in the uterus. The

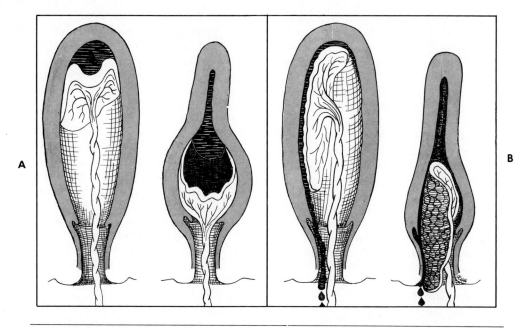

Fig. 7-10 Placental expulsion. **A,** Schultze mechanism. **B,** Duncan mechanism.

blood distends the uterus and stimulates it to contract, changing it from a soft spongy mass to a firm round ball that rises up in the now relaxed abdominal wall. The uterus should remain contracted and firm. If it relaxes, serious blood loss can occur within a few minutes. External massage of the fundus or dome of the uterus through the abdomen stimulates the sensitive muscle to contract, squeezes the blood sinuses closed, and controls hemorrhaging.

Uterine regression

The heavy uterus may fall to either side or back into the abdominal cavity. For this reason, some authorities advise the mother to lie on her abdomen when resting until the uterus regresses to its prepregnant state, about 4 to 6 weeks (Fig. 13-4). After 10 days the uterus has usually descended into the true pelvis and can no longer be felt in the abdomen. Nerve

reflexes initiated in the nipples by the sucking infant stimulate the pituitary gland to secrete oxytocin, which causes the uterus to contract. For this reason, uterine regression is speeded up by breast-feeding.

▶ KEY CONCEPTS

1. Mechanism of labor is the process by which the baby is born; it involves the passageway, passenger, and fetal position.
2. The passageway is the mother's funnel-shaped pelvis, which is composed of four bones joined by fixed joints; pelvis has a brim or inlet, cavity, and outlet; outlet is bordered by two ischial spines, symphysis pubis, and sacral tip.
3. Fetal skull is widest part of passenger, it is composed of seven bones joined by sutures, or membranous spaces, with an anterior and posterior fontanel; compression of skull at birth causes temporary molding of the head.
4. Positions of baby are *lie*—relationship of spinal column of baby to spinal column of mother;

presentation—relationship of general area of baby to outlet (cephalic, breech, shoulder); *attitude*—relationship of fetal parts to one another (flexion, extension); *positions*—relationship of designated point on baby to mother (occiput, sacrum, mentum, brow, bregma); *station*—relationship of presenting part to ischial spines of mother.

5. Before onset of labor the following occur: *lightening*—dropping of baby before contractions begin; *bloody show*—passage of operculum; *breaking of bag of waters*—amniotic membrane rupture.

6. Onset of labor results from many causes. Indications of true labor are regular contractions, shortening of intervals between contractions, contractions becoming more intense and last longer, discomfort spreading from back to abdomen, walking intensifying contractions, and cervix dilating and effacing.

7. Phases of uterine contractions are increment, acme, decrement. Duration is beginning of increment to beginning of next increment. In the process the fundus thickens and lower segment retracts with each contraction, making cavity smaller.

8. Abdominal muscles help with expulsion; to prevent cervical tearing, they should not be used to push until cervix is dilated.

9. Stages of labor are *first*—onset to cervical dilation (10 cm), includes latent and transition stages; *second*—cervical dilation to birth; *third*—birth to placental expulsion; *fourth*—placental expulsion to continuous contraction of uterus.

10. Mechanism of labor involves descent, flexion, internal rotation, extension, restitution, external rotation, placental expulsion, (shiny Schultze and dull Duncan), and uterine contraction.

■ ANNOTATED SUMMARY

I. Anatomical relationships
 A. The passageway—the mother's pelvis—funnel-shaped and composed of four bones
 B. The passenger—the baby
  1. Fetal skull—widest part of baby; composed of seven bones
  2. Fetal shoulders—nearly as wide as head
  3. Fetal body—relatively narrow
 C. Positions of the baby within the mother
  1. Lie and presentation—lie is the relationship of fetal and maternal spinal columns, can be transverse or longitudinal; presentation is the area of baby's body that is toward the outlet
  2. Presenting part—the part of the baby that will come out first
  3. Attitude—the relationship of fetal parts to one another
  4. Positions—the relationship of some designated point on the presenting part to the mother's pelvis, such as LOA
  5. Correlation of positions—lie, presentation, and presenting part
  6. Stations—relationship of the presenting part to the level of the ischial spines

II. Process of labor
 A. Before labor begins
  1. Lightening (dropping)
  2. False labor—Braxton Hicks' contractions
  3. Vaginal discharge and show
  4. Rupture of amniotic membrane
 B. Onset of labor
  1. Causes—several factors
  2. True labor—signs are regular contractions, with shortening intervals between each one, increased duration and intensity of contractions; back to abdomen discomfort; walking causes increased intensity of contractions; cervical dilation and effacement progress.
 C. Power of labor—combination of uterine and abdominal muscles
  1. Uterine contractions—phases, duration, intervals
  2. Abdominal muscle contractions
 D. Stages and duration
  1. First stage—onset to complete dilation
  2. Second stage—complete dilation to birth
  3. Third stage—birth to placental expulsion
  4. Fourth stage—placental expulsion to end of danger of hemorrhage
 E. Mechanism of labor
  1. Descent
  2. Flexion—head flexes toward chest

3. Internal rotation—head turns on shoulders
4. Extension—chin lifts up after passage under pubic bone
5. Restitution—head is free
6. External rotation—head rotates to normal position
7. Placental expulsion—Schultze's and Duncan's mechanisms
8. Uterine regression

● *STUDY QUESTIONS AND LEARNING ACTIVITIES*

1. Immediately after delivery the baby's head may be a strange shape. What is this called? Why does it happen and when, if ever, will the baby's head become round?
2. Define the following terms: lie, presentation, attitude, presenting part, station, and position.
3. What is a "bloody show"? What causes it and what does it mean?
4. The "bag of waters" is the lay term for what? What are its functions during labor?
5. What are the physical reasons for the woman relaxing and *not* using her abdominal muscles to push until the cervix is dilated?
6. When do each of the stages of labor begin and end? What are some of the factors that influence the length of each stage?
7. What causes the placenta to become dislodged from the endometrium?

REFERENCES

Bobak IM, and Jensen MD: Essentials of maternity nursing: the nurse and the childbearing family, ed 2, St Louis, 1987, The CV Mosby Co.

CHAPTER 8

Nursing Care During Labor

VOCABULARY

Amniotomy
Auscultation
Induction
Leopold's maneuvers
Lightening
Nursing process
Palpation
Transition stage

LEARNING OBJECTIVES

- Describe hospital admission procedures and their rationales.

- List the items included on the nursing history and state the reasons they are important.

- Describe how to time contractions accurately.

- Describe the information to be gained by Leopold's maneuvers.

- Discuss the significance of the FHR and describe intermittent and continuous monitoring.

- Identify the advantages and disadvantages of external and internal fetal monitoring and the information that can be gained from a fetal and a maternal monitor.

- Describe the methods, purpose, and patient care for the induction of labor.

- List the four basic desires of laboring women as identified by Lesser and Keane.

- Describe the role of a lay support person during labor and birth.

- Explain the reasons for attention to the food and fluid intake, elimination, position, and pain control of the laboring woman.

- Define the nursing process and list the steps relative to care of a laboring woman.

- List the danger signals that might occur during the first or second stage of labor.

- List the signs of impending delivery.

As the months of pregnancy pass, the expectant couple looks forward with increasing anticipation to the time the woman will go into labor. Many couples have attended preparation-for-childbirth classes together and visited the delivery suite where their baby will be born. Ideally, the mother has had adequate prenatal care and is in good health.

Sometime during that last month the baby descends into the pelvis. This change, called *lightening,* lightens the mother's load and makes breathing easier. The cervix softens and is described as "ripe." The woman has been instructed to notify the physician or midwife if contractions start and become regular, if the bag of waters breaks, or if she passes a mucous show. And one day, something begins to happen.

The woman notices a dull, low backache. After a time it intensifies at intervals, girdling her pelvis from the front to the back. The uterus becomes painlessly firm for a few seconds and then relaxes. This is the beginning of labor. The contractions come closer and closer together. Each one lasts a few seconds longer and seems to be more forceful than the last. When the contractions are coming at 10-minute intervals, the woman reports her symptoms by telephone. She is told to go to the hospital, which will be notified of her coming.

The time has arrived at last. For weeks the

suitcase has been packed. The expectant parents proceed to the hospital.

GENERAL HOSPITAL ADMISSION

When the mother enters the hospital, the admitting clerk obtains general information such as name, address, telephone number, nearest relative, who or what insurance will cover the hospital cost, and attending physician. An identification bracelet is placed on her wrist, and the woman is seated in a wheelchair and wheeled to the delivery suite (Fig. 8-1). If delivery seems imminent, hospital routines are adjusted accordingly.

If the mother has been receiving prenatal care through the hospital clinic, the accumulated record of her history and physical examination is sent to the delivery suite on her admission to the hospital. Records of private clients are brought to the hospital at the direction of physicians.

Many hospitals offer alternate birthing facilities (Fig. 8-2) that are homelike in decor in which fathers and family members may participate in the birth. The mother is attended by nurses and her midwife or physician, but both labor and delivery occur in the same room and surgical intervention is kept to a minimum. If complications develop, the resources of the hospital are immediately available.

DELIVERY SUITE ADMISSION
Establishing rapport

No matter how well prepared the mother may be, she is anxious and excited now that the time for delivery has come. It is important for the admitting nurse to establish rapport with the woman during the initial interview, data collection, and preparation process. A relationship of trust and mutual respect serves as a basis for cooperation throughout labor.

Clothing and valuables

The nurse escorts the mother to the assigned labor room and helps her undress and

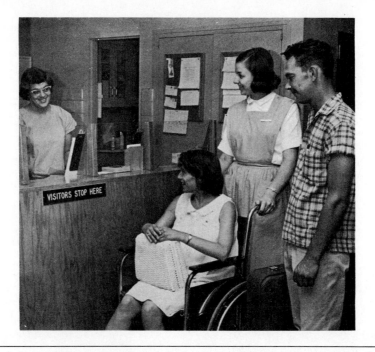

Fig. 8-1   Mother arrives for admission to the delivery suite with the father.

put on a hospital gown. Clothing may have to be listed on a special form if it is not sent home with the support person.

Valuables such as jewelry and money should be sent home or placed in the hospital safe. Any rings that are to be worn should be taped in place to prevent loss. Contact lenses or reading glasses are best placed in their cases when the woman is not using them. Dentures are removed before delivery if general anesthesia is given to prevent their being swallowed, aspirated, or lost.

Data collection
Initial interview and nursing history

As the admitting nurse assists the mother to undress, data collection begins and should include the following:

1. Contractions—when they began, their frequency, and their duration
2. Show and/or bleeding—if, when, and how much
3. Amniotic membrane—intact or ruptured and when (if there is a question, test with Nitrazine tape)
4. Expected date of confinement (due date)
5. Blood type (A, B, AB, or O and Rh factor)
6. T (number of term infants), P (number of preterm infants), A (number of abortions), L (number of living children)
7. Food and fluids—time and amount
8. Allergies to foods or drugs
9. Knowledge base and expectations for participation of labor coach
10. Name of physician who will care for newborn infant
11. Plans for feeding infant—breast or bottle

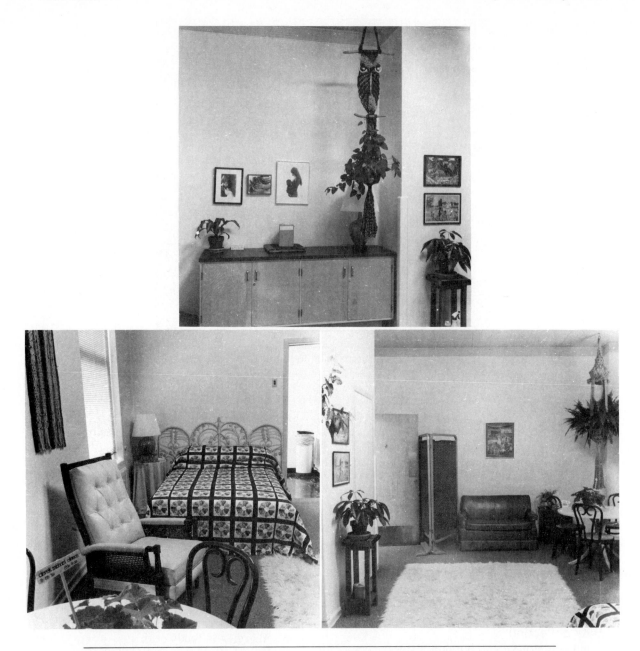

Fig. 8-2   Alternative birthing center. Homelike atmosphere is created for uncomplicated labor and birth in Alternative Birth Center at Mount Zion Hospital and Medical Center in San Francisco. Hospital delivery suite, intensive care nursery, and staff are in immediate facility to meet any emergency situation. *From Jensen, M, and Bobak, IM: Maternity and gynecologic care: the nurse and the family, ed. 3, St. Louis, 1985, The CV Mosby Co.; courtesy Mount Zion Hospital and Medical Center, San Francisco, Calif.)*

12. Other pertinent questions (see Fig. 8-3, sample nursing history form)

Hospital regulations, routines, and the locations of bathrooms, telephones, and other conveniences are explained at this time. It is important to tell the mother what to expect next, where her support person or labor coach will be, and when to expect her physician. Remember that the language and customs of hospitals are foreign and frightening. The mother has a right to respectful explanations.

Physical examination

A physical examination provides valuable data on which to base nursing care. It involves inspection, auscultation (listening), and palpation (feeling). Physical examination may be carried out by more than one person and should be adjusted to the progress of labor. It includes evaluation of vital signs, uterine contractions, abdomen, vaginal examination (including cervical dilation), and fetal heart tones.

Vital signs. Blood pressure elevations over 140/90 may indicate preeclampsia. Temperature elevation may indicate either infection or dehydration. Elevation of pulse and respirations may indicate infection, stress, or dehydration.

Uterine contractions. Do not call contractions "pains." The character of the uterine contractions provides valuable information about the progress of labor. A continuous account of their duration, frequency, and force is kept by the nurse from the time of admission until delivery.

To time contractions accurately, place a hand on the bare skin of the patient's abdomen over the fundus of the uterus. Press the fingertips lightly down into the skin and wait for the muscle to contract. When the muscle begins to firm, start timing. The contraction may start even before the patient notices it. As the uterus becomes firm, note the *intensity*—whether it becomes moderately firm as a bas-

ketball or really hard as a baseball. After the uterus reaches its peak, it begins to relax. When it has completely relaxed, note the time, but continue to feel the muscle. When the next contraction begins, note the time again. Remember the three phases of uterine contractions: increment, acme, and decrement (see p. 148). The *frequency* is the time from the increment (beginning) of one contraction to the increment of the next. The *duration* is the time from the increment to the decrement (end) of the same contraction (Fig. 8-4). In some centers an external fetal-maternal monitoring device is attached immediately on admission (Fig. 8-10).

If the patient is admitted in early labor, contractions may be many minutes apart. For this reason, any contractions that occur during the admitting process should be palpated and the time noted.

Abdominal inspection and palpation. Preliminary explanation to the mother, privacy, and adequate lighting are all necessary. Unless the fetus is surrounded by an unusually large amount of amniotic fluid or is blanketed by a thick layer of maternal fat, the experienced examiner usually can feel fetal parts through the uterine and abdominal walls. Valuable information about the degree of engagement, lie, attitude, activity, and even the presenting part are obtained in this way.

Before palpating the mother's abdomen the nurse first inspects it to observe its general shape and size and whether there is any obvious fetal movement.

Standard palpation of the abdomen is carried out by using the four Leopold's maneuvers. They are:

First maneuver: palpate the uterine fundus to determine what part of the fetus lies in the upper part of the uterus. The head is hard and round and can be moved from side to side on the neck. A fetal head in the fundus indicates a breech presentation.

Second maneuver: palpate in a downward

ADMISSION DATE_____ TIME _____ a.m.
                                                      p.m.
☐ Direct admit   ☐ Transport   ☐ other   ☐ Ambulatory
                                             ☐ Wheelchair

Reasons for admission
☐ Onset of labor   ☐ Spontaneous abortion
Observation/evaluation   Cesarean section
   ☐ Fetal status   ☐ Primary ☐ Repeat
   ☐ Medical complication   Induction of labor
   ☐ Obstetric complication   ☐ Elective ☐ Indicated
☐ Other_____
Detail
Reasons

Patient Care Data
Contractions on admission   ☐ None

Frequency _____ Duration _____ Quality _____
                                    a.m.
   Began on _____ at _____ p.m,

Membranes on admission   ☐ Intact
                                         a.m.
   ☐ Ruptured date _____ at _____ p.m.

   Fluid was ☐ Clear ☐ Meconium ☐ Foul smelling
Vaginal bleeding   ☐ None
   ☐ Normal show   ☐ Bleeding (describe) _____

Patient has:
   ☐ Dentures   ☐ Glasses
   ☐ Contact lenses   ☐ _____
                                    a.m.
Last oral intake _____ at _____ p.m. ☐ Fluids ☐ Solids
Current Medications ☐ None ☐ Vitamins
      Name/type of medication   Last taken
   _____   _____
   _____   _____

Patient plans:
Yes   Yes
☐ Private room   ☐ Father in delivery
☐ LeBoyer   ☐ Circumcision for boy
☐ ABC   ☐ Breast feeding
☐ Lamaze   ☐ Bottle feeding

Baby's name _____
Baby's physician _____
Special visitor _____
Procedures: ☐ Prep ☐ Enema (results)_____
                                                      a.m.
Physician notified _____ time _____ p.m.

      BY _____ R.N.

SIGNIFICANT PRENATAL DATA ☐ None

Blood Type	RH	Serology	Rubella

Allergies/sensitivities ☐ None
Food/milk _____   Reaction _____
Drug _____   Reaction _____
Sibling Allergies _____

Admission Physical Examination   Race:

Ht.	Wt.	Bp.	Temp.	Pulse	Resp.

OB History · Complications: _____
_____

T		A		L		E		A	
P		L		M		D		G	
				P		C		E	

Fetal evaluation	Presentation
Weight gain _____	☐ Vertex
FHR _____	☐ Face/brow
Station _____	☐ Breech (type)_____
Effacement _____	☐ Transverse lie
Dilatation _____	☐ Compound

PRE-ANESTHESIA INFORMATION

	YES	NO	FOR ANESTHETIST ONLY
Recent anemia			Consent Signed ☐
Swollen ankles/fingers			Blood Pressure _____
Kidney trouble			Hemoglobin ____ Gm% _____
Headaches			EKG _____
Sinus drip or recent "cold"			Other Lab _____
Stuffy nose			Anesthesia Plan Local ☐
Do you have asthma?			Gen ☐ Spinal ☐ Stand by ☐
Do you smoke? Amt: ½ pk 1 pk More			
Do you drink alcohol drinks? Amt per day · 2 drinks/less ☐ 4 drinks ☐ More ☐			Signed _____
Do you have a cough? Constant ☐ In a.m. only ☐			Date _____
Have you had convulsions, epilepsy, seizures? If yes, explain			
Heart trouble			

Have you ever received a blood transfusion?	Yes	No
Would you refuse a blood transfusion?	Yes	No

ADDRESSOGRAPH

Obstetric Admitting Record

Fig. 8-3   Sample admitting record on which information gained from initial interview and examination is recorded.

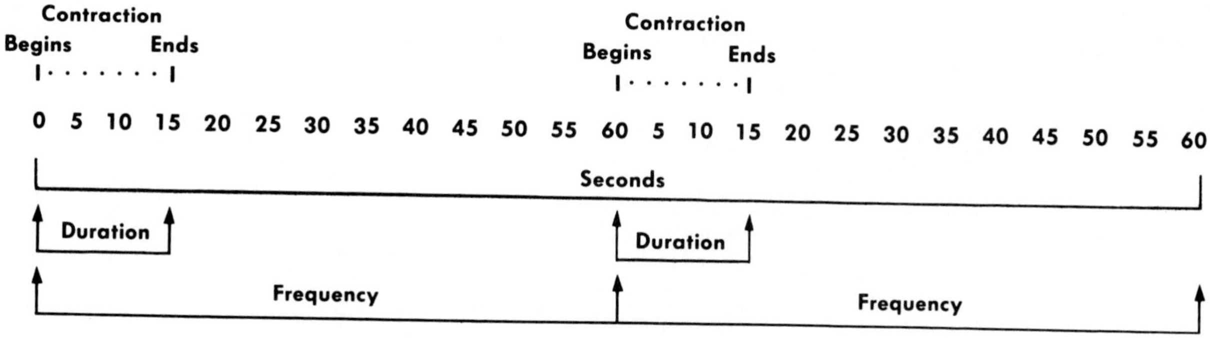

Fig. 8-4   Timing contractions. In this example contractions occur every 60 seconds (frequency) and last 15 seconds (duration).

direction on the two sides of the uterus. A smooth, long side indicates the fetal back; lumps that move indicate fetal feet and hands.

Third maneuver: Place one hand over the symphysis pubis and feel for the presenting part. If the head is not engaged, it can be felt above the symphysis pubis.

Fourth maneuver: Turn and face the woman's feet. To confirm that the head is presenting, press down on both sides of the uterus, about 2 inches above the symphysis pubis. This maneuver is to feel for the baby's brow, which should be on the side opposite from where the back was palpated (Fig. 8-5).

Vaginal examination. The vaginal examination is performed to assess five factors: (1) cervical dilation, firmness, and effacement; (2) amniotic membrane status; (3) presentation; (4) position; and (5) station. It is done with a sterile glove after the vulva has been thoroughly cleansed. The cervix and presenting part of the fetus are felt directly by the gloved fingers of the examiner. This method is more accurate and less painful than rectal examinations, and clinical studies indicate no significant increase in infections when aseptic technique is carried out.

For the first vaginal examination, sterile water may be used, since lubricants can alter the

Nitrazine paper test used to diagnose ruptured membranes.

When there is frank bleeding, vaginal examinations must never be performed by nurses because if a placenta previa exists it might be dislodged and a fatal hemorrhage result. The physician may do the examination in the operating room so that immediate cesarean birth can take place if necessary.

For the examination, the patient lies on her back with a pillow under her head and her knees flexed and separated. As she is being positioned, she should be told she will be examined internally to determine her progress in labor and that the procedure is uncomfortable but not painful.

Fetal heart rate. The fetal heart rate (FHR) or fetal heart tone (FHT) is a sensitive gauge of fetal status, especially as it relates to uterine contractions. Normally the FHR ranges between 120 and 160 beats per minute. A sudden rise or fall in rate, prolonged periods above or below normal, or slowing after a contraction indicates fetal distress.

Fetal heart rate is counted by a number of devices. It can be monitored both intermittently and continuously.

Intermittent monitoring. In low-risk pregnancies the FHR is counted every 15 minutes dur-

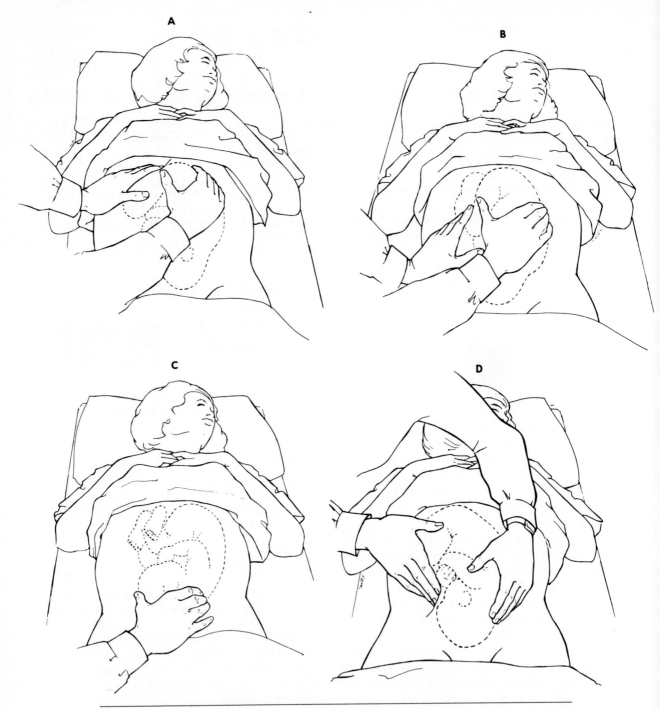

Fig. 8-5   Leopold's maneuvers. *(From Jensen, MD, and Bobak, IM: Maternity and gynecologic care: the nurse and the family, ed. 3, St. Louis, 1985, The CV Mosby Co.)*

ing the first stage of labor and checked every 5 minutes during the second stage of labor. Periodically throughout labor it should be counted during two successive contractions and a full 3 minutes after the second one. The FHR should be checked during, immediately after, and 10 minutes after any stressful event, such as rupture of the membranes or administration of spinal anesthetic.

The time, rate, position, and regularity of the FHR are recorded in the mother's chart. It is customary to use a large cross to represent the four quadrants of the woman's abdomen centered on her navel and to place a small x on the corresponding spot where the fetal heart was heard, with the beats per minute written beside the x. If irregularity was noticed, the word *irregular* is charted beside the rate. A regular fetal heart tone of 136 beats per minute heard in the left lower quadrant of the woman's abdomen would be recorded as follows:

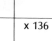

x 136

Devices used for intermittent monitoring include the DeLee fetoscope (Fig. 8-6), weighted fetoscope (Fig. 8-7), and various instruments that use the Doppler principle (Fig. 8-8). The device must be placed firmly against the mother's bare skin over the baby's torso. Obviously, the position of the fetus will determine the location at which the sound is heard best. To locate the sound, begin at the umbilicus and move in a widening circle until the area of maximum density is found (Fig. 8-9). Some nurses mark the spot with an X for future use.

To avoid mistaking the uterine souffle (throb of the mother's heart heard in large maternal blood vessels) for the fetal heartbeat, first count the mother's radial pulse (wrist) and then listen to the fetal heart. Normally the fetal heart rate is much faster than the moth-

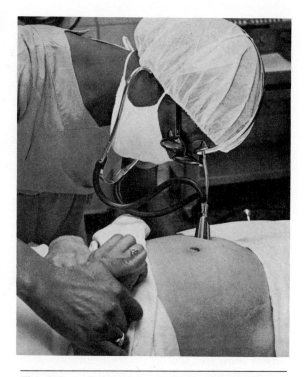

Fig. 8-6   DeLee fetoscope. Nurse's hands are free to check the mother's pulse while listening to the fetal heart tones.

er's and does not beat in time with hers.

Continuous monitoring. Continuous monitoring of fetal heart tones and uterine contractions is accomplished with a device called an electronic monitor (Fig. 8-10). It provides immediate information about the baby's condition. With this information early signs of fetal distress are noted and appropriate measures initiated. Continuous electronic monitoring is indicated if either the mother or the fetus is considered high risk (see box on p. 108). When continuous monitoring is to be used, admission procedures such as enemas or perineal preparation are done before the monitoring equipment is attached.

Methods. Continuous fetal and maternal monitoring can be done externally or internally or by a combination of both methods.

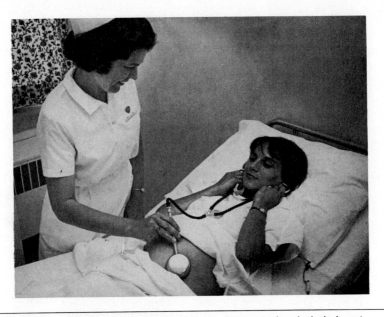

Fig. 8-7   Weighted fetoscope. Mother listens to her baby's heart.

Leads from the mother carry information to the electronic monitor where the fetal heartbeat and uterine contractions are displayed on an oscilloscope and recorded on a recording strip.

External monitoring consists of an ultrasound system to pick up and to amplify fetal heart tones and a pressure-sensitive gauge strapped against the abdominal wall to measure tension when the uterus contracts (Fig. 8-10). The advantage of external monitoring is that it does not require rupture of the membranes and can be used for tests of fetal status, such as the oxytocin challenge test (OCT). It can also be used during early labor (Fig. 8-11).

Internal monitoring consists of a scalp electrode by which a tiny wire is attached to the scalp of the fetus to record the FHT. A soft, polyethylene, saline-filled catheter is placed inside the uterus to record the frequency, duration, and intensity of contractions and the resting tonus of the uterus (intrauterine pressure between contractions) (Fig. 8-12). The advantage of internal monitoring is its accu-

racy. The disadvantage is that it is an invasive procedure that requires rupture of the amniotic membrane, which increases the risk of infection.

Information obtained. Because uterine contractions cause repeated stress to the fetus, signs of fetal distress may first appear as changes in the FHR relative to uterine contractions. The value of electronic monitoring is that it gives simultaneous information about the FHR and uterine contractions.

FHR is noted in six categories relative to uterine activity:

1. Baseline beats per minute (bpm). Before labor or between contractions; normal is 120 to 160 bpm.
2. Baseline variability. Amount baseline FHR varies from minute to minute; normal varies from 6 to 10 bpm. Less than 3 to 5 bpm indicates central nervous system depression associated with fetal hypoxemia.
3. Periodic FHR, acceleration. FHR during uterine contraction; normal is 15 bpm or more above baseline.

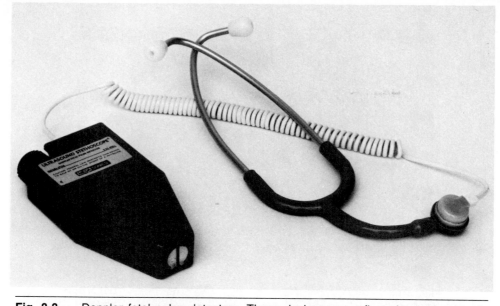

Fig. 8-8   Doppler fetal pulse detectors. These devices use reflected sound waves to detect fetal heart activity. The instrument can be plugged into another headset or amplifier for those nearby to hear. *(Courtesy MedSonics, Inc., Mountain View, Calif.)*

4. Periodic FHR, early deceleration. FHR just after peak of the contraction as the fetal head is compressed; normal follows the same pattern as the contraction, but should not drop below 100 bpm.
5. Periodic FHR, late deceleration. Indicates uteroplacental circulatory insufficiency or placental hypoperfusions.
6. Periodic FHR, variable deceleration. Indicates compression of the umbilical cord, which causes decreased oxygen supply to fetus (Fig. 8-13).

Laboratory tests

Although policies differ from hospital to hospital, most require urine and blood tests when the patient is admitted. The admitting nurse is responsible for collecting a clean, midstream urine specimen. A laboratory technician usually collects the blood for tests that are indicated on special laboratory test forms. Urine testing, as has been mentioned, may be done in the delivery suite by the staff or in a central laboratory. Laboratory technicians perform

blood tests. These tests may include hemoglobin, Rh factor, type determination, clotting time, complete blood counts, and occasionally a serology test for syphilis.

Treatment

Preparation of the vulva, collection of a urine specimen, and an enema if ordered, are usually done before fetal monitoring devices are attached. Nurses should explain what they are about to do and provide privacy.

Preparation of perineal area. Strictly speaking, the perineum is only that space between the vagina and anus, but in obstetrics the general area from the pubis to and including the skin around the anus is referred to by this term. The "peri prep" means to soap and then shave hair from this region. A "mini-prep" excludes pubic hair (Fig. 8-14), and sometimes shaving is entirely omitted.

The purpose of preparation is to provide as nearly an aseptic field for delivery as possible by removing bacteria-harboring hair. The shave should be done with a minimum of dis-

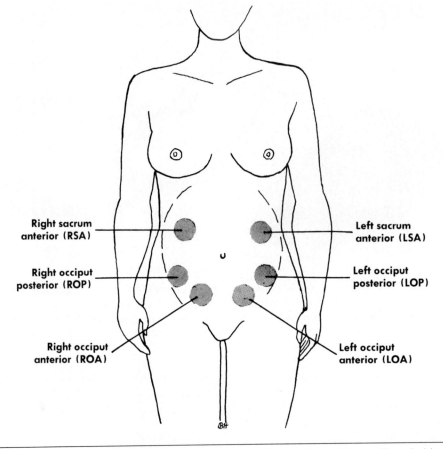

Fig. 8-9 Areas on the mother's abdomen where the fetal heart tone will probably be heard most clearly according to the position of the baby.

comfort to the patient. The principle to remember is to move from the clean to the dirty. This means that shaving strokes should be downward toward the anus and that the anal area should be done last. Equipment for this procedure will differ from hospital to hospital, but the principle and purpose are the same for all. To accomplish these objectives, the following suggestions may be helpful.

1. Provide adequate light
2. Soften the hair by soaping generously and by using warm water
3. Use a new razor blade

4. Separate the legs widely while shaving down to the perineum, then turn the patient on her side, flex the thighs at the hips, and proceed to shave the anal area
5. Use a gauze square to hold the skin taut
6. Shave with the grain of the hair—always toward the anus, never from the anus toward the vagina and urethra
7. Wash off the soap and then check for thoroughness
8. Discard the razor in a safe receptacle

Urine specimen. The best time to collect a clean urine specimen is immediately after

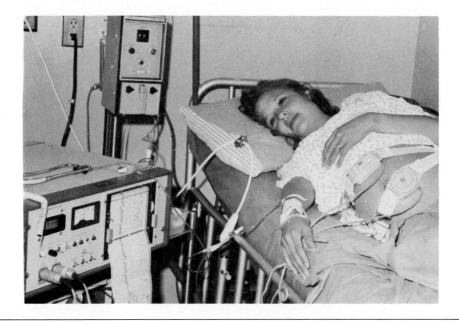

Fig. 8-10 Electronic monitor. Leads transmit fetal heart tones and uterine contractions to an oscilloscope and strip chart. External monitoring is shown here.

cleansing and shaving the vulva and before the vaginal examination. The woman voids either into a bedpan or over the toilet and a midstream specimen is caught in a paper cup. The specimen is labeled and sent to the laboratory for examination for sugar, acetone, and albumin. In some hospitals nurses perform these tests in the treatment room and records their findings on the admission record.

Enema. The woman may involuntarily defecate during the expulsive phase of labor if there is feces in the lower bowel. To prevent such contamination, a low small-volume enema sometimes is prescribed. Enemas are contraindicated with premature labor or bleeding.

To administer an enema, the mother should be lying on her left side in a Sims' position while the solution is introduced slowly into the rectum. The woman is allowed to expel the enema on the toilet if she has not been sedated, her membranes are intact, her contrac-

tions are light to moderate, and she does not feel dizzy. The nurse should stay nearby, ready to help her back to bed. The time, results, and reaction of the patient to the enema are recorded on the chart.

INDUCTION

Initiating or stimulating labor is done for medical, surgical, and personal reasons. It is done by amniotomy and administration of drugs.

Amniotomy

Perhaps the most common physical procedure used to initiate labor is transcervical amniotomy, or artificial rupture of the membranes. Before it is performed the physician checks to see if the cervix is soft, partially effaced, slightly dilated, and if the presenting part is engaged. The simple, painless procedure is done by a hook or other sharp instrument passed over the gloved finger into the

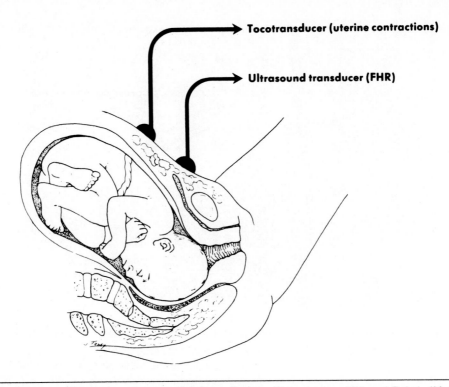

Tocotransducer (uterine contractions)

Ultrasound transducer (FHR)

Fig. 8-11 External noninvasive fetal monitoring. *(From Jensen, MD, and Bobak, IM: Maternity and gynecologic care: the nurse and the family, ed. 3, St. Louis, 1985, The CV Mosby Co.)*

cervix. The warm amniotic fluid flows out, sometimes with considerable force. The nurse immediately should inspect the perineum to see if there is a prolapsed cord. Fetal heart tones are checked immediately and again in 10 minutes.

Drugs

Labor-inducing drugs stimulate uterine muscle contractions. Effective dosage is highly variable. Overdosage may cause uterine tetany or rupture. For these reasons, these potent drugs are administered by means of an intravenous infusion pump with a piggyback setup so that the induction solution can be turned off and the vein kept open with a second solution. Pitocin, a natural oxytocin, and Syntocinon, a synthetic oxytocin, are the

drugs of choice. Prostaglandin may also be used. Intramuscular and intranasal administration are not recommended. During induction the baby's condition is checked closely by means of a fetal monitor.

CONTINUING SUPPORT

The admission of the maternity client is complete when all initial care has been given and recorded on the chart, the physician or midwife has been notified, and the woman is situated in her room. Continuing support now becomes the chief concern of the nurses.

Basic desires of the mother

Four major desires of the woman in labor have been identified by nurse researchers Lesser and Keane. They are:

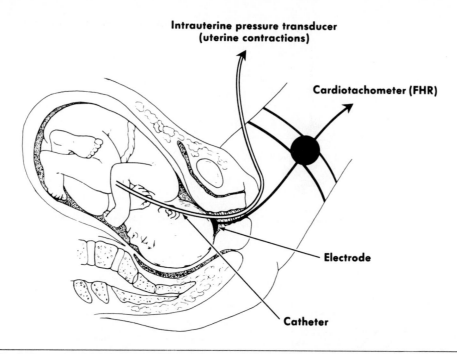

Intrauterine pressure transducer
(uterine contractions)

Cardiotachometer (FHR)

Electrode

Catheter

Fig. 8-12   Internal invasive fetal monitoring (membranes ruptured and cervix dilated). *(From Jensen, MD, and Bobak, IM: Maternity and gynecologic care: the nurse and the family, ed. 3, St. Louis, 1985, The CV Mosby Co.)*

1. To be sustained by another human being
2. To have relief of pain
3. To be assured of a safe outcome for both herself and her baby
4. To have attendants accept her personal attitude toward and behavior during labor

To sustain the woman in labor, nurses should try to convey a feeling of continuous presence with her, even if they cannot actually remain in the room every minute of the labor. It was suggested by Lesser and Keane that this feeling of presence be achieved in the following ways:

1. For the time nurses are with the woman, they should concentrate completely on that one person. This makes it possible for them to listen attentively to her every word and to make better observations of all the many unspoken gestures and expressions that convey so much meaning.
2. Nurses should make physical contact by washing the woman's face, rubbing her back, and holding her hand. This seems to provide real, tangible evidence that someone cares and is doing something specific to prove it.
3. Nurses should take the woman into their confidence by explaining why they cannot stay, where they are going, and when they expect to be back. They should provide a means to call them when needed.

Support person's role

The husband or other support person can play an important role for the laboring woman. If the support person has attended prenatal

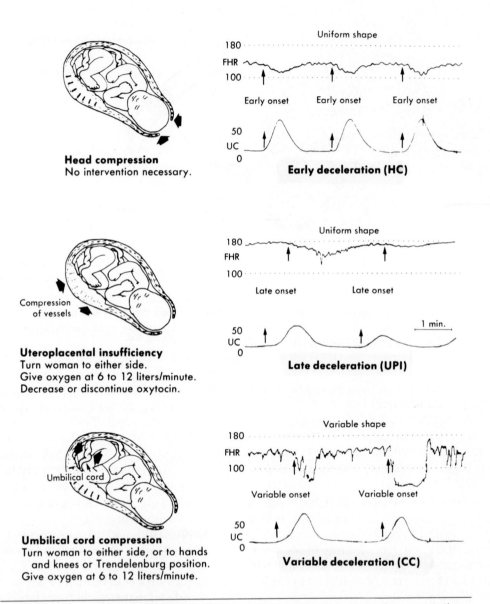

Head compression
No intervention necessary.

Early deceleration (HC)

Uteroplacental insufficiency
Turn woman to either side.
Give oxygen at 6 to 12 liters/minute.
Decrease or discontinue oxytocin.

Late deceleration (UPI)

Umbilical cord compression
Turn woman to either side, or to hands
and knees or Trendelenburg position.
Give oxygen at 6 to 12 liters/minute.

Variable deceleration (CC)

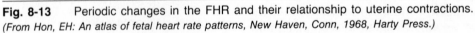

Fig. 8-13 Periodic changes in the FHR and their relationship to uterine contractions.
(From Hon, EH: An atlas of fetal heart rate patterns, New Haven, Conn, 1968, Harty Press.)

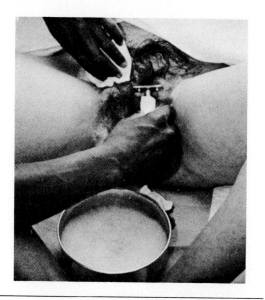

Fig. 8-14   Perineal preparation.

classes with the mother, he or she can give informed assistance. The support person can time the mother's contractions, rub her back, encourage her to rest between contractions, and remind her of breathing techniques. The support person can hold her hand, wash her face, and give her undivided attention.

Nurses must remember that they are responsible for the mother and baby even when a knowledgeable support person is present. They establish rapport with the mother and continuously monitor the progress of labor.

Teaching and coaching

It has been found that fear of the unknown contributes to the pain of labor. This is one of the chief reasons for prenatal classes. If the woman in labor has not attended these classes or availed herself of literature, the nurse will need to explain, coach, and teach her a great deal in a short period of time.

To teach a woman the entire physical process of labor and delivery during the few hours

that she is laboring is a big order. It cannot be done in detail, but certain important aspects can be clearly and simply explained. These should be appropriate to the phase of each stage of labor as the woman meets it. For instance, during the long first stage of labor, while the cervix is gradually effacing and dilating, the nurse can explain that the opening to the womb must be gradually pulled open by the contracting uterine muscles.

After the cervix is fully dilated, the nurse can explain that now the mouth of the womb is open and the mother can help the baby to be born by pushing down. The episiotomy can be explained as a controlled cut in preanesthetized soft tissue of the mother to prevent tearing and to hasten delivery. The expulsion of the placenta can be described as the afterbirth slipping out with one last contraction. All women especially primigravidas, appreciate the obvious interest in their welfare that such explanation indicates.

Food and fluids

As a general rule, solid foods should not be given during active labor, since food stays in the stomach much longer than fluids and digestion is greatly slowed during labor. At the same time the stress of labor, the contractions, and certain medications may produce nausea. Together these factors—a full stomach and nausea—may cause vomiting, with the danger of aspiration of food particles into the lungs.

On the other hand, it is important to avoid dehydration. For this reason, many physicians encourage the woman to take clear liquids throughout labor. If the woman becomes nauseated, an intravenous infusion of 5% lactated Ringer's solution may be prescribed. In some hospitals, intravenous fluids are routinely prescribed for all women in labor.

Elimination

The bladder should be emptied at frequent intervals throughout labor, at least every 2 hours. A careful record is kept of the amount and time of each voiding. If the woman is unable to void and her bladder becomes distended, the descent of the baby into the pelvis may be hampered. A full bladder can be palpated just above the pubis (Fig. 8-15). It is painful and greatly increases the discomfort of labor, but because of labor contractions, the woman may not recognize the origin of her discomfort. The nurse must keep a careful check of this important need.

If the woman has had an enema on admission, her lower bowel will be empty. Therefore, if the woman says that she needs to defecate again, the nurse should take a careful look at the perineum. There is a good possibility that the baby is ready to be born. Pressure of the baby's head on the perineum stimulates reflex nerve pathways, causing an urge to defecate.

Positioning and activity

Some authorities believe that if a woman in labor squats or walks, the cervix will dilate and efface more rapidly. There is evidence that if the woman can completely relax her abdominal muscles, labor will proceed more easily.

It is important to do all that is possible to promote relaxation and comfort.

Probably the most comfortable position for the mother is the one in which she usually sleeps. Pillows artfully placed at the back, under the abdomen, and between the knees may also help. Rubbing the back and sponging the perspiration-covered face are most comforting, since they help to convey concern in a tangible way. The support person can help with these measures. Because the pressure of the uterus on the vena cava and other major vessels can slow venous return of blood, the mother never should lie flat on her back. Doing so may cause *supine hypotensive syndrome* (Fig. 8-16).

Bathroom privileges and ambulation about the labor room are usually permitted unless the mother is sedated or precipitate (rapid) delivery is likely. After the membranes have ruptured, delivery may occur very quickly; patients whose membranes have ruptured should remain in bed. In the absence of a specific prescription, a common-sense approach should be applied to the question of ambulation. If there is *any* question about safety, bed rest is the wisest choice.

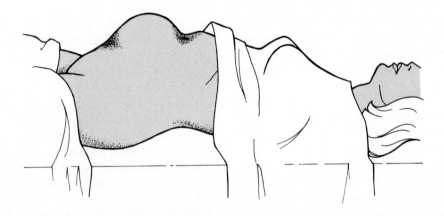

Fig. 8-15   A full bladder impedes descent of fetus. It can be observed and felt above symphysis pubis.

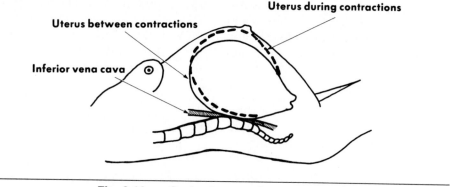

Fig. 8-16   Supine hypotensive syndrome.

Most labor room beds are equipped with buttocks pads that can be changed easily and quickly whenever they become soiled. It is important to keep the woman clean and dry not only to make her more comfortable but also to reduce the possibility of contamination of the birth canal.

Control of pain

The tolerance for pain varies greatly. Some women experience pain only during birth of the baby's head, while others become almost frenzied with pain early in labor. Pain during labor and delivery is caused by emotional tension, pressure on nerve endings, stretching of tissues and joints, and hypoxia of the uterine muscle during and after strong contraction. Cephalopelvic disproportion and other causes of difficult birth (dystocia) greatly increase labor pain.

Natural childbirth methods were originally designed to reduce fear and control the pain associated with labor. Their focus has broadened to include a holistic view of the mother and family unit, but their primary emphasis continues to be pain reduction. Using muscle-stretching exercises, relaxation techniques, breathing, and coaching behaviors, these methods prepare a woman for childbirth. Some popular methods are described in Chapter 5.

Nurses who work in birthing suites need to know the terminology and techniques of the natural childbirth methods practiced in their locale. They must assess the mother's physical and mental status objectively, however, and be prepared to offer medications as prescribed by a physician when necessary.

Drugs that control pain are called analgesics and anesthetics. See Chapter 9.

PROGRESS OF LABOR

Although each woman and each labor is different from the next, the progress and pattern of labor are essentially the same.

The first stage of labor is usually characterized by a rather long *latent period*, during which the cervix is effacing and contractions are relatively mild and infrequent. This is followed by the *active phase*, the last part of which is called the *transition phase*. Then the contractions become harder and more frequent until the cervix is completely effaced and dilated. These contractions continue uninterrupted until the presenting part presses on the perineum. The pressure causes an involuntary response in the woman to push the baby out at birth.

After the cervix is dilated, the second stage being. In multiparas it usually is rather short.

Primigravidas, on the other hand, may have a long second stage that lasts over an hour. This information is used by nurses to plan appropriate nursing care.

NURSING SUPERVISION

During the long latent phase of the first stage of labor, contractions may be mild enough to allow the woman to sleep, read, knit, or converse with her support person or nurses. As labor moves through the transition phase into the active phase, nursing supervision intensifies. It may be shared by a number of persons on the obstetric team. This supervision, called the *nursing process*, includes data collection, assessment and planning, implementation, and evaluation. The practical-vocational nurse participates in these functions to various degrees. All members of the team provide the mother with warmth and genuine concern. If a support person is present and so desires, he or she is included in as much of the care as possible.

Data collection

The following nursing observations are made during the first stage of labor:
1. Contractions are observed for duration, intensity, and frequency every 30 minutes or oftener.
2. Vital signs, including temperature, pulse, respirations, and blood pressure, are taken frequently.
3. Vaginal discharge is observed for color, amount, consistency, sudden change, and presence of placental tissue. The perineum is inspected for umbilical cord or fetal parts.
4. Fetal heart tone is monitored for rate, position, intensity, and change every 15 to 30 minutes or more often.
5. Voiding is checked every 2 hours. A full bladder can impede the progress of labor and increase discomfort.

6. Fluid intake is checked. If there is nausea or possible complications, an intravenous infusion of water or lactated Ringer's solution is started. The infusion then becomes another item for observation.
7. Food intake is limited during active labor; if permitted, appetite and intake are observed.
8. Mood and general level of activity are observed.
9. Discomfort of any type and its location, duration, intensity, and character are noted. Backache, headache, leg cramps, chest pain, continuous abdominal pain, and discomfort with contractions are all significant observations.
10. Skin color, abrasions, rashes, or unusual configuration are noted, because they may indicate undiagnosed disorders.

Danger signals

Nurses should note any observation of the following danger signals:
1. Changes in fetal heart tone—speeding up, slowing down, weakening, irregularity developing
2. Vaginal bleeding of any amount
3. Vaginal discharge of black or green meconium, unless breech presentation is expected
4. Continuous uterine contraction (tetany) or unusual contour
5. Umbilical cord or some fetal part other than the head presenting on the perineum

Signs of impending delivery

The following signs and subjective experiences indicate delivery is near:
1. Contractions more frequent and of longer duration
2. Bloody show increasing
3. Rupture of the membranes

4. Increasing restlessness
5. Nausea and vomiting
6. Mustache of perspiration
7. Bulging perineum
8. Anal dilation
9. Increasing backache
10. Rectal pressure
11. Abdomen too painful to touch
12. Grunts or cries, "My baby is coming!"
13. Uncontrollable desire to bear down

Assessment and planning

As the nurse's level of preparation and experience increases, so does the ability to assess the importance of observations and plan appropriate actions. One of the great values of the team approach is that observations are shared, consultation is immediately available, and a plan for action can be taken without delay.

Implementation

The nursing care plan that results from the observations and assessments is ongoing; its implementation is continually adjusted to the needs of the laboring woman. The midwife or physician is kept informed of the progress of labor. If complications arise, they are dealt with immediately. The mother is supported and encouraged as the wonderful moment of birth draws near.

Evaluation

Evaluation of nursing interventions for their effectiveness in meeting needs and solving problems is essential. Such evaluation provides a feedback loop. For example, after an analgesic drug is administered to the mother, her level of pain and the effect of the drug on the FHR are monitored and new interventions planned, if necessary.

▶ *KEY CONCEPTS*

1. Admission to general hospital, then to delivery suite, involves establishing rapport, checking valuables and clothing, collecting essential data, laboratory testing, physical examination, and initial treatment.
2. Physical examination includes measurement of vital signs, inspection of vaginal discharge, palpation of fetal position and uterine contractions, and auscultation of fetal heart tones.
3. Contractions are evaluated manually and by monitor for duration, frequency, and force.
4. Fetal position is assessed using Leopold's four maneuvers.
5. Fetal heart tones are assessed for rate, position, and regularity, assessment may be intermittent or continuous, internal or external.
6. Perineal preparation may be "mini" or omitted; enema may be omitted and is contraindicated with premature labor or vaginal bleeding.
7. Induction of labor may be by amniotomy or with intravenous administration of Pitocin or other drugs.
8. Basic desires of mother during labor are to be sustained, to have pain relief, to be assured of a safe outcome, and to be given unconditional acceptance.
9. Continuing support, coaching, and care during labor are provided by support persons, nurses, midwife, and physician, it includes attention to fluids and foods, elimination, activity, positioning, pain control, and progress of labor.
10. Danger signs are FHR changes, vaginal bleeding, vaginal discharge of meconium unless breech, uterine tetany, fetal part or cord on perineum.

■ *ANNOTATED SUMMARY*

I. Initial care
  A. General hospital admission—same as for all clients
  B. Delivery suite admission
    1. Establishing rapport—a relationship of trust between mother and nurses
    2. Clothing and valuables—accounted for or sent home
    3. Data collection
      a. Initial interview and nursing history—pertinent information is gathered
      b. Physical examination—involves inspection, auscultation, and palpation

(1) Vital signs
(2) Uterine contractions—frequency, duration, and intensity
(3) Abdominal inspection and palpation—Leopold's maneuvers
(4) Vaginal examination
  c. Fetal heart rate—normal range, 120-160 bpm
(1) Intermittent monitoring—for low-risk fetuses
(2) Continuous monitoring—for high-risk fetuses
  (a) Methods—external (noninvasive), internal (invasive)
  (b) Information obtained—relation of uterine contractions to fetal heart rate
  d. Laboratory tests—blood and urine
  e. Treatment
(1) Preparation of perineal area—cleanliness
(2) Urine specimen—tests for albumin, sugar, and acetone
(3) Enema—cleansing and stimulating; contraindicated with premature labor or bleeding
  C. Induction—to intensify contractions or initiate labor
    1. Amniotomy
    2. Drugs
II. Continuing support
  A. Basic desires of the mother—to be sustained, to have relief of pain, to be assured of a safe outcome, to have acceptance
  B. Support person's role—to provide informed assistance
  C. Teaching and coaching—important to reduce fear and pain
  D. Food and fluids—food withheld during active labor, but not liquids; IV fluids necessary if mother cannot tolerate oral fluids
  E. Elimination—full bladder hampers descent of fetus; defecation may contaminate sterile field at birth
  F. Positioning and activity—relaxation of abdominal muscles enhances uterine muscle effectiveness; supine hypotensive syndrome can be avoided by positioning mother off back
  G. Control of pain—natural childbirth methods now popular; nurses need to know those used in their region and when to administer prescribed drugs
III. Progress of labor
IV. Nursing supervision—follows the nursing progress
  A. Data collection—contractions, vital signs, vaginal discharge, FHR, voiding, fluid intake, food, mood, discomfort/pain, and skin
    1. Danger signals—FHR change, vaginal bleeding, vaginal discharge, uterine tetany, umbilical cord or fetal part other than head presenting on perineum
    2. Signs of impending delivery—13 signs
  B. Assessment and planning
  C. Implementation
  D. Evaluation

● **STUDY QUESTIONS AND LEARNING ACTIVITIES**

1. Describe the signs and symptoms of beginning labor.
2. What information should be obtained from the woman in labor on admission?
3. The fetal heart rate is an important indicator of the baby's condition. How is it counted and recorded? What is the normal range? What does a sudden change in the fetal heart rate indicate?
4. What three factors should be reported when observing uterine contractions?
5. According to Lesser and Keane, the mother has four major desires in labor. What are these desires, and how should the nurse meet them?
6. Describe two ways labor is induced.
7. What does a negative OCT mean?
8. The laboring woman tells the nurse she just felt a gush of warm water. What has probably happened? What nursing observations and care should be carried out immediately?
9. Describe the five danger signs of labor and their significance.
10. List five signs and symptoms of imminent delivery.

REFERENCES

Davis E: A guide to midwifery: heart and hands, ed 2, Santa Fe, NM, 1986, John Muir Publications.

Jensen MD, and Bobak IM: Maternity and gynecologic care: The nurse and the family, ed 3, St Louis, 1985, The CV Mosby Co.

CHAPTER 9

Nursing Care During the Birth

VOCABULARY

Analgesia
Anesthesia
Apgar score
Ataraxia
Narcotic antagonist
Pudendal block
Saddle block

LEARNING OBJECTIVES

- Compare psychophysical and pharmacologic measures to control discomfort in labor

- State nursing implications of sedatives, ataractics, narcotics, and narcotic antagonists

- Define anesthesia and describe nursing care for general and regional anesthesia

- Differentiate between injection sites of: saddle, epidural, caudal, pudendal, and paracervical blocks and local infiltration of the perineum

- Describe two areas reserved for births in the hospital and discuss their relative advantages and disadvantages

- Describe nursing care of a woman just before delivery, including perineal preparation, positioning, recordkeeping, and attention to the woman's needs

- Describe nursing care of the mother and immediate care of the infant after the birth

- Describe the Apgar scoring method for evaluating the newborn's general condition and parent-baby interaction developed by Gray

CONTROL OF DISCOMFORT

Childbirth is rarely free from discomfort. With modern measures, however, safety for the baby and reasonable comfort for the mother are possible. These measures are psychophysical and pharmacologic. (Table 9-1).

Terminology

Some of the terms associated with relief of the discomforts of childbirth are:

amnesia—loss of memory

analgesia—absence of normal sensations of pain

anesthesia—partial or complete loss of sensation with or without loss of consciousness; it may be general or regional

ataraxia—state of mental calm and tranquility

hypnotics—drugs that cause insensibility to pain and partial or complete unconsciousness; they include sedatives, analgesics, anesthetics, and intoxicants

narcosis—an unconscious state produced by narcotics

narcotic antagonists—drugs that displace opioids from receptor sites; they can reverse, for example, respiratory depression caused by morphine

sedation—state of calm or sleepiness

Psychophysical measures

A number of nonpharmacologic methods to control the discomfort of childbirth have been developed. The most common ones, discussed in Chapter 5, include Dick-Read, psychoprophylaxis (Lamaze), Bradley, hypnosis, and acupuncture/acupressure. These alternatives require varying degrees of cooperation and preparation by the mother.

The advantages of these methods are that the baby is not affected, the birth process is not slowed, and the mother remains aware and in some control. Their main disadvantage is that they require preparation and participation by the mother in the context of a normal birth process. When the mother is unprepared or when complications arise, these measures cannot be used or they are inadequate. If complications should arise and psychophysical measures prove inadequate, pharmacologic measures are used. It is important to assure the woman that she has not "failed" because she needs medication to relieve her discomfort.

Pharmacologic measures
Analgesia

A variety of drugs are used to provide relief of painful sensations, including sedatives, ataractics (potentiators, tranquilizers), narcotics, and narcotic antagonists.

Sedatives, such as secobarbital and pentobarbital, are barbiturate drugs that produce sleep. They are used to relieve anxiety and induce sleep during early labor. If sedatives are given too close to delivery, the baby will be born sleepy, with depressed pulse and respirations.

Ataractics are drugs that potentiate analgesic drugs to enhance their effectiveness. Promethazine (Phenergan), propiomazine (Largon), hydroxyzine (Vistaril), and promazine (Sparine) are commonly used. Ataractics intensify narcotic effects, including central nervous system depression in the baby and, if given near delivery cause the baby to be born with depressed pulse and respirations.

Narcotics such as meperidine (Demerol), alphaprodine (Nisentil), and morphine produce excellent analgesia. However, they are potent central nervous system depressants. If they are administered intramuscularly there is a 30 to 45 minute waiting period for relief, drug doses must be relatively high, and the fetal heart rate is depressed. If narcotics are given intravenously, smaller doses are possible and will give immediate relief

Table 9-1 Psychophysical and pharmacologic measures to control discomfort

Measure	Action and area affected	Maternal concerns	Effects on fetus	Nursing considerations
Psychoprophylaxis	Analgesia, whole mind/body	Prior training needed; no drugs	None	Pain controlled, not eliminated
Hypnosis	Analgesia, whole mind/body	Prior training needed; no drugs	None	Reinforcement required
Sedatives: Secobarbital Pentobarbital	Sedation, whole mind/body	Sleep, not pain relief	Hypoactivity, sleepiness	Check FHR for fetal bradycardia
Ataractics: Promethazine Propiomazine	Tranquilizer, potentiator of narcotics	Reduce anxiety, nausea	Hypoactivity, sleepiness	Check FHR for fetal bradycardia
Narcotics: meperidine alphaprodine	Analgesia, whole mind/body	Potent, rapid if given IV; may hasten progress of labor	Hypoactivity, sleepiness	Check FHR for fetal bradycardia; check cervical dilation
Narcotic antagonists: levallorphan naloxone	Counteract respiratory depression of narcotics	Withdraws analgesic effect of narcotic	Prevents respiratory depression	Not effective against barbiturates or ataractics
General anesthetics: nitrous oxide methoxyflurane halothane	General anesthesia inhalant inhalant inhalant	Loss of consciousness	Respiratory depression	Keep client NPO if being considered Check FHR for fetal bradycardia
thiopental	intravenous	No postpartum nausea	Sleepiness	Check uterus for postpartum atony
Regional anesthestics: bupivacaine	Nerve root block: saddle	Given in one dose just before birth	May slow FHR	Check FHR, mother's BP for hypotension
chloroprocaine	epidural/caudal	Prevents pushing, may slow labor, cause postpartum headache	May slow FHR	Check FHR, mother's BP for hypotension
	Peripheral nerve block: Pudenal	Effect limited to perineum/lower vagina	May slow FHR	Check FHR, mother's BP for hypotension
	Local infiltration	Effect limited to perineum	No effect	Explain to and support mother

to the mother and affect the fetus less; they can be administered at any stage of labor (Petree, 1985).

Narcotic antagonists reverse the central nervous system depression caused by narcotics. They are, by themselves, potent analgesics. Two narcotic antagonists commonly used in obstetrics are levallorphan (Lorfan) and naloxone (Narcan). These drugs are useful particularly when a mother has been given an intramuscular narcotic and birth comes more quickly than expected. Narcotic antagonists *do not* reverse the depressant effects of barbiturates or ataractics. If given to narcotic addicts, these drugs cause instant withdrawal symptoms and reversal of pain relief.

Anesthesia

Anesthesia, or loss of sensation, is achieved by the administration of various drugs. These drugs may be administered generally or regionally.

General anesthesia affects the brain and central nervous system, causing generalized insensitivity to stimuli and varying degrees of relaxation. The drugs are administered by inhalation or intravenous infusion. They give immediate pain relief but render the woman unconscious, so that she misses participation in and satisfaction from the birth event. In addition, various amounts of the drugs reach the baby by way of maternal circulation and act upon the fetal nervous system.

General anesthetics are administered by an anesthetist at the time of delivery and are continued until the perineal repair is complete. The woman is monitored closely until she is fully awake; monitoring includes assessment of vital signs, level of consciousness, and other postpartum concerns. Interventions include maintaining an open airway and giving reassurance.

Regional anesthesia renders areas of the body insensitive to pain and other stimuli. The areas affected depend on the nerves involved (Fig. 9-1). When a nerve root is injected with an anesthetic, as in saddle, epidural, or caudal blocks, large areas of the body are anesthetized. When individual nerves are injected, as in pudendal blocks, only the distribution of those nerves is affected. When tissue is infused with an anesthetic drug in solution, nerve endings in that location are anesthetized (Fig. 9-2).

Saddle block anesthesia usually is administered in the delivery room near the end of the second stage of labor and before the woman is draped for the birth. The woman is positioned with her back arched and her head flexed down on her chest (Fig. 9-3). A blood pressure cuff is placed around her upper arm, and an initial, baseline reading is made before the procedure. The physician selects the site, cleanses it, administers a local anesthetic into the skin, and inserts the spinal needle. The drug is injected slowly and the needle is removed. Blood pressure readings and level of anesthesia are checked frequently thereafter. Then the woman is placed in lithotomy position for delivery. Her head should be slightly elevated.

After delivery, the woman who has had a saddle block anesthetic requires special care because her lower extremities will remain paralyzed and insensitive for 2 to 4 hours. Her legs are lifted together from the supports. She will need help to transfer from the delivery table to the gurney and from the gurney to her bed. She should be encouraged to roll from side to side, but she should be discouraged from raising her head for the next 24 hours, to prevent postspinal headache.

Caudal and epidural anesthesia are administered near the end of the first stage of labor. A blood pressure cuff is placed on the upper arm and a baseline reading taken. The woman is placed in a Sims', or knee-chest, position.

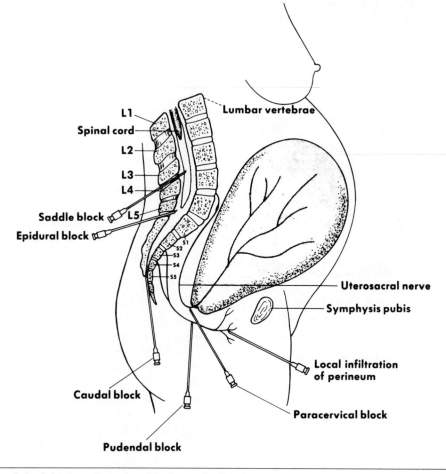

Fig. 9-1 Injection sites of regional anesthetics.

The physician anesthetizes the skin, inserts the needle, and introduces the drug into the sacral hiatus. If repeated injections are anticipated, a polyethylene catheter is inserted through the needle and left in place after the needle is removed. In this way, continuous caudal anesthesia can be maintained for several hours. Special care must be taken to secure the catheter in place. Blood pressure and level of anesthesia are monitored frequently until sensation and motor activity have returned.

THE BIRTH
Birthing areas of the hospital

In the modern hospital, two areas are reserved for births: delivery rooms and alternative birthing centers.

Delivery rooms are like surgical suites. They are designed to be as aseptic and functional

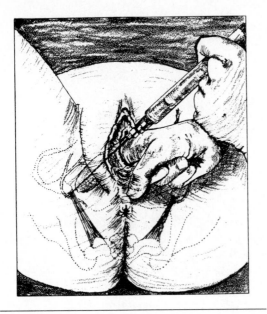

Fig. 9-2 Pudendal block. *(From Ingalls, AJ, and Salerno, MC: Maternal and child health nursing, ed 5, St Louis, 1987, The CV Mosby Co.)*

as possible. Only necessary equipment that is in working order and that can be readily cleaned is kept in delivery rooms. Personnel who enter them wear clean garments, caps over their hair, and masks when sterile fields are open. Those who "scrub in" don sterilized gowns and gloves. When a delivery room is to be used, the mother stays in a labor room until birth is imminent, and then she is transferred to the delivery room.

Alternative birthing centers are homelike rooms, usually in proximity to a delivery room. For uncomplicated pregnancies, both labor and birth take place in an alternative birthing center (Fig. 8-2). When birth is imminent a sterile field is provided, and the process of birth goes on without interruption.

Labor to delivery room

When a mother is in active labor in a labor room, the attending nurse keeps the super-

vising nurse informed of her progress. The supervising nurse, in turn, keeps the physician or midwife informed. Most midwives and many physicians remain with the mother after labor becomes active and decide when she is ready to go to the delivery room. As a general rule, multiparas go to the delivery room when the cervix is fully dilated, primigravidas when the perineum bulges, and all clients when signs of impending delivery appear.

When a mother labors on a regular bed, she must be moved to a gurney for transport to the delivery room. In the delivery room she must be moved from the gurney onto the delivery table. Some hospitals use the more portable recovery room beds for labor. When the client on this type of bed is ready for delivery, she is wheeled into the delivery room where she slides over onto the delivery table. This eliminates one transfer.

The move from her labor room bed to the delivery table may be a frightening experience for the mother. She may fear that the baby will come before she gets there, or worse, while she is en route. To reduce some of this anxiety, the mother should be taken to the delivery room in plenty of time. Although there are occasions when delivery comes suddenly, an attempt is usually made to get the woman to the delivery room before the actual birth, because sterile supplies and necessary equipment for mother and baby are all there. Every effort should be made to reduce nervous chatter and anxious motion.

Although the last-minute rush to the delivery room is undesirable for both client and personnel, so is a long wait by the mother on the thinly padded, narrow delivery table or birthing chair. Once she is taken to the delivery room, the mother is not left alone, even for a minute.

Preparation for the birth

The mother and baby are the center of activities within the delivery room. Since the

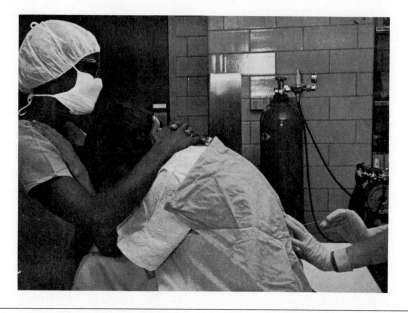

Fig. 9-3 Position for saddle block anesthesia. Patient sits on the side of the table with her feet resting on a stool. Nurse hold the patient's head down, arching the back.

mother is having strong and frequent contractions, anesthesia is one of the considerations. If a spinal anesthesia is to be given, it is administered before the woman is positioned for the birth (Fig. 9-3). If there is to be no anesthesia, the mother is placed in position immediately. If present, the anesthetist usually sits at the head of the delivery table to monitor the mother's vital signs and administer an anesthetic if necessary. If no anesthetist is present, the circulating nurse is responsible for monitoring the mother's vital signs and the FHR, ministering to the mother, and assisting the physician or midwife. If a support person is present, that person stands near the head of the table to encourage and coach the mother.

Positioning and perineal cleansing

Positions for delivery are dorsal recumbent, lithotomy, side-lying, and knee-chest. In the *dorsal recumbent* position, the head of the bed is at a 35- to 45-degree angle, the mother's knees are bent, and her feet are flat on the table. This position facilitates the mother's pushing efforts and keeps the weight of the uterus off of her major blood vessels (Fig. 9-4). *Lithotomy* position is used most often when some surgical intervention is needed, such as when forceps are used. The legs are covered with ether socks and then lifted together into the stirrups. The head of the table may be raised somewhat. *Side-lying* and *knee-chest* positions are used most often when the birth takes place in a regular bed, as in home birth.

As soon as the mother is positioned, her perineum is cleaned with antiseptic solutions, using downward strokes toward the rectum.

When the mother has been cleansed, the sterile back table and basins are uncovered (Fig. 9-5). Sterile drapes are placed under the buttocks and over the legs and abdomen, leaving only the vaginal orifice, perineum, and rectum exposed. It should be remembered that if a sterile drape covering an unsterile surface becomes wet it is no longer sterile, because moisture allows bacteria to pass through the fibers.

Assisting the physician or midwife

The physician or midwife dons a scrub suit, mask, and cap and then scrubs as for surgery. After entering the delivery room, the physician or midwife is helped into a sterile gown and gloves (Fig. 9-6) and then moves to the foot of the delivery table or birthing chair in front of the back table. The light is adjusted and a stool provided. Various special supplies, medications, forceps, and suture materials may be requested at this time. They should be placed on the back table or given directly to the physician or midwife without contaminating the sterile field.

Recordkeeping

An accurate record of birth is very important for medical-legal purposes. Usually it is kept on a specially prepared form that includes such information as the time events occurred, premedications and anesthetic given, position and condition of the baby at birth, type of forceps (if used), a description of the episiotomy (if performed) and its repair, and a description of the placenta. Not only is this important chronicle of the birth kept for the mother's chart, but in many hospitals a copy also is kept on the infant's chart. The birth record provides physicians with valuable information for future care of the child and also is used in preparing the birth certificate.

If an anesthetic is administered, the anesthetist keeps a separate record that becomes part of the mother's chart.

Most hospitals also keep a cumulative record of all deliveries in a large ledger-like volume. This record is especially valuable in preparing statistical studies and reports, such as the number of twin and single births in a given period of time.

Nursing care of the mother

In the midst of all the busy preparation by delivery room personnel, the mother continues to experience strong uterine contractions. She may need coaching to help her make the most of them.

Traditionally, the *Valsalva breathing method,* which requires the woman to hold her breath and push, has been encouraged. Currently, a modified Valsalva is suggested, to avoid the maternal and fetal anoxia. In the modified method, the mother takes several deep breaths and then holds her breath for 5 seconds. Then, through slightly pursed lips, she exhales slowly every 5 seconds. She takes another breath and continues the exhale breathing and pushing as long as the contraction is present. When the contraction is over the mother lets herself go limp, relaxing completely. Indeed, this is hard labor. To avoid exhaustion, she may need to simply pant during some of the contractions.

Blood pressure, pulse, and ability of the mother to react and cooperate are indicators of her condition. Occasionally a woman may become nauseated during this stage of labor, especially if her labor started shortly after a large meal. An emesis basin is kept ready for such an emergency.

Preparation of the outlet

As the presenting part moves toward the outlet, the midwife or physician prepares the soft tissue by stretching it manually (Fig. 9-7, *A*). An anesthetic drug may also be injected into the perineal skin or the pudendal nerve root to provide a larger area of numbness to pain (see Fig. 9-2).

At first the presenting part is only visible during the height of each contraction. But as the head descends further, the perineum and

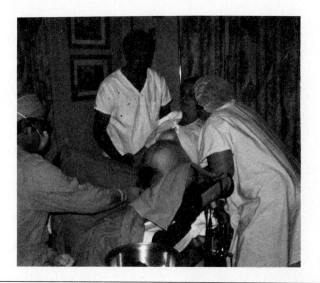

Fig. 9-4 Dorsal recumbent position for labor facilitates pushing efforts. *(From Sumner, PE, and Phillips, CR: Birthing rooms: concept and reality, St Louis, 1981, The CV Mosby Co. Used with permission from the Labadorf family.)*

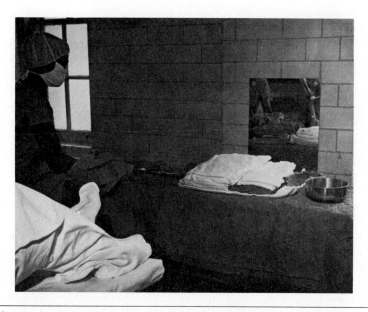

Fig. 9-5 Sterile delivery pack opened on back table. Drapes and supplies are made ready for use.

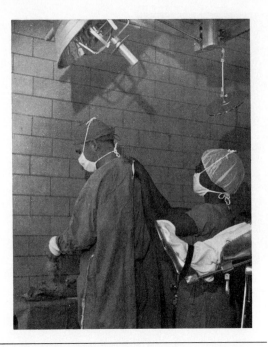

Fig. 9-6 Nurse assists the midwife or physician to don sterile gown and gloves.

vulva are stretched open and the baby's hair and scalp bulge outward so that the vulva and perineum seem to form a crown on the baby's head—hence the apt description *crowning* (Fig. 9-7, *B* and *C*).

To prevent the delicate vulvar and perineal tissue from being torn at the height of the contraction, the physician or midwife may slip a blunt-ended scissors between the baby's head and the perineum and with one motion enlarge the opening by a controlled cut of the tissue. This cut is called an *episiotomy* and may be made directly downward toward the midline or to the left or right, laterally.

Birth of the baby

The way is now open for the baby to pass. With one or more contractions the head slips out, followed by the shoulders and then the body (Fig. 9-7, *D* to *H*). The baby is born. The

time is noted. A lusty, spontaneous cry usually announces the birth. If there is mucus and amniotic fluid in the baby's nose and mouth, the midwife or physician may help remove it with a rubber bulb syringe. The baby may then be placed across the mother's abdomen to clamp and cut the cord (Fig. 9-8).

The mother needs constant encouragement during the last expulsive contractions, both by word and by deed. She may need help from the labor coach or nurse to know when to pant, when to push, when to blow out air through her open mouth, and when to use pursed lips.

During the second stage of labor the fetus is being squeezed down into and through the pelvis. This is harsh treatment, and it is important to know how the baby is faring. The fetal heart rate gives an indication. It is checked frequently and reported to the physician or midwife.

Expulsion of the placenta

As the infant is delivered, the uterus contracts down as much as is possible with the placenta still within the cavity. The greatly reduced uterine surface causes the placenta to begin to separate. There is then a latent or quiet period of a few seconds to a few minutes during which bleeding occurs behind the placenta, distending the uterus and stimulating the uterus to contract. Some physicians prescribe an oxytocic drug for the mother immediately after delivery to cause the uterus to contract at once, freeing the placenta for expulsion. As the uterus contracts, it is lifted forward in the abdominal cavity. The cord is grasped with one hand and the fundus of the uterus is massaged with the other (Fig. 9-9). The placenta usually slips out into the waiting basin. The time and mechanism (Duncan's or Schultze's) (see Fig. 7-7) are noted.

The placenta is carefully inspected to be sure that it is whole. If pieces remain within the uterus, it cannot clamp down completely,

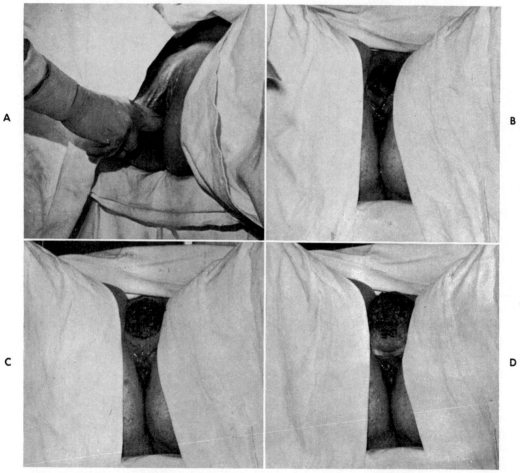

Fig. 9-7 Vertex delivery. **A,** Stretching the soft tissues. **B,** Crowning. **C,** Perineum taut. **D,** Head extends.   *Continued.*

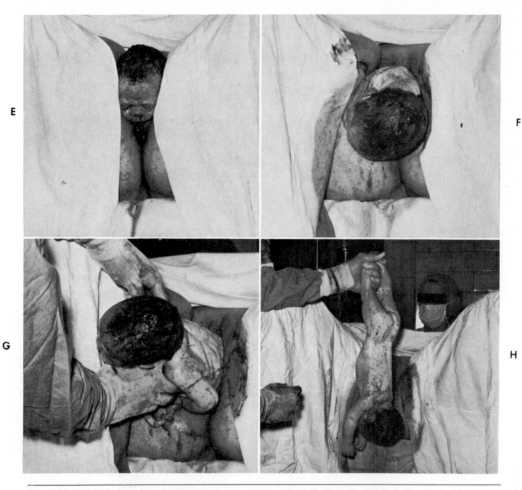

Fig. 9-7, cont'd Vertex delivery. **E,** Face exposed. **F,** External rotation. Shoulder emerges. **G,** Body slips out. Note umbilical cord. **H,** Birth complete.

and serious hemorrhage may result. When the physician or midwife is satisfied that the whole placenta has been expressed, the mother is given an injection of an oxytocic drug, such as methylergonovine (Methergine) or Pitocin.

Immediate care of the baby

Immediately after birth the baby may be bathed in warm water, in what Leboyer termed "birth without violence—gentle birth" (Fig. 9-10). The warm water, like the amniotic fluid, provides security and warmth after the

trauma of the birth process. The support person may do this as the nurse and mother look on.

Some mothers wish to put the baby to breast soon after birth. It is a time of great emotion as the mother, father, and infant initiate their family relationship (Fig. 9-11).

The baby's welfare is of prime importance. Warmth and safety from falls are vital. A stockinette cap is put on the baby's head to reduce heat loss from evaporation. If the baby is having difficulty breathing, resuscitation efforts

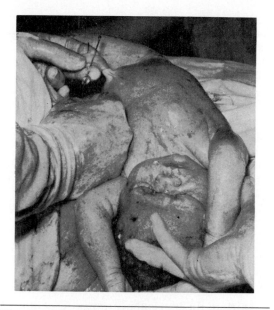

Fig. 9-8 Clamping the cord with a Hesseltine clamp. Baby rests on mother's abdomen.

are begun immediately. These measures are discussed in detail in Chapter 11.

Evaluation
General condition

A standardized means of evaluating the condition of a newborn is of great value. Although several systems have been devised, the one Dr. Virginia Apgar described in 1953 has been widely accepted. It consists of five observations made at 1-, 5-, and 30-minute intervals after birth. A value of 0 to 2 is given for each

observation, and the values are then added, giving a total Apgar score (Table 9-2). A baby in excellent condition would score 9 to 10; a dead baby would score 0. Most babies score 7 or better. Generally, premature babies, those born after long labors, and those born in breech or abnormal positions have lower scores than full-term babies born in the occiput anterior position after normal labors.

Parent-baby interaction

Concern with the roots of child abuse has led to studies of the interaction, or *bonding*, between parents and infants. This early claiming process is affected by the expressed attitudes of staff members, the physical environment of the delivery suite, and the parents' feelings about the new baby. Observations of how the mother looks, what she says, and what she does in the perinatal period have proved to be accurate predictors of child abuse. A standardized means of evaluating parent-child bonding was devised by Gray and associates in 1975 (Table 9-3). It consists of three observations made in the delivery suite during and immediately after the infant's birth and again during the first 2 to 3 days of the postpartum period. A value of 1 to 4 points is given for each observation, and the values are totaled for each period. A highly positive interaction would total 10 to 12 for each period. A strongly negative interaction would be a score of 3 to 6. Follow-up counseling for low-

Table 9-2 Apgar scoring chart for newborn babies

Sign	Score		
	0	1	2
Color	Blue, pale	Body pink, extremities blue	Completely pink
Heart rate	Absent	Below 100	Over 100
Respiratory effort	Absent	Irregular	Good, crying
Muscle tone	Limp	Some flexion of extremities	Active motion
Reflex irritability (catheter in nostril)	None	Grimace	Cough, sneeze

Table 9-3 Scoring chart for parent-baby interaction*

| Bonding score | How mother acts regarding her baby | | |
	Looks	Says	Does
1 Strongly negative, inappropriate 2 Mildly negative, inappropriate 3 Mildly positive, appropriate 4 Strongly positive, appropriate	General appearance: depressed, fearful, angry, apathetic ↓ Joyful, exuberant, happy, enthusiastic, serene, beaming	Makes disparaging remarks about baby and husband; expresses hostility or disappointment in baby's sex or looks ↓ Talks directly to baby, using baby's name; expresses positive reactions	Focuses attention on self; turns away from baby; cries ↓ Reaches out for, cuddles, examines, establishes eye contact with baby

*Modified from Gray J, Cutler C, Dean J, and Kempe CH: Perinatal assessment of mother-baby interaction. In Helfer RE, and Kempe CH: Child abuse and neglect: the family and community, Philadelphia, 1976, Ballinger Publishing Co.

scoring parents is indicated to prevent child abuse and teach nurturant parenting.

The physician or any other person in the delivery room may make the observations. The scores should be recorded on the delivery room record and on the baby's chart.

When the midwife or physician is satisfied that the infant is in good condition or when the care of the infant has been turned over to another responsible person, attention then turns to the mother.

Inspection and repair

The midwife or physician carefully examines the cervix and vagina for tears that may have occurred during birth, since hemorrhages can result from enlarged blood vessels in the area. Tears or lacerations are classified according to the depth of tissue involved. A *first-degree laceration* is one that involves only superficial layers of tissue; a *second-degree laceration* involves deeper layers; and a *third-degree laceration* includes muscle. If a tear is discovered, it is repaired, as is the episiotomy. Suture material that will dissolve without being removed is used for these repairs.

During the episiotomy repair the mother usually rests quietly on the birthing bed; she is not uncomfortable because the anesthetic has desensitized her perineal area. The uterus should be a firm ball beneath her now flaccid abdominal muscles. The mother may be talkative and excited or she may be serenely calm, holding the infant or watching with interest as the nurse places matching identification bands on her baby and herself.

Continuing care of the mother and infant

When the midwife or physician has finished the repair, a final check is made to see that the mother and baby are in satisfactory condition. The soiled drapes are removed from the mother, old blood is washed away with the cleaning supplies at hand, and dry, sterile perineal pads are put in place with a T binder. A warm, clean gown and blanket add greatly to the mother's comfort just before she is transferred from the delivery room.

When birth occurs in an alternative birthing center, the new family remains there during the fourth stage of labor. If there are no complications, when the condition of both mother

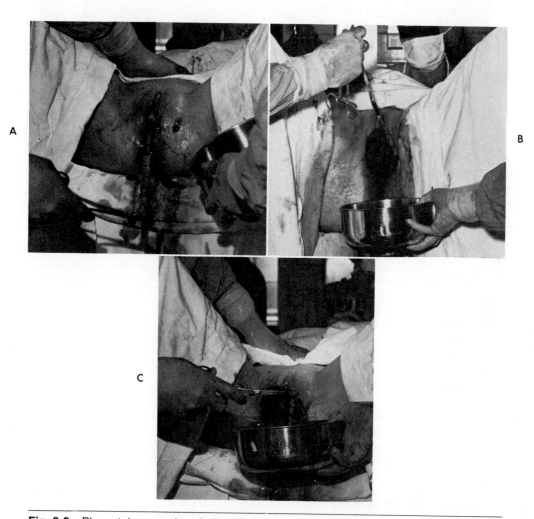

Fig. 9-9 Placental expression. **A,** Physician grasps the cord with one hand and massages the uterine fundus with the other. **B** and **C,** Placenta slips out into waiting basin.

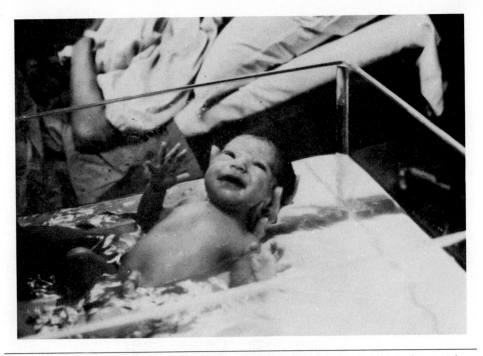

Fig. 9-10 Leboyer method of "gentle childbirth." Father bathes infant while mother watches. *(From Jensen, MD, and Bobak, IM: Maternity and gynecologic care: the nurse and the family, ed 3, 1985, St Louis, The CV Mosby Co.)*

and infant has stabilized, they are discharged to their home. If the mother and infant are to remain in the hospital in a rooming-in arrangement, both mother and baby occupy a single room together. If rooming-in is not available or desired, the baby is taken to the newborn nursery and the mother moved to a recovery unit where she is closely observed.

Follow-up responsibilities of the nurse

After a birth the delivery room is stripped of all soiled instruments, linen, and supplies and is washed with antiseptic solution. It is then set up for reuse. Antepartum and delivery records are completed, and the mother's chart is made ready for postpartum recording. Hospital bookkeeping forms and other records of the delivery also are completed.

■ ANNOTATED SUMMARY

I. Control of discomfort
   A. Terminology—words associated with discomfort control
   B. Psychophysical measures—Dick-Read, psychoprophylaxis, Bradley, hypnosis, acupuncture/acupressure
   C. Pharmacologic measures
     1. Analgesia—sedatives, ataractics, narcotics, narcotic antagonists
     2. Anesthesia—general, regional
II. The birth
   A. Birthing areas of hospitals—delivery rooms, alternative birthing centers
   B. Labor to delivery room—multiparas: when cervix is dilated; primiparas: when perineum is bulging; all mothers: with signs of impending delivery
   C. Preparation for the birth
     1. Positioning and perineal cleansing
     2. Assisting the physician or midwife

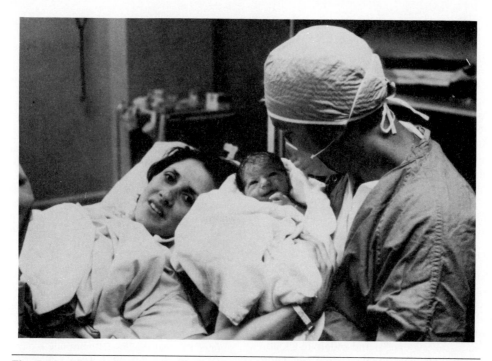

Fig. 9-11 Mother, father, and new baby form a new family. *(From Jensen, MD, and Bobak, IM: Maternity and gynecologic care: the nurse and the family, ed 3, St Louis, 1985, The CV Mosby Co.)*

3. Recordkeeping
4. Nursing care of the mother
5. Preparation of the outlet
D. Birth of the baby
E. Expulsion of the placenta
F. Immediate care of the baby—Leboyer bath; baby to breast; protection from falls or heat loss; resuscitation if necessary
G. Evaluation
   1. General condition using Apgar
   2. Bonding using interaction score
H. Inspection and repair
I. Continuing care of mother and infant
J. Follow-up responsibilities of nurse

▶ *KEY CONCEPTS*

1. Psychophysical and pharmacologic measures make modern childbirth safe and help reduce discomfort.
2. Terms associated with relief of discomfort include amnesia, analgesia, anesthesia, ataraxia, hypnotics, narcosis, narcotic antagonists, and sedation.
3. Psychophysical measures used today include Dick-Read, psychoprophylaxis, Bradley, hypnosis, acupuncture/acupressure.
4. Pharmacologic measures used today include analgesics (sedatives, ataractics, narcotics, narcotic antagonists) and anesthesia (general and regional).
5. Birthing areas of hospitals are delivery rooms maintained as surgical suites and alternative birthing centers maintained as homelike areas where support persons and mother remain throughout labor and birth if there are no complications.
6. When delivery room is used multiparas go there when fully dilated, primiparas go when perineal is bulging, and all mothers go whenever signs of impending delivery appear.

197

7. Responsibilities of nurse include the mother, baby, physician or midwife, support person, and recordkeeping.
8. During birth nurses coach mother using modified Valsalva breathing, monitor vital signs, and give support.
9. Evaluation of infant's condition at birth by Apgar scoring; of parent-baby interaction by Gray bonding scale.
10. Nursing care of mother includes cleansing, comforting, providing warmth, and monitoring.
11. Other nursing duties include recordkeeping; cleaning and setting up delivery room for reuse.

● *STUDY QUESTIONS*

1. As a general rule, multiparas go to the delivery room at what stage of labor? When are primiparas usually taken to the delivery room?
2. How does regional anesthesia differ from general anesthesia? Describe the nursing care for a mother receiving caudal and saddle block anesthetics. What observations should be made during the administration of a general or regional anesthetic?
3. What is the first order of concern immediately after the baby is born?
4. After the episiotomy repair, what nursing care is given to the mother?
5. Apgar scoring is done by whom, how many times, and at what intervals? What are the five categories assessed?

REFERENCES

Clark JB, Queener SF, and Karb VB: Pharmacological basis of nursing practice, ed 2, St Louis, 1986, The CV Mosby Co.

Ingalls AJ, and Salerno MC: Maternal and child health nursing, ed 6, St Louis, 1987, The CV Mosby Co.

Jensen MD, and Bobak IM: Maternity and gynecologic care: the nurse and the family, ed 3, St Louis, 1985, The CV Mosby Co.

Klaus MH, and Kennell JH: Parent-infant bonding, ed 2, St Louis, 1981, The CV Mosby Co.

Leboyer F: Birth without violence, New York, 1975, Alfred A Knopf, Inc.

Phillips CR, and Anzalone JT: Fathering: participation in labor and birth, ed 2, St Louis, 1982, The CV Mosby Co.

Sumner PE, and Phillips CR: Birthing rooms: concept and reality, St Louis, 1981, The CV Mosby Co.

CHAPTER 10

Complications of Labor and Birth

VOCABULARY

Cephalopelvic disproportion
Dystocia
Effleurage
Grief work
Multiparity
Tocolytic drugs
Trial labor

LEARNING OBJECTIVES

- Discuss problems caused by fear as they affect labor and birth, relating goals of nursing interventions.

- Describe hypertonic and hypotonic dysfunctional labor patterns, and prolonged labor, its complications, and nursing interventions.

- Compare precipitous labor and precipitous delivery; state common causes, dangers, assessment, and nursing interventions for precipitous labor.

- Describe preterm labor, contributing factors, and the major concerns associated with premature rupture of membranes (PROM); discuss nursing assessment and interventions.

- Describe a pathological retraction ring, explaining why it obstructs labor and problems created by cephalopelvic disproportion.

- Describe fetal distress, its assessment, and interventions.

- Discuss the implications of macrosomia and hydrocephaly for the mother and fetus and describe two malpositions that complicate delivery and explain why.

- Discuss assessment of multiple pregnancies, prenatal and delivery consequences, and typical interventions.

- Describe interventions for intrauterine fetal death, discussing the experience of loss and grief as it relates to fetal death, identifying stages of grieving and nursing interventions.

- Compare placenta previa and abruptio placentae; describe nursing assessments and interventions for each condition.

- Indentify common maternal conditions associated with prolapsed cord and explain emergency nursing interventions.

- Describe factors that contribute to hydramnios, resulting complications, and its assessment.

- Describe amniotic fluid embolism and disseminated intravascular coagulation, stating dangers and interventions.

- Describe causes of third-stage, and fourth-stage hemorrhage.

- Discuss methods of inducing labor and nursing interventions.

- Discuss episiotomy, its purpose, placement, and postoperative care.

- Describe types of version and use of forceps, stating purposes and nursing interventions.

- Discuss cesarean birth, its incidence, indications, complications, common problems, and nursing interventions.

The successful completion of pregnancy and birth of a baby involves the combined functioning of four factors (Olds and others, 1988):

1. *Psyche* is the woman's mental and emotional processes.
2. *Power* is the muscular force of uterine and abdominal muscles.
3. *Passageway* is the vagina, introitus, and bony pelvis.
4. *Passenger* is all the products of conception.

Complications sometimes arise to disrupt the normal birth process, however, and surgical procedures may be performed in an attempt to conclude the pregnancy successfully.

COMPLICATIONS OF THE PSYCHE
Description

Ignorance leads to fear, which greatly complicates the birth process. Fear produces nervous and endocrine responses that result in sodium retention, potassium excretion, and reduction of glucose needed by the contracting uterus. These responses also lead to secretion of epinephrine, which inhibits myometrial activity, and release of norepinephrine, which leads to uncoordinated or increased uterine activity. Increased physical distress and ineffective labor creates a vicious cycle, causing even more fear and discomfort.

Nursing research indicates that pain and loss of control are the most unpleasant factors of labor (Butane, 1973, and others). Women who participate in prenatal classes benefit by maintaining better control, using fewer medications, manifesting more positive attitudes, and experiencing anticipation rather than fear (Genest, 1982).

Assessment

When a woman arrives at the delivery suite, it is important to assess her preparation for the birthing process. Cultural and religious factors influence her expectations, values, and responses. Women who are prepared for childbirth and accompanied by a support person often demonstrate joyful and even euphoric feelings during the birth process. Those who have not prepared for childbirth are more likely to be anxious and exhibit their fears in a wide range of behaviors, from stoic silence to hysterical crying.

Interventions

The goal of nursing interventions is to reduce fear and assist the woman to maintain control. To that end, the nurse:

1. Gives positive verbal encouragement
2. Provides information about the progress of labor
3. Offers specific instructions about breathing, relaxation, and body posture
4. Physically contacts the woman with back rubbing, effleurage, holding, and face washing
5. Provides nonjudgmental acceptance of the woman's responses
6. Maintains a calm, reassuring presence

COMPLICATIONS OF THE POWER

Rhythmical contractions of the uterine myometrium are the means by which the fetus is expelled. These contractions are affected by contractile proteins, energy resources, and ionic exchange of electrolytes, and endocrine sources. Disruption in any of these factors may result in ineffective, *dysfunctional labor* with hypertonic or hypotonic patterns. Prolonged, precipitous, and preterm labor also may occur. There may be premature rupture of the membranes, dystocia (difficult labor) resulting from retraction rings, and uterine rupture or inversion.

Hypertonic labor
Description

Hypertonic labor usually occurs in the latent phase of labor, with an increase in frequency of contractions and a decrease in their intensity. Contractions are extremely painful because of uterine muscle cell anoxia, but are ineffective in dilating and effacing the cervix, which leads to maternal exhaustion. Contractions may interfere with uteroplacental exchange and lead to fetal distress and even death.

Interventions

Management of hypertonic labor includes bed rest and sedation to promote relaxation and reduce pain. Oxytocin is *not* administered to a woman suffering from hypertonic uterine activity because it is likely to increase the abnormal labor pattern. If the hypertonic pattern continues and develops into a prolonged latent phase, the possibility of cephalopelvic disproportion or fetal malpresentation is investigated. If not present, amniotomy and oxytocin infusion may be instituted.

Potential problems of hypertonic labor include dehydration, urinary ketones, maternal exhaustion, and fetal distress. Therefore the nurse maintains a record of intake and output, checks urinary ketones every 2 hours, assesses the woman's level of fatigue and the fetal heart rate (FHR), and administers analgesics as needed.

Hypotonic labor
Description

Hypotonic labor is defined as less than three contractions of mild to moderate intensity occurring in a 10-minute period during the active phase of labor. Cervical dilation and fetal descent slow greatly or stop. Such labor occurs when uterine fibers are overstretched from large babies, twins, hydramnios, or many pregnancies (multiparity). Hypotonic labor also may occur when drugs such as meperidine are given in the latent phase of labor or when bowel or bladder distention is present. Although painless, such labor leads to maternal exhaustion, stress, intrauterine infection, and postpartum hemorrhage. Prolonged labor may lead to fetal sepsis.

Interventions

Management of hypertonic labor includes assessment of the mother's vital signs, level of exhaustion, hydration, and FHR. The physician assesses the adequacy of the mother's pelvic measurements and fetal maturity. If these measures are within safe limits, the physician may perform an amniotomy to stimulate the labor process or administer oxytocin via an infusion pump to improve the quality of uterine contractions. Nursing care for these interventions is described on p. 218.

Potential problems of hypertonic labor include dehydration, urinary ketones, maternal exhaustion, and fetal distress. Therefore the nurse maintains a record of intake and output, checks urinary ketones every 2 hours, assesses the woman's level of fatigue and the fetal heart rate (FHR), and administers analgesics as needed.

Prolonged labor
Description

Labor that lasts more than 24 hours is termed prolonged. Usually the first stage of labor is extended; active and latent phases are prolonged; and the cervix fails to dilate within a reasonable time. To prevent complications, early recognition and treatment are vital.

Complications of prolonged labor include maternal exhaustion, infection, and hemorrhage from uterine atony, uterine rupture, or lacerations of the birth canal. Forceps delivery or cesarean birth may be necessary. Fetal distress may result from impaired blood supply and reduced oxygen, causing fetal asphyxia. Premature rupture of the membranes (PROM) increases the risk of infection and prolapse of the cord if the presenting part fails to descend and engage. Soft tissue injury or cerebral trauma may result from continuous and intense pressure on the fetal head or from forceps delivery.

Interventions

Interventions for prolonged labor are based on the causes. Nursing actions include (1) monitoring the status of the mother and fetus; (2) providing hydration, comfort measures, and prescribed medications; and (3) helping the couple cope with frustration and anxiety. Following delivery, the mother is monitored for signs of hemorrhage, shock, and infection. The neonate is observed for signs of sepsis, cerebral trauma, and cephalohematoma.

Precipitous labor
Description

Precipitous labor is labor that lasts less than 3 hours. *Precipitous delivery* is delivery that occurs with little or no warning; it may or may not be associated with precipitous labor.

The most frequent causes of precipitous labor are lack of resistance by maternal tissues, hyperactive uterine contractions, and a small fetus in a favorable position. Such labor is seen more often in women who are multiparous, have a history of precipitous labors, or have large pelvic measurements.

If the cervix is effaced and the tissues resist stretching, lacerations of the birth canal, uterine rupture, and amniotic fluid embolism may occur. Postpartal maternal hemorrhage may result from stretched uterine fibers. The fetus may suffer hypoxia from decreased periods of uterine relaxation and cerebral trauma from the rapid labor. If the birth is unattended, the baby may suffer from lack of care during the first few minutes of life and experience suffocation or aspiration.

Assessment

Women at risk for precipitous labor are those who have: (1) a history of rapid labor, (2) accelerated cervical dilation and fetal descent, (3) uterine contractile patterns with no relaxation between contractions, or (4) pain that seems out of proportion to the contractions.

Interventions

At-risk women are monitored closely and attended constantly, to provide rest and comfort. The physician or midwife is kept informed of unusual contraction patterns. If an accelerated labor pattern develops while a woman is receiving oxytocin it is stopped immediately. The woman is turned on her left side to promote blood supply to the uterus, and oxygen is started at once. Preparations for delivery are made. If birth cannot be halted, nurses must *never* hold a woman's legs together. Such action may damage the fetal head.

Preterm labor
Description

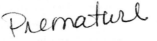

Preterm labor is defined as rhythmical uterine contractions that produce cervical change between 26 and 37 weeks' gestation. Such labor is treated as an obstetrical emergency. Factors that contribute to preterm labor are infection, multiple fetuses, hydramnios, pregnancy-induced hypertension, abdominal surgery or trauma, fetal death, uterine bleeding or abnormalities, incompetent cervix, and PROM. Other maternal factors include socioeconomic status, less than 18 years or more than 40 years of age, smoking more than 10 cigarettes per day, and previous premature delivery. Preterm labor is of special concern because before week 37 of gestation, fetal mortality increases, primarily because of respiratory system immaturity.

Assessment

Assessment of preterm labor includes determination of (1) cervical dilation and whether or not the membranes have ruptured, (2) presence of severe preeclampsia and hemorrhage, and (3) fetal age and condition by ultrasonography. Labor is *not* stopped if one or more of the following are present: (1) cervical dilation of 4 cm or more; (2) ruptured membranes; (3) hemorrhage; (4) severe preeclampsia/eclampsia; (5) fetal anomalies,

distress, or death; and (6) maternal insulin-dependent diabetes, hyperthyroidism, or cardiac pathology.

Interventions

Treatment to stop preterm labor (inhibition therapy) is indicated if:
1. Membranes are intact.
2. No maternal or fetal contraindications exist.
3. Fetus weighs 500 to 2,499 gm.
4. Fetal lungs are immature.
5. Cervical dilation and uterine irritability progresses.

This therapy consists of bed rest in the left lateral position, sedation, hydration, and administration of *tocolytic drugs* such as terbutaline and ritodrine. The mother and fetus are monitored closely because these drugs may cause palpitations, tachycardia, dyspnea, tremor, headache, anxiety, and pulmonary edema.

When preterm labor cannot be arrested, preparations are made for delivery. Glucocorticoid administration initiates the maturation of preterm lung membranes. If a drug such as dexamethasone is given to the mother more than 24 hours before delivery, the incidence of respiratory distress syndrome of the neonate may be reduced by 50%. Cesarean birth is considered if fetal presentation is breech or transverse. When vaginal delivery is chosen, analgesia is minimized and every effort is made to reduce fetal trauma. Qualified personnel are present at the birth to care for the preterm infant.

Nurses give emotional support to the couple, keeping them informed of the progress of labor, treatment plan, and status of their baby.

Premature rupture of the membranes
Description

Premature rupture of the membranes (PROM) is the spontaneous rupture of the amniotic membranes 1 hour or more before the onset of labor. The cause is not known, but some evidence suggests that bacteria or irritating maternal secretions may dissolve the amniotic membrane. Second-trimester PROM may be caused by a cervix that does not remain contracted (incompetent).

The major concerns associated with PROM are preterm labor and ascending intrauterine infection. Mortality for preterm neonates is 30%. The leading cause of death is infection, usually of the respiratory tract. Prolapsed cord and malpresentation further jeopardize the preterm fetus.

Assessment and interventions

Management of PROM depends on the presence or absence of infection and the gestational age of the fetus. Nitrazine paper is used to test for amniotic fluid and microscopic examination for pathogens. If infection is present, antibiotics are prescribed for the mother and the fetus is delivered immediately, regardless of age.

When maternal infection is not present and gestation is more than 34 weeks, labor may be induced. If gestation is less than 34 weeks, efforts are directed toward maintaining the pregnancy. If gestation is between 26 and 32 weeks, tocolytic therapy may be attempted. Its purpose is to delay labor long enough for the fetal lungs to mature with administration of glucocorticoids. (See previous section on preterm labor).

Nurses monitor vital signs and describe the character of the amniotic fluid, uterine activity, fetal responses to labor, and hydration. Comfort measures and emotional support are provided as nurses prepare the mother for possible cesarean birth, a preterm neonate, and potential loss of the fetus.

Uterine retraction rings

With each contraction during normal labor, the upper uterine segment becomes thicker and shorter as the fetus descends. In the process, the muscle of the lower uterine segment expands, becoming thinner and longer to accommodate the fetus. The boundary between these two segments, a ridge on the inner surface of the uterus, is called a *physiological retraction ring.*

A *pathological retraction ring* is an exaggerated form of a physiological retraction ring. The most common type is Bandl's ring, which results from excessive retraction of the upper uterine segment and overdistention of the lower uterine segment. A Bandl's ring may occur when fetal descent is prevented by malposition, CPD, or maternal tumors that block the downward movement of the fetus. Bandl's ring obstructs labor because part of the fetus is above the ring and part is below. As the ring rises with further uterine contractions, the lower uterine segment becomes even more distended and may rupture. Cesarean birth then is necessary.

Uterine rupture
Description

Uterine rupture is the tearing of an intact uterine muscle or of a previous uterine scar after the fetus is viable. *Complete rupture* involves all three muscle layers and may be caused by a weakened cesarean scar, obstetrical trauma, mismanagement of oxytocin induction, obstructed labor, uterine defects, or external trauma.

Signs and symptoms of complete rupture include excruciating pain and cessation of contractions. Vaginal hemorrhage may appear but usually is not profuse. Massive internal hemorrhage may occur with profound shock and death. The fetus may be forced into the abdomen, where it becomes excessively active as it faces asphyxia. FHR becomes erratic and then absent as the baby dies.

Interventions

Emergency laparotomy is performed with complete rupture. Usually the uterus is removed, and attempts are made to save the baby. When the mother's physical needs are met, nurses focus on meeting the couple's emotional needs. If the fetus does not survive, the couple are encouraged to hold the infant and are offered grief counseling. If the uterus is spared, women are advised to have cesarean births with future pregnancies.

COMPLICATIONS OF THE PASSAGEWAY

Even when there are no problems with the psyche or power, successful birth cannot occur if the passageway is *contracted* (too small) or if it is blocked by an obstruction such as a tumor.

Contractures of the bony pelvis
Description

A contracted pelvis is one in which the bony funnel of the woman's pelvis is too narrow at some point for the fetus to pass through. Contractures may be of the inlet, midpelvis, and outlet. Before pregnancy, pelvic measurements can be made using clinical and x-ray pelvimetry. During pregnancy, sonography is used to measure the fetal head in relation to the pelvis.

When pelvic measurements are large enough for the fetus to pass, they are termed *adequate*. When measurements are minimal in one or more places, they are described as marginal pelvis if the infant has a moderately small head, is in a normal position, and contractions are forceful. When measurements are marginal, the physician may decide to allow a *trial labor* for a few hours. Then, if the baby descends normally, vaginal delivery may be accomplished, and the woman is spared major surgery. If there is little or no progress in the baby's descent, cesarean birth is performed.

Fetal head–to–maternal pelvis discrepancy is termed *cephalopelvic disproportion (CPD)*.

When CPD is so great that it is impossible for the fetus to pass, no amount or length of labor will permit delivery. Maternal implications of such labor include PROM, uterine rupture, and necrosis of maternal soft tissue from pressure of the fetal head. Fetal implications include prolapsed cord if the fetal head has not entered the inlet, extreme molding of the skull with possible fracture, and intracranial hemorrhage.

Assessment and interventions

Assessment of the adequacy of a woman's pelvis is done before and throughout pregnancy and during labor. CPD is suspected when labor is prolonged, cervical dilation and effacement are slow, and engagement of the presenting part is delayed. Contractions are monitored as well as the FHR. Trial labor is allowed to continue only as long as dilation and descent progress. If there is no progress, cesarean birth is performed.

The couple may need support to cope with the stress of a complicated labor. They are kept informed and participate in the decision regarding cesarean birth.

Tumors

Another cause of *dystocia* (difficult labor) is the presence of tumors that partially or totally block the passageway. Tumors may be in utero, on the cervix, in the vagina, on the ovary, or in nearby tissue (see Fig. 6-3). Such tumors may be unknown until the woman receives antepartal care. Once discovered, treatment is planned based on the size, position, and type of tumor; the woman's age; number of previous pregnancies; and the weeks of gestation. Treatment may be (1) immediate surgical excision, (2) a trial labor at term with the possibility of cesarean birth, (3) a planned cesarean birth at term, or (4) a cesarean birth followed by a hysterectomy.

COMPLICATIONS INVOLVING THE PASSENGER

Delivery may be complicated by problems of the fetus, placenta, cord, or amniotic fluid and when any of these is in an unusual position.

Problems of the fetus

Fetal distress

Description and assessment. The fetus becomes distressed when it is not receiving enough oxygen by way of maternal-fetal circulation. Such hypoxia may be caused by such factors as problems of the uterus, cord, placenta, and fetus. Initial signs are deceleration (slowing) of the FHR, meconium-stained amniotic fluid, and fetal hyperactivity. Fetal scalp blood samples show a pH of 7.2 or less. Prolonged fetal hypoxia may lead to mental retardation, cerebral palsy, and even death.

Interventions. Initial interventions include changing the mother's position and administering oxygen by mask at 7 L per minute. Fetal monitoring is begun if not already being done, and scalp blood samples are taken. If the fetal condition does not improve rapidly, cesarean birth is performed.

When performing so many activities for the baby, nurses may fail to give emotional support to the laboring woman and her partner. It is important to comfort them and keep them informed. If they had prepared to share in the birth experience, they may be deeply disappointed if a cesarean birth becomes necessary.

Excessive size (macrosomia)

Description and implications. Few babies weigh more than 10 pounds (4,536 g) at birth, which is fortunate because a larger size greatly complicates delivery. Largeness is associated with a number of factors, including inheritance, maternal diabetes, and numerous pregnancies.

Implications of macrosomia for the mother involve distention of the uterus, which causes overstretching of uterine fibers. This leads to dysfunctional labor, chance of uterine rupture, and increased incidence of postpartum hemorrhage. Labor may be prolonged, and surgical procedures at delivery may be more extensive.

Implications for the fetus include cerebral trauma from forceful contact with the mother's bony pelvis. Also, a more difficult delivery may result in fetal asphyxia, cord compression, nerve damage of the overstretched neck, and cerebral trauma.

Assessment and interventions. During antepartal care, the mother's pelvis and size of the growing fetus are assessed. Fetal size is estimated by palpating the crown-rump length of the fetus in utero. Ultrasound pelvimetry may give further information. Whenever the uterus appears excessively large, hydramnios, oversized fetus, or multiple fetuses are considered as possible causes.

When CPD caused by a large fetus is known before labor, cesarean birth is planned. If shoulder dystocia occurs at delivery and birth cannot take place otherwise, the physician may fracture the clavicle to save the baby's life.

Large neonates are inspected carefully after delivery for fractures, cephalohematoma, and Erb's palsy. The nursery staff is alert for signs of neurological damage.

Hydrocephaly

Description and assessment. Hydrocephaly literally means "water head." It is an abnormal condition in which cerebrospinal fluid collects within the fetal head, causing progressive enlargement of the cranium and underdevelopment of the brain.

Antepartal abdominal palpation may alert the physician to the possibility of a breech position. A sonogram is done to evaluate the cranium. With a vertex presentation, vaginal examination reveals wide suture lines between the cranial bones and a globular-shaped head. Outlook for these babies is poor. Other congenital malformations, such as spina bifida and myelomeningocele, often accompany hydrocephaly. The neonate is severely brain damaged and may die during or after delivery from malformations and infections.

Interventions. Because the head is larger than the birth canal, vaginal delivery is impossible with hydrocephaly. If labor is allowed to continue without medical intervention, uterine rupture may result. The treatment of choice is *craniocentesis* (withdrawal of cerebrospinal fluid) to collapse the fetal skull before a. vaginal delivery.

With a vertex presentation craniocentesis is accomplished when the cervix is dilated 3 cm by inserting a large-gauge needle into the fetal ventricle. With a breech presentation it is done using ultrsonic guidance. If cesarean delivery is performed, craniocentesis is performed through the abdominal incision before the fetus is removed to prevent incisional enlargement.

The couple needs information and much empathetic support as they face the difficult decisions regarding delivery. They may need help to cope with the crisis and deal with their grief.

Multiple pregnancies

Description. In Chapter 3 the mechanism that produces multiple pregnancies is described. *Monozygotic twins* are identical because they develop from fertilization of one ovum. *Dizygotic twins* result from the fertilization of two separate ova. They are not identical and may not be of the same sex. Heredity, age, parity, and fertility drugs influence the incidence of dizygotic twinning. Fetal anomolies occur more often in multiple pregnancies.

Assessment. Initial maternal assessment includes a family history of twinning or use of fertility drugs. At each prenatal visit fundal height, FHR, and fetal movement are assessed. If twins are suspected, sonography is used for conclusive evidence. Occasionally, multiple pregnancies are not diagnosed until the time of delivery.

During pregnancy these women experience more physical discomforts, such as backaches and dyspnea. They have a higher rate of abortions, pregnancy-induced hypertension (PIH), anemia, third-trimester bleeding from placenta previa, and hydramnios. During labor, complications include preterm labor, uterine dysfunction, and abnormal fetal presentations. Abruptio placentae can occur when membranes rupture in the presence of hydramnios. Multiple pregnancies create many fetal problems. Labor is usually preterm, resulting in a high incidence of prematurity and respiratory distress syndrome.

Intervention. During labor mother and fetuses are monitored closely. An external electronic monitor is applied to each fetus. Sometimes an internal monitor is applied to the presenting twin and an external one to the other.

Ideally the largest fetus is delivered through a vertex presentation and is the first to be born. If the first is a breech presentation or the smaller twin, delivery is complicated. The position of the second twin must be assessed quickly. Cesarean birth is recommended if fetal distress, CPD, placenta previa, or severe PIH is present, or if prior cesarean deliveries have occurred. When there are more than two fetuses, cesarean birth is planned because the risks of vaginal delivery are so great.

When multiple births are expected, delivery room preparations are made for each neonate. Neonatal specialists may attend.

Malpositions and malpresentations

Even when the fetus is of normal size and the birth canal is adequate, delivery may be complicated if the baby's position in relation to the mother's pelvis is abnormal. In 9 of 10 deliveries the position of the baby at birth is *occiput anterior.* That is, the face is toward the mother's back and the occipital bone is toward the mother's pubis. Unless there are other problems of size or uterine power, this fetal position allows the baby to pass through the irregular birth canal with least difficulty.

Any other position or presentation complicates delivery to some degree and is termed a *malpresentation* or *malposition.* (See Table 7-1 for a summary of various positions and presentations that occur.) Two positions of special concern are occiput posterior and breech presentation.

Occiput posterior position. Occiput posterior position is one of the most common obstetrical problems. When in this position, the fetus must rotate 135 degrees to occiput anterior. As a result, labor is prolonged. Dilation and descent are slowed, and the woman experiences intense back pain because the fetal head presses on sacral nerves. If the physician decides to deliver the baby in the posterior position, forceps may be used and a large mediolateral episiotomy performed (see Fig. 10-4).

Breech presentation

Breech presentation occurs in 3% to 4% of all pregnancies (Fig. 10-1). The cause is not known, but it seems to be related to an ability of the fetus to move freely within the uterus. This is thought to be true because breech presentation is associated with preterm birth, placenta previa, hydramnios, multiple pregnancies, and fetal defects of the cranium.

If vaginal delivery takes place, labor is prolonged because the head cannot act as an effective dilating wedge. Lacerations, tears, and a large episiotomy may result. The cord is more likely to prolapse. The fetus is at increased risk to suffer intercranial hemorrhage; spinal cord injuries caused by stretching and manipulation; bleeding into kidneys, liver, and spleen; brachial plexus palsy; and fracture of the arms. Because the largest part of the baby

delivers last, it is almost too late to save the baby if problems develop. For this reason, version at 37 weeks' gestation may be attempted. (See later section on version.) If it is not possible to turn a fetus to a vertex presentation, cesarean birth may be performed.

Intrauterine fetal death

Description and assessment. Intrauterine fetal death (IUFD), once called *stillbirth,* is associated with preeclampsia/eclampsia, abruptio placentae, placenta previa, diabetes, infection, congenital anomalies, and isoimmune disease.

The first sign of fetal death—cessation of fetal movement—is followed by a gradual decrease in signs and symptoms of pregnancy. Fetal heart tones are absent, sonography shows no heart movement, and radiography indicates overriding fetal cranial bones, called Spalding's sign.

Spontaneous labor begins in 75% of the cases within 2 weeks. Because prolonged retention of the fetus may lead to disseminated intravascular coagulation (see later section), labor is induced with prostaglandin or oxytocin.

Interventions. When IUFD has been confirmed, parents are invited to participate in making decisions about the labor and delivery of the fetus. This gives them some control in an uncontrollable situation. Following are the various issues to be addressed.

Timing of labor and delivery. Parents may wish to "get this thing over" immediately. However, those who have experienced IUFD recommend that labor be delayed for a few days to allow parents to acknowledge the reality of the situation, to inform their family and friends, and to gather a support system. Thus they can handle one crisis at a time rather than coping with birth and death all at once.

Support person in labor. Mothers are encour-

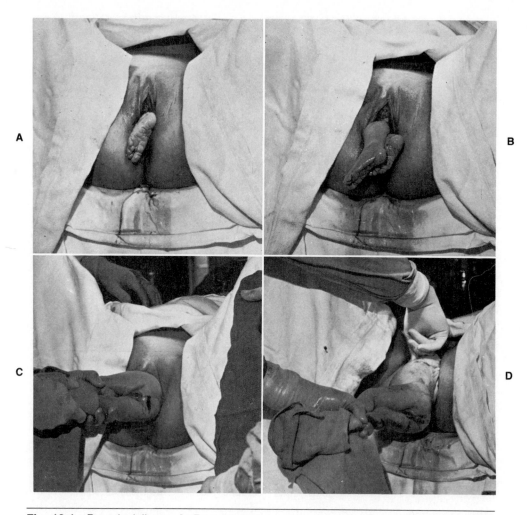

Fig. 10-1 Breech delivery. **A,** Foot presents on the perineum. **B,** Second foot emerges after the physician brings it down. **C,** Buttocks appear in the left sacral transverse position. (Note meconium at baby's rectum.) **D,** Body emerges.

aged to invite a support person to be with them just as if the baby were alive.

Analgesia and anesthesia during labor. Medications are offered to relieve pain but not to interfere with grieving. Grieving is facilitated if the parents are able to acknowledge the reality of the birth and confirm the loss. They are encouraged to see and hold the baby.

Room arrangements. Some mothers want to be in a room where they can express their grief privately. Others prefer a roommate who may help facilitate the grieving process. Some mothers want to be on a postpartum unit; others do not. They should be given a choice when possible.

Naming the baby. Parents are encouraged to

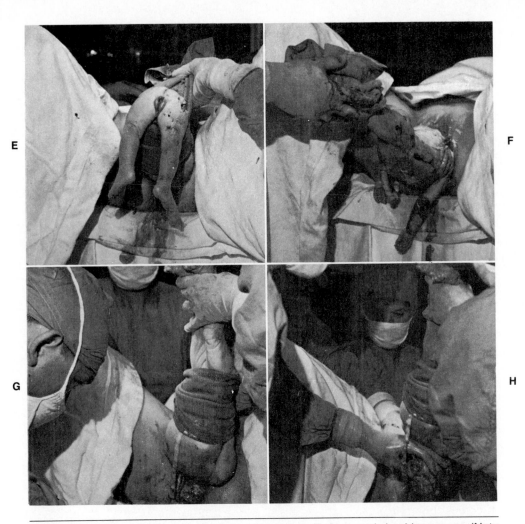

Fig. 10-1, cont'd. **E,** Nurse lifts body in a towel sling. **F,** Arms and shoulder appear. (Note umbilical cord.) **G,** Delivery of the head. **H,** Birth completed.

name the baby. They thus acknowledge the status, identity, and reality of the child.

Taking a picture. Although it may seem morbid at the time, taking a picture of the baby is recommended. In future years this photograph may be a source of great comfort.

Autopsy. Parents are encouraged to have an autopsy performed. This may help reduce guilt feelings in those who think they may have done something wrong.

Memorial services. These serve a valuable function in confirming the importance of the baby's life and the reality of the death. It is vital that mothers be included in planning such services and that they are delayed until mothers are home from the hospital.

Husbands, grandparents, older children. Many men in our society do not know how to express grief. As a result, they may become isolated and misunderstood. They should be encouraged to express their feelings and share them with the mother. Thus, instead of grief creating a wedge between the parents, it helps bond them together. Grandparents, too, are encouraged to express their sadness. They may be deeply grieved by the death and saddened by the sorrow it has brought the parents. Older children should be told about the death in an age-appropriate way.

Returning home after delivery with empty arms. For the mother, this may be the most painful time of all. The new items for the baby she collected now must be put away. She may feel a sense of emptiness for weeks or even months. This is especially true for those who have no other children.

Seeing pregnant women and babies. This is an almost universally painful experience for women whose babies have died. Often women report that just when they begin to accept the baby's death and readjust their lives, the sight of a newborn or pregnant woman triggers intense grief.

Anniversary of the baby's birth and death. By the end of the first year most parents think they have their feelings pretty well under control. Then comes the anniversary of their baby's birth and death. All the memories return, along with the feelings that accompanied the loss. Thereafter, special days and events are always remembered by, for example, "if John were alive" thoughts: he would be starting school, graduating from college, getting married, and so on. No one ever forgets a baby who died.

Future pregnancies. When another pregnancy is attempted, the mother wonders, "Will it happen again?" After experiencing a perinatal death, mothers often feel strangely detached after the birth of a healthy child. Many days or even weeks may pass before the woman allows herself to accept and feel love for the new baby.

Loss and grief

Parents of infants who die in the perinatal period suffer a devastating experience. During pregnancy they had begun to identify with and become attached to the baby. Suddenly the child is lost. Often their grief is as intense as that experienced when older children die. Couples who experience abortion, whether spontaneous or induced, also may experience great grief. This is especially true of those who have undergone therapeutic abortion because of genetic defects.

Parents who experience the loss of babies born with serious defects have a particularly difficult time coping. Unlike a death, their loss goes on and on. There is no funeral, no special support, and no acknowledgement by others. They may hold themselves responsible, and thoughtless relatives and friends may enforce that guilt.

People experience grief when they lose something they identify with and value. Their sadness is acutely painful. Intellectually they know that the loved object is lost and their attachments should be withdrawn, but they are not willing to let go. *Grief work* is the process by which individuals acknowledge loss and withdraw attachment from the loved object.

In the grieving process people exhibit typical behaviors and feel characteristic emotions. These have been grouped together into variously named stages. Labels and numbers assigned to these stages differ, but they all describe the same feelings and behaviors, including (1) shock and denial, (2) anger and bargaining, (3) disorientation and depression, and (4) reorganization and acceptance.

Shock and denial. When told of the baby's death, parents first reaction usually is one of shock, numbness, disbelief, and denial. Physical symptoms may appear, such as weakness, palpitations, loss of appetite, and tightness of the chest. Parents feel empty and alone.

Interventions. Allow parents to see and hold their dead baby or stillborn infant and give factual information to help them grasp the reality of the loss. Provide physical comfort, accurate empathy, warmth, and genuineness.

Anger and bargaining. Some authors call this the searching stage because parents seek reasons for the death. They look for what they might have done differently. Their powerlessness to change the circumstances creates anger, which parents may project on staff members, women who delivered healthy babies, each other, and themselves.

Interventions. An angry person wants to be heard. Do not answer confrontive anger with a similar response. Instead, listen with empathy and genuine concern. Let parents know that their feelings are normal and part of the grieving process.

Disorientation and depression. The predominant emotion during this stage is sadness. Grievers are preoccupied with the loss; they weep and withdraw. Parents may have difficulty returning to normal patterns of living. Physiological postpartal depression that normally appears 24 to 48 hours after delivery may compound the grief depression for mothers of fetuses or neonates who die.

Interventions. Refer parents to a support group with other grieving persons before discharge from the hospital. Give them information about usual postpartal depression to help them gain a sense of normalcy.

Reorganization and acceptance. The final stage of grief involves acceptance of the loss and a return to normal activities of daily living. This highly individual course of action may take many months. It requires *grief work,* the process of experiencing the painful truth of the loss, letting go of the lost object, and reorganizing life without the lost one. Emotional energy is withdrawn from the deceased and reinvested in new relationships and activities.

Interventions. Nurses may see patients during this stage of the grieving process on an outpatient basis, perhaps as they return for checkups or even prenatal care. Acknowledge their loss as significant and encourage and support them in their new endeavors.

Problems of the placenta and cord
Placenta previa

Description. Placenta previa is a condition in which the placenta is implanted in the lower uterine segment (Fig. 10-2, *A*). As the uterus contracts and dilates in the later weeks of pregnancy, placental villi tear from the uterine wall, exposing uterine sinuses and allowing bleeding. The amount of bleeding depends on the number of sinuses exposed. Placenta previa is described as *complete* (placenta totally covers internal os), *partial* (small portion of placenta covers internal os), and *marginal* (placental edge is attached near, but not covering, internal os).

Placenta previa occurs in about one of 167 deliveries and is more common in multiparas. One placenta previa in five completely covers the internal os. Because of the placement of the placenta, the presenting part cannot engage and a transverse lie of the fetus typically occurs.

Assessment. The primary symptom of placenta previa is painless bleeding in the third trimester. The fetus is not affected unless profuse hemorrhage and maternal shock occur. Diagnosis can be made by vaginal examination, but this is highly dangerous and not attempted unless emergency cesarean equipment is set up in advance. Indirect diagnosis is determined by ultrasound scan.

Interventions. If the pregnancy is less than 37 weeks' gestation, nursing care includes:
1. Bed rest
2. No vaginal or rectal examinations

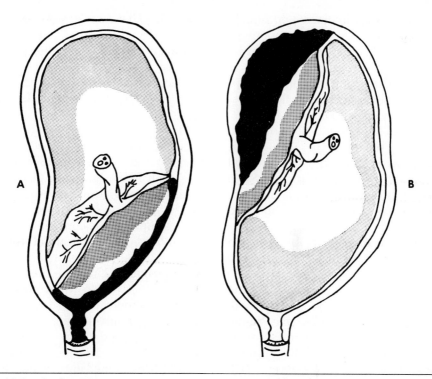

Fig. 10-2 A, Complete placenta previa in which placenta covers the internal uterine mouth. (Baby not shown.) **B,** Abruptio placentae in which hemorrhage is hidden. (Baby not shown.)

3. Regular assessment of blood loss, uterine contractility, pain, FHR, and vital signs and laboratory tests of blood and urine.

4. Intravenous fluids (Ringer's lactate)

5. Two units of cross-matched blood availabe for immediate transfusion

6. Ongoing encouragement and communication with the woman and her family about her condition.

At 37 weeks' gestation, delivery is performed by cesarean birth or induction depending on the degree of previa. A vaginal examination is performed in the delivery room with a *double setup,* in which equipment for both vaginal

and cesarean birth is made ready. The baby's blood cell volume, erythrocyte count, and hemoglobin are checked immediately. Oxygen and blood are administered as needed. The mother and her partner are kept informed and supported as they cope with this unexpected event.

Abruptio placentae

Description. Abruptio placentae is a premature separation of the placenta from the wall of the uterus (Fig. 10-2, *B*). It occurs in about one of 140 pregnancies and is considered a catastrophic event. In seven of 1,000 cases, separation is severe and maternal or fetal death may occur from hemorrhagic shock. Women who have had five or more pregnancies and those with preeclampsia/eclampsia, a renal condition, or vascular disease are at greatest risk. A serious complication of abruptio placentae is disseminated intravascular coagulation (see later discussion).

The three types of abruptio placentae are *covert* (placenta separates in the center, and bleeding is concealed), *overt* (blood passes from under placenta, causing visible vaginal bleeding), and *placental prolapse* (total separtion of placenta with massive bleeding).

Assessment. In partial *overt* abruptio placentae vaginal bleeding occurs but there is no increase in uterine pain. With *covert* abruptio placentae no vaginal bleeding appears, but the abdomen becomes extremely tender, rigid, and boardlike. Sudden changes may signal complete separation of the placenta. Assessment includes uterine irritability, fundal height for a sudden increase, bleeding, FHR, fetal activity level, amniotic fluid for meconium staining, and signs of maternal shock.

Interventions. In mild cases of placental separation when gestation is near term, labor may be induced and the fetus delivered vaginally. If induction is unsuccessful, cesarean birth is performed. In moderate to severe separation, cesarean birth is performed after fibrinogenemia is treated with intravenous plasma or cryoprecipitate. When severe hemorrhage occurs, cesarean birth and hysterectomy are done to save the lives of mother and baby. They are given intensive nursing care in a specialized unit. Emotional support and information are needed by the woman and her family to help cope with this life-threatening, unexpected outcome.

Prolapse of the cord

Description. When the umbilical cord passes out of the uterus ahead of the presenting part, it is said to have *prolapsed* (Fig. 10-3). When this occurs, the cord is compressed between the maternal pelvis and the presenting part with each contraction. As a result, fetal circulation is seriously impaired and fetal distress develops, with a mortality rate of 20% to 30%.

Maternal conditions associated with prolapsed cord include breech presentation, transverse lie, extra long cord, contracted inlet, small fetus, low-lying placenta, hydramnios, and twin gestation. Any time the inlet to the pelvis is not closed and the membranes rupture, the cord may wash down into the birth canal in front of the presenting part.

Interventions. Until the presenting part has engaged, all women whose membranes have ruptured should remain on bed rest. At the time of spontaneous rupture or amniotomy, FHR is assessed for a full minute. If fetal bradycardia appears during labor, the woman should be examined immediately for prolapsed cord.

If a loop of cord is discovered, the nurse's gloved fingers are held in the vagina, and attempts are made to lift the fetal head off the cord until the physician arrives. The woman is instructed to assume the knee-chest position, or the bed is adjusted to a Trendelenburg's position. The woman then is transported to the delivery or operating room in that position.

A prolapsed cord is not always visible on the perineum. It may lie beside or just in front of the presenting part. Under no circumstances, however, should attempts be made to replace the cord in the uterus. This could seriously damage the cord and greatly increase the chance of intrauterine infection.

Vaginal delivery may be attempted if the cervix is fully dilated, membranes have ruptured, presentation is vertex, and measurements are adequate. However, cesarean birth is the method of choice. Calm, knowledgeable ac-

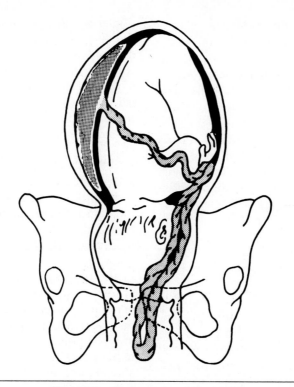

Fig. 10-3 Prolapsed umbilical cord.

tion by nurses in such an emergency situation helps reassure the mother and her partner.

Abnormalities of the cord

Several abnormalities of the cord can seriously affect the fetus. These include absence of an umbilical artery, velamentous insertion, and variations in cord length, knots, and loops.

Congenital absence of an umbilical artery. This is found in 25% of fetuses with anomalies. For this reason, immediately after the cord is cut, it is inspected to determine whether there are three vessels. If only two are present, the baby is examined closely for other birth defects.

Velamentous insertion. In this condition vessels of the umbilical cord divide some distance before they reach the placenta. (Velamentous means "resembling a veil.") Because they are unprotected, these vessels may tear or prolapse during delivery, causing fetal hemorrhage or asphyxia. Any sign of fetal distress is investigated immediately and appropriate action taken.

Cord length variations. An umbilical cord may be shorter or longer than the average length of 55 cm. Short cords are associated with cord rupture and abruptio placentae, but they rarely cause direct complications. Long cords tend to twist, tangle, and knot and may wrap around the baby's neck. Problems do not usually arise until labor, when fetal bradycardia appears. Repositioning the mother may be enough to relieve the cord compression. If discovered at delivery, the midwife or physician must take quick action to untangle the cord.

Problems of the amniotic fluid and bleeding

Hydramnios

Description. Hydramnios occurs when there is more than 2,000 ml of amniotic fluid in utero. The exact cause is unknown. A contributing factor may be overactivity of the specialized amnion cells of the placenta. These cells produce most of the amniotic fluid.

Hydramnios often accompanies fetal abnormalities that affect the swallowing mechanism. In the second trimester the fetus begins to swallow amniotic fluid and urinate. The condition also is found in neurological disorders in which the fetus is thought to urinate excessively because of overstimulation of cerebrospinal centers.

Hydramnios is associated with multiple pregnancies, maternal diabetes, and Rh sensitization. This condition leads to premature delivery, malpresentation, prolapsed cord, and abruptio placentae, thus increasing the incidence of perinatal mortality.

Most cases of hydramnios are *chronic,* in which fluid volume increases gradually. In *acute* cases the volume increases rapidly in a few days, creating great maternal discomfort. Milder forms of hydramnios produce fewer symptoms and are more common. When the amount of fluid is more than 3,000 ml the mother experiences shortness of breath and edema of the lower extremities from compression on the vena cava. Overstretched fibers may cause uterine dysfunction during labor and an increased incidence of postpartum hemorrhage.

Assessment. During prenatal care hydramnios is suspected if fundal height increases out of proportion to gestational age. The nurse has difficulty hearing the FHR and palpating the fetus. The mother's abdomen appears extremely taunt. Sonography shows large spaces between the fetus and uterine wall and may reveal fetal defects and multiple pregnancies.

Interventions. If the mother is dyspneic and in pain, she may be hospitalized. A transabdominal or vaginal amniocentesis is performed with the aid of sonography. Efforts are made to remove the fluid slowly to prevent abruptio placentae. Nurses offer support by explaining the procedure and may assist in interpreting sonographic findings.

Amniotic fluid embolism

Description. Amniotic fluid embolism is the accidental infusion of amniotic fluid into the mother's bloodstream under pressure from the contracting uterus. Amniotic fluid containing fetal vernix, lanugo, meconium, and mucus enters maternal blood sinuses through defects in the placental attachment. These particles of fetal waste become emboli in the mother's general circulation, causing acute respiratory distress, circulatory collapse, hemorrhage, and cor pulmonale as they block the vessels of her lungs. The particles stimulate abnormal coagulation, initiating disseminated intravascular coagulation (see next section). Maternal death rate is extremely high.

Assessment and interventions. In the course of hard labor the mother suddenly experiences acute respiratory distress and circulatory collapse. Emergency measures are instituted immediately, including cardiopulmonary resuscitation (CPR), an intravenous line for central venous pressure (CVP) monitoring, and blood transfusions. Efforts are made to save the fetus by immediate delivery. Labor and delivery nurses assist the code team, care for the neonate, and provide family members with comfort and information about the status of the mother and infant.

Disseminated intravascular coagulation

Description. Disseminated intravascular coagulation (DIC) is an acute abnormal stimulation of the normal coagulation process. The normal clotting process is a balance between clot formation and dissolution. In DIC the balance is disrupted. The abnormal stimulation of coagulation results in widespread thrombi formation that eventually exhausts clotting factors and platelets and activates the process that dissolves fibrogen. Major bleeding results. Acute conditions that initiate DIC include amniotic fluid embolism, abruptio placentae, sepsis, shock, respiratory distress syndrome (RDS), mismatched blood, and fat embolism.

Intervention. Patients are transferred to intensive care units where specialized nursing can be provided.

Third-stage and fourth-stage hemorrhage

Postpartum hemorrhage is defined as a loss of blood in excess of 500 ml in the first 24 hours following delivery. This is most often caused by uterine atony, lacerations of the vagina and cervix, retained placenta, retained placental fragments, and placenta accreta.

Uterine atony. Uterine atony (relaxation of the uterine muscle) following delivery is expected following the birth of multiple fetuses, macrosomia, hyramnios, dysfunctional labor, oxytocin stimulation during labor, and anesthesia that produces uterine relaxation. Hemorrhage from uterine atony is slow and steady rather than sudden and massive. Blood may escape from the uterus and collect in the vagina. The pulse and blood pressure may not change until blood loss is significant.

Lacerations. Lacerations of the cervix or vagina cause bright-red vaginal bleeding that persists in the presence of a well-contracted uterus. Nursing observations are reported to the physician, who inspects the cervix and vagina. If lacerations are found, they are sutured.

Retained placenta. Hemorrhage may occur after the delivery of the baby and before delivery of the placenta. To hasten placental separation, the physician manually removes the placenta by inserting a gloved hand into the uterus and placing the other hand externally on the fundus. If hemorrhage continues, the same medical interventions instituted for uterine atony are carried out.

Retained placental fragments. These fragments are the major cause of late postpartum hemorrhage. To prevent this type of hemorrhage, the placenta is inspected carefully after delivery for missing pieces or unusual blood vessels. When these are noted, or if heavy bleeding persists in the presence of a contracted uterus, the physician inspects the uterine cavity and removes retained placental fragments.

Placenta accreta. This is the attachment of chorionic villi directly to the uterine muscle so that the placenta cannot separate normally after delivery of the baby. Placenta accreta may be total, partial, or focal and causes serious hemorrhage. Hysterectomy may be necessary to save the woman's life.

Interventions. After delivery of the placenta, the fundus is palpated to ensure that it is firm and well contracted. If it is not firm, vigorous massage is instituted. Oxytocics such as methylergonovine (Methergine) and oxytocin (Pitocin) may be given. If bleeding persists, the physician undertakes bimanual intrauterine compression. Intravenous oxytocin is administered at a rapid rate, blood transfusions may be ordered, and oxygen at 4 to 7 L per minute is given by face mask.

After the physician checks the uterine cavity for retained placental fragments and the cervix and vagina for lacerations, nurses check the fundus frequently to see that it remains contracted. Vital signs are assessed, as is amount of bleeding. Nursing and medical interventions are explained to the woman and her partner, who are encouraged to voice their concerns.

OPERATIVE OBSTETRICS

Operative obstetrics refers to surgical procedures used to treat the complications of pregnancy, labor, and delivery. The most common procedures are induction of labor, episiotomy, version, use of forceps, and cesarean birth.

Induction of labor

For most mothers, the time when labor begins is not critical. For others, however, this time may mean life or death. Induction of labor is the use of physical or chemical stimulants to initiate or intensify uterine contractions. It is done for women who have diabetes mellitus, chronic hypertensive disease, renal disease, histories of precipitous labors (less than 3 hours), PROM, severe preeclampsia/eclampsia, and abruptio placentae. Labor also is induced with severe fetal hemolytic disease, for postterm pregnancy, when the fetus has died, and for the convenience of the mother or physician. Before induction is attempted, cervical readiness and fetal maturity are assessed.

The most frequently used methods of induction are amniotomy, oxytocin infusion, and prostaglandin administration.

Amniotomy

Description. Amniotomy is purposeful cutting of amniotic membranes to release the fluid. When the cervix is ready and the fetal head is against the lower uterine segment, amniotomy effectively initiates labor in 80% of women within 24 hours. Advantages are that contractions are similar to those of spontaneous labor, fetal monitoring is facilitated, and color and composition of amniotic fluid can be evaluated. Disadvantages are that labor may not begin, the cord may prolapse, and infection may ascend.

The painless procedure is performed in the labor bed by the physician using a sterile instrument. Amniotic fluid immediately flows from the uterus.

Interventions. A nurse auscultates the FHR before and after amniotomy and attends the mother during the procedure. The vagina is examined immediately thereafter to check for a prolapsed cord. Bed pads are changed frequently thereafter because amniotic fluid continues to drain throughout labor.

Oxytocin infusion

Description. Intravenous infusion of oxytocin is an effective method of initiating uterine contractions. Pitocin, 10 units, is added to 1 L of intravenous fluid (usually Ringer's lactate), providing a mixture 10 mU of oxytocin per milliliter. An intravenous line is started with nonmedicated fluid, and the oxytocin bottle is connected to the line. An external monitor may be attached to the mother's abdomen to provide continuous data about the FHR and contractions.

Dosage is prescribed by the attending physician and is increased gradually. The goal is to achieve contractions of good intensity every 2 to 3 minutes, each of which lasts 40 to 50 seconds.

Oxytocin induction is not entirely risk free. Too-rapid infusion rates may overstimulate the uterus. This may compromise the fetus because of decreased placental perfusion and cause a rapid labor with danger of cervical tears, perineal lacerations, or uterine rupture. Water intoxication may occur if large doses are given in an electrolyte-free solution over prolonged periods.

Assessment and interventions. Baseline data on the mother and fetus are obtained before the oxytocin infusion begins, again every 15 minutes, and before each increase in dosage. These data include the mother's vital signs, contractions, cervical dilation, effacement, station, urinary output, and FHR.

Prostaglandin administration

Description. Prostaglandin is administered both as an intravenous infusion and as an intravaginal gel. The gel also is used for ripening the cervix. Because prostaglandin administration is effective, free of side effects, and non-invasive, some authorities believe it will replace amniotomy and oxytocin as the method of choice for induction of labor.

Assessment and interventions. As with other methods of induction, baseline data about the mother and fetus are obtained before the infusion or gel application is begun. During induction, assessment is made of urinary output, cervical dilation, effacement, station, and fetal status. The woman is kept informed of the progress of labor.

Episiotomy
Description

An episiotomy is a surgical incision of the perineum that extends down from the vaginal orifice (Fig. 10-4). The incision is made just as the presenting part begins to crown and usually is repaired immediately after placental expulsion. An episiotomy is done to reduce stretching of perineal tissues and to decrease trauma to the fetal head during delivery. Some authors dispute the benefits of episiotomy and recommend against its routine use.

The most typical incisions are midline or left or right mediolateral. Midline episiotomy is preferred when the perineum is of adequate length and no difficulty is expected. The incision is easily repaired, less blood loss occurs, and it heals with less discomfort. The major disadvantage is that a midline incision may extend through the anal sphincter and rectum. A mediolateral episiotomy provides more room and is less likely to extend into the rectum. However, there is greater blood loss, a

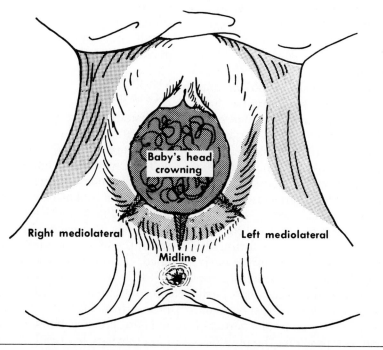

Fig. 10-4 Episiotomy. Three typical lines of incision.

longer healing period, and more postpartum discomfort.

Because sutures used to repair episiotomy are of absorbable material, they do not need to be removed and no dressing is applied.

Assessment

The episiotomy site is inspected every 15 minutes during the first hour after delivery and then on a daily basis. The site is assessed for tenderness, redness, swelling, and evidence of a hematoma.

Interventions

Ice packs help relieve pain and swelling during the first 8 hours. Thereafter, warm sitz baths and dry heat help increase circulation to the area and promote healing. Analgesic sprays and oral analgesics may be prescribed. The mother is given instructions on hygienic perineal care. Healing time depends on the type and extent of the episiotomy incision.

Version

Description

Version is the turning of a fetus within the uterus. It may occur naturally, or version may be done manually by the physician to facilitate delivery. There are three recognized types: external (cephalic), internal (podalic), and combined (internal and external) version.

External (cephalic) version is the use of external abdominal manipulation to rotate the fetus from a breech or transverse to a cephalic position. Version is done at 37 weeks' gestation after a tocolytic drug such as ritodrine has been given to relax the uterus. During the version the fetus is monitored continuously. Approximately 90% of fetuses remain in vertex position, thus avoiding a cesarean birth.

Internal (podalic) version is direct fetal manipulation to rotate the fetus from a vertex or transverse to a breech position. The physician reaches up into the uterine cavity, grasps one or both feet, and draws them through the cervix. Podalic (foot) version is an emergency measure used to deliver a second twin, when the cord has prolapsed, or when immediate delivery is required.

Combined version is the use of both internal and external version to turn a fetus into a more favorable position for delivery. In this procedure one hand is placed on the abdomen to provide external pressure, and the other hand is inserted up into the uterine cavity to the fetus. Combined version is an emergency measure used when immediate delivery is required, such as with a prolapsed cord.

Interventions

Nursing care during external version includes assessing the mother's blood pressure every 5 minutes and continuously monitoring the fetus. These assessments are continued for 30 minutes after the version. After internal version the woman is observed closely for signs of hemorrhage because trauma to the uterus may interfere with its ability to contract.

Use of forceps

Description

Obstetrical forceps are double-bladed instruments designed to grasp the fetal head. They were invented in the sixteenth century by the Chamberlen family of England. Since that time many different forceps have been created, each named by its designer, such as Piper's, Elliot's, and Kjelland's.

Forceps are used (1) to hasten delivery when the life of the mother or fetus is threatened, (2) to shorten the second stage of labor, or (3) to intervene when regional or general anesthesia has affected the woman's ability to push effectively.

There are two types of forceps deliveries: *outlet* (when the head is visible on the perineum) and *midforceps* (when the fetal head is above the ischial spines). Outlet forceps are advocated for delivery of preterm infants. Midforceps use is rare because it is associated with cerebral damage and neonatal depression.

The use of forceps requires a completely dilated cervix, ruptured membranes, vertex or face presentation, and an engaged head, preferably on the perineum. The physician must know the exact position and station of the fetal head.

Interventions

If the woman is awake, the nurse explains what the physician will do. The woman is encouraged to maintain breathing techniques and asked not to push during application of the forceps. The nurse monitors contractions. With each contraction the woman pushes as the physician provides traction. FHR is monitored continuously until delivery. Fetal bradycardia may occur temporarily from head compression as traction is applied to the forceps.

The infant may have a scalp bruise from the blades of the forceps. Parents are told of the bruise and assured that it will disappear in a few days. Neonates are observed closely for signs of Erb's palsy or cerebral trauma.

Cesarean birth
Description

Cesarean birth is the delivery of a baby through an abdominal and uterine incision. It has been known for centuries, but only in modern times has the procedure become relatively safe. Therefore cesarean birth is performed for more and more reasons with less and less danger. In 1980 one of every six babies was delivered by cesarean birth. However, this is major surgery, and the decision to use this method of delivery is made only after careful consideration. The most typical reasons for cesarean birth are fetal distress, breech presentation, dystocia, and prior cesarean surgery.

Cesarean births have two to four times the maternal mortality of vaginal deliveries, primarily because of underlying medical conditions and anesthesia accidents. Complications for the woman include infection, hemorrhage, blood clots, and surgical injury to the bladder or intestines. Risks to the fetus of a traumatic vaginal delivery are weighed against maternal risks of cesarean surgery. If possible, cesarean birth is avoided when the fetus is dead or too small to survive outside the uterus.

Common incisions for cesarean birth are low-segment transverse and low-segment or fundal classical (Fig. 10-5). Low-segment incisions reduce the risk of uterine rupture in future labors. Before their widespread use, surgeons followed the dictum that "once a cesarean, always a cesarean." However, vaginal birth after cesarean (VBAC) is becoming increasingly common. In 1982 Lavin and others found that when women with nonrecurring indications were allowed a trial labor, 74.2% had successful vaginal deliveries. In general, such deliveries are less expensive and safer for both mother and baby, and mothers are more satisfied.

When a mother who has had cesarean birth wants to deliver vaginally, a "trial labor" may be undertaken. She must be in good health, and her medical history must be available. The fetus must be in vertex position with no CPD or other complications. The birthing center must be able to provide fetal and maternal monitoring, blood transfusions, anesthetic services, and physician availability.

Interventions

Preparation for childbirth classes. This should include the possibility of a cesarean birth not as "abnormal," but as an alternative when problems arise. Information is given about cesarean births, including roles of significant others, anesthesias, delivery room, interaction with the baby, immediate recovery,

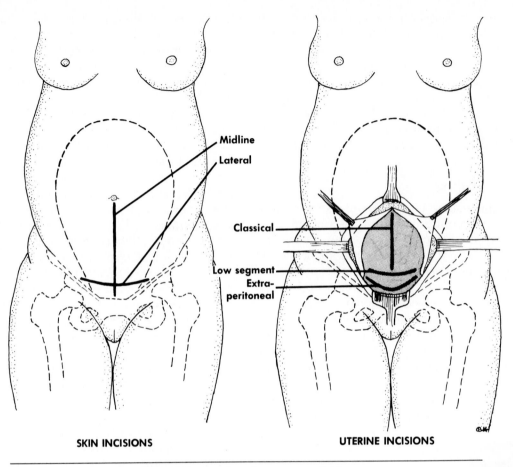

Fig. 10-5 Incisions for cesarean births.

and postpartum period. When couples know in advance that a birth will be by cesarean, they are encouraged to attend precesarean birth classes, where they may discuss their fears and negative experiences.

Preparation for an emergency cesarean birth. When couples are advised in advance of the possible need for a cesarean birth, they respond more positively than when the news comes as a surprise (Affonso and Stichler, 1980). They have a sense of control over the birth experience and therefore feel less power-

lessness and helplessness. By being told in advance, parents can process the information and summon the strength to face the crisis. Nurses need to explain procedures before beginning them, tell mothers why they are doing them, and inform mothers what they can expect to feel.

Standard preoperative measures include:
1. Nothing by mouth
2. Abdominal and perineal shave from nipple line to pubis
3. Indwelling catheter to dependent drainage

4. Signed operative permit
5. Two units of whole blood ready for administration
6. Intravenous line in place
7. Preoperative medications
8. Infant preparations: warmer, resuscitation and suction equipment, and notification of the pediatrician

Delivery. Fathers are no longer excluded from the operating suite. In fact, their presence leads to more positive evaluations of the birth experience. Also, mothers require less postpartum pain medication, experience less loneliness, and are less anxious about their babies.

Two types of anesthesia are used for cesarean birth: general and conduction (spinal and epidural). Nurses provide continuous emotional support to parents during the procedure. When the surgical team is ready, nurses connect the suction and record the actual time the incision is made and infant delivered. Just as the infant is born, they administer oxytocin intravenously to the mother. They then assist the pediatrician with physiological support of the neonate. When the neonate's condition is stable, the baby is shown to the mother if she is awake. Circulating nurses assist with placing a dressing on the incision and pads to the perineum. The mother is covered with a fresh, warm blanket and moved to the recovery room.

Postpartum recovery period. Care after a cesarean birth includes both postoperative and postpartum care. Assessment for potential complications associated with conditions in both areas are made together with appropriate interventions. In addition, when maternal disease exists, assessment and interventions relative to that condition are made.

Nursing care plan for cesarean birth

Problem: maternal powerlessness, helplessness, sadness, anger

Interventions: Integrate cesarean birth infor-

mation into childbirth preparation classes.
  - Encourage expression of feelings.
  - Maximize couple's opportunities to make decisions.
  - Avoid "last minute" approach.
  - Communicate effectively.
  - Provide privacy.
  - Use therapeutic touch and eye contact.
  - Relate birth events to mother if she was not awake.
  - Include father in birth experience.
  - Serve as father's support system.

Problem: recovery from surgery
Intervention:
  - Assess vital signs every 5 minutes until stable, then every 15 minutes for an hour, then every 30 minutes for 8 hours.

Problem: fluids and nutrition
Interventions:
  - Maintain intravenous infusion flow rate.
  - Check patency and inspect intravenous site for redness and swelling.
  - Give ice chips for first 24 hours, then advance diet as bowel sounds return.

Problems: bladder drainage
Interventions:
  - Connect indwelling bladder catheter to dependent drainage.
  - Usually, remove catheter 1 to 2 hours after intravenous fluids are discontinued.
  - Measure output on first two voidings.
  - Check bladder for distention.

Problem: hemorrhage and blood loss
Interventions:
  - Assess lochia and incision.
  - Evaluate firmness and position of fundus (may be palpated from side of abdomen to avoid discomfort).
  - Check hemoglobin and hematocrit levels on first postoperative day.

Problem: pain
Interventions:
  - Administer pain medication as needed.
  - Assess vital signs before administration.
  - Monitor maternal use if breast-feeding.

- Place mother in comfortable position.
- Teach women to splint incision when coughing or deep breathing.

Problem: nausea and vomiting
Interventions:
- Administer antiemetic as needed.
- Check vital signs before administration.

Problems: incisional healing
Intervention:
- Inspect incision for redness, swelling, drainage, bruising, and tissue separation.

Problem: bowel function
Interventions:
- Listen for bowel sounds.
- Assist progressive ambulation.
- Administer bowel softener as needed.

Problem: pulmonary status
Intervention:
- Turn patient, splint incision, and have patient cough and deep-breathe every 2 hours for 24 hours.

Problem: bonding
Interventions:
- Provide early opportunities for parent-infant interaction.
- Maintain mother's comfort.
- Provide information about baby (sex, weight, etc.) as soon as possible.
- Discuss woman's feelings about the cesarean birth and her role as mother.

Problem: information about self-care and infant care
Interventions:
- Provide education about self-care and infant care.
- Stress handwashing.

Nursing care evaluation. Following cesarean birth, the mother is discharged after the nurse determines that:

1. Mother is in good physical and emotional state with no sign of infection.
2. Involution is proceeding normally.
3. Bonding has begun between infant and parents.

4. Mother understands aseptic self-care and infant care.

▶ *KEY CONCEPTS*

1. Complications caused by fear during labor and delivery can be reduced by information, instruction, emotional support, and specific physical interventions.
2. Hypertonic and hypotonic contractions and prolonged labor may lead to maternal exhaustion, dehydration, and fetal distress.
3. Precipitous labor lasts less than 3 hours. The most common causes are lack of resistance by tissues, contractions, and small fetus. At-risk women are monitored closely and turned on left side to promote blood supply to uterus. Preparations are made for delivery.
4. Preterm labor (26 to 37 weeks' gestation) is an obstetrical emergency because of high fetal mortality. Inhibition therapy includes bed rest, sedation, hydration, and tocolytic drugs.
5. Premature rupture of membranes (PROM) leads to preterm labor and intrauterine infection. Interventions include monitoring vital signs, uterine activity, hydration, and fetus and providing comfort and emotional support.
6. Bandl's ring is a pathological retraction ring that obstructs fetal pathway and may lead to uterine rupture.
7. Uterine rupture is life threatening to both mother and fetus and causes severe pain and stops contractions. Emergency laparotomy is required, usually with hysterectomy.
8. Contractures of pelvis may cause cephalopelvic disproportion and obstruct birth. Cesarean birth is necessary.
9. Fetal distress is indicated by slowing of FHR, meconium-stained amniotic fluid, and fetal hyperactivity. Interventions include turning mother to left side to relieve pressure on blood vessels, increasing oxygen to fetus, monitoring fetus, and supporting mother.
10. Macrosomia (fetus larger than 10 pounds) causes overstretched uterine fibers and leads to dysfunctional labor, uterine rupture, and postpartum hemorrhage.
11. Hydrocephaly, often associated with congenital

defects, causes brain damage. If vaginal delivery not possible, craniocentesis is necessary. Nurses give parents emotional support and information.

12. Multiple pregnancies complicate delivery and are associated with a high incidence of prematurity. Cesarean birth is required if more than two babies are born.

13. Occiput posterior (OP) position and breech presentation complicate delivery. If in OP position, fetus must rotate 135 degrees to be born. If in breech presentation, version at 37 weeks' gestation or cesarean birth may be preferred to breech vaginal delivery.

14. Intrauterine fetal death (IUFD) is associated with maternal disease and fetal defects; first sign is cessation of movement. No FHR and Spalding's sign are present. Nurses involve the parents in decisions about timing of induction; give support; and provide information on analgesia, room assignment, naming baby, taking infant's picture, autopsy, memorial services, returning home, grief process, and future pregnancies.

15. Loss and grieving process follows stages of shock and denial, anger and bargaining, disorientation and depression, and reorganization and acceptance. Grief work is the process of letting go of a lost object.

16. Placenta previa (complete, partial, or marginal) causes painless bleeding in third trimester. Before 37 weeks' gestation, nurses provide bed rest and continuous monitoring. After 37 weeks, labor induction or cesarean birth is necessary.

17. Abruptio placentae (covert, overt, or placental prolapse) is premature separation of the placenta. Interventions include induction of labor with vaginal delivery or cesarean birth; hysterectomy may be necessary.

18. Prolapsed cord may occur whenever pelvic inlet is not closed and membranes rupture. Nurses monitor FHR for fetal bradycardia and check perineum, especially after amniotomy. If cord prolapsed, mother is placed in knee-chest or Trendelenburg's position until vaginal or cesarean birth is performed.

19. Abnormalities of cord include absence of umbilical artery (found in 25% of infants with defects), velamentous insertion (veil like divided umbilical vessels), and length variations (more or less than 55 cm).

20. Hydramnios (amniotic fluid more than 2,000 ml) leads to prolapsed cord, premature delivery, malpresentation, and abruptio placentae. Mother may be hospitalized and amniocentesis performed.

21. Amniotic fluid embolism is accidental infusion of amniotic fluid into mother's bloodstream through defects in placental attachment. Particles become emboli causing acute respiratory distress and disseminated intravascular coagulation (DIC).

22. DIC is life-threatening stimulation of coagulation process with widespread thrombi formation followed by serious bleeding. DIC requires intensive nursing care.

23. Third-stage and fourth-stage hemorrhage may be caused by uterine atony, lacerations of birth canal, retained placenta, and placenta accreta (attachment of villi to uterine muscle). Nurses monitor and report vital signs and blood loss. The physician makes the diagnosis and treats according to the cause.

24. Induction of labor depends on cervical readiness and fetal maturity. This is done for various reasons using amniotomy, oxytocin, or prostaglandin.

25. Episiotomy (midline or mediolateral) is performed at delivery to enlarge vaginal opening. Nurses assess for hematoma, tenderness, redness, and swelling; at first treat with ice, then local heat until incision is healed.

26. Version (external, internal, and combined) involves turning the fetus in the uterus and is performed to obtain better fetal position for delivery. Nurses monitor mother's blood pressure and the fetus.

27. Forceps (outlet and midforceps) are instruments used to grasp the fetal head during delivery. Nurses monitor FHR and contractions; infant may have scalp bruises.

28. Cesarean birth is done in one of six births for fetal distress, breech, dystocia, and prior cesarean births, although vaginal birth after cesarean (VBAC) is becoming common. Inter-

ventions include presenting the possibility of cesarean birth in prenatal classes so that parents are less upset if cesarean is required; allowing fathers in surgery with mothers; using spinal and general anesthesias; and addressing postoperative and postpartum care problems. These problems involve maternal powerlessness, surgical recovery, fluids and nutrition, bladder drainage, blood loss, pain, nausea and vomiting, incisional healing, bowel function, pulmonary status, bonding, and self-care and infant care information.

■ **ANNOTATED SUMMARY**

I. Complications of the psyche
  A. Description—fear causes physical distress and ineffective labor, producing cycle of fear
  B. Assessment—preparation, culture, religion, support person
  C. Interventions—positive encouragement, information, instructions, physical contact, acceptance, presence
II. Complications of the power
  A. Hypertonic labor
    1. Description—painful but ineffective contractions; may lead to fetal distress
    2. Interventions—bed rest, sedation; assess for potential dehydration, maternal exhaustion, fetal distress
  B. Hypotonic labor
    1. Description—fewer than three contractions in 10 minutes; caused by overstretched uterine fibers
    2. Interventions—investigate CPD and fetal malpresentation; assess for urinary distention, maternal exhaustion, infection
  C. Prolonged labor
    1. Description—labor lasting more than 24 hours; complications: maternal exhaustion, infection, and hemorrhage from uterine atony or rupture; fetal distress, PROM; soft tissue injury and cerebral trauma of fetus
    2. Interventions—monitor mother, fetus; provide hydration, comfort measures, emotional support
  D. Precipitous labor

1. Description—labor less than 3 hours; precipitous delivery not necessarily associated; caused by hyperactive contractions, small fetus, lack of resistance
    2. Assessment—at-risk women: history, cervical dilation, fetal descent, contractions, pain
    3. Interventions—monitor woman, provide comfort, turn woman on left side, never attempt to halt birth
  E. Preterm labor
    1. Description—rhythmical uterine contractions that produce cervical change at 26 to 37 weeks' gestation; obstetrical emergency because of increased fetal mortality
    2. Assessment—cervical dilation, presence of hemorrhage or preeclampsia, fetal age
    3. Interventions—inhibition therapy: bed rest, sedation, hydration, tocolytic drugs, close monitoring of mother and fetus; if delivery inevitable, glucocorticoids given to mother 24 hours before delivery to initiate lung maturity in neonate
  F. Premature rupture of the membranes (PROM)
    1. Description—spontaneous rupture of membranes 1 hour or more before onset of labor; complications: infection, prolapsed cord, malpresentation of preterm fetus
    2. Assessment and interventions—test fluid with nitrazine paper, test for pathogens: antibiotics prescribed; if gestation at 26 to 32 weeks: tocolytic therapy; if more than 34 weeks: labor induced; nurses monitor vital signs, uterine activity, hydration, fetus; give support and comfort
  G. Uterine retraction ring—physiological and pathological; Bandl's ring is common pathologic type: obstructs labor, blocking downward movement of fetus; cesarean birth required
  H. Uterine rupture
    1. Description—tearing of uterine muscle layers, (complete or partial); excruciat-

ing pain, cessation of contractions, massive internal hemorrhage, fetal death

    2. Interventions—emergency laparotomy, usually hysterectomy; grief counseling

III. Complications of the passageway

  A. Contractures of the bony pelvis

    1. Description—narrowing of inlet, mid-pelvis, or outlet; x-ray pelvimetry, sonography, or trial labor used to decide adequacy; cephalopelvic disproportion (CPD): fetal head–to–maternal pelvis discrepancy may cause prolonged labor, PROM, uterine rupture, prolapsed cord, fetal damage

    2. Assessment and interventions—assessment done before pregnancy and during labor; trial labor and cesarean birth if necessary; support couple

  B. Tumors—may be located in various places; surgical excision, trial labor at term with possible cesarean birth

IV. Complications involving the passenger

  A. Problems of the fetus

    1. Fetal distress

      a. Description and assessment—caused by hypoxia, evidenced by slowing of FHR, meconium-stained amniotic fluid, hyperactivity, blood pH 7.2 or less

      b. Interventions—change mother's position, give oxygen by mask, monitor fetus, prepare for emergency cesarean birth

    2. Excessive size (macrosomia)

      a. Description and implications—fetus more than 10 pounds complicates delivery; associated with maternal diabetes, inheritance, multiparity; maternal implications: prolonged labor, uterine rupture, postpartum hemorrhage; fetal implications: asphyxia, cerebral trauma, cord compression, nerve damage

      b. Assessment and interventions—prenatal measurements, ultrasound pelvimetry; cesarean birth planned with known CPD; nursery staff assesses infant for neurological damage

    3. Hydrocephaly

      a. Description and assessment—abnormal collection of cerebrospinal fluid in fetal head; sonogram confirms; prognosis poor, severe brain damage

      b. Interventions—craniocentesis; vaginal or cesarean birth; grief counseling

    4. Multiple pregnancies

      a. Description—twins or more

      b. Assessment—sonography, FHR, movement; mothers have more complications, often preterm labor

      c. Interventions—monitor closely during pregnancy; electronic monitoring during labor; cesarean delivery for more than twins and with complications

    5. Malpositions and malpresentations

      a. Occiput posterior position—fetus must rotate 135 degrees to be born; prolonged labor, often with forceps and large episiotomy

      b. Breech presentation—3% to 4% of pregnancies, associated with placenta previa, hydramnios, multiple pregnancies; labor prolonged if vaginal delivery; version at 37 weeks or cesarean birth preferred

    6. Intrauterine fetal death (IUFD)

      a. Description and assessment—"stillbirth"; signs: no fetal movement or FHR, Spalding's sign on radiography; labor begins in 2 weeks in 75% or is induced to prevent DIC

      b. Interventions—parents participate in decisions: timing of labor, support person, analgesia, room assignment, naming baby, taking picture, autopsy, memorial services, other family members, returning home, anniversary, future pregnancies

    7. Loss and grief—loss of infant is devastating regardless of cause; grief work, a process of withdrawing attachment: shock and denial, anger and bargaining, disorientation and depression, reorga-

sion, reorganization and acceptance

B. Problems of the placenta and cord
 1. Placenta previa
   a. Description—placenta implants in lower uterine segment (complete, partial, or marginal); 20% complete, interferes with engagement, more transverse lies
   b. Assessment—painless bleeding in third trimester
   c. Interventions—less than 37 weeks: bed rest, no vaginal or rectal examinations, monitor fetus, prepare transfusion blood; give support; at 37 weeks: cesarean birth or labor induction depends on degree of previa; prepare vaginal examination with double setup
 2. Abruptio placentae
   a. Description—premature separation of placenta (covert, overt, and placental prolapse)
   b. Assessment—uterine irritability, fundal height, bleeding, FHR, activity level, amniotic fluid for meconium, maternal shock
   c. Interventions—mild: induce labor if possible, if not, cesarean birth; moderate: cesarean; severe hemorrhage: cesarean and hysterectomy; intensive nursing care, emotional support
 3. Prolapse of the cord
   a. Description—cord passes out ahead of presenting part, compressed at each contraction, 20% to 30% fetal death rate
   b. Interventions—bed rest after membranes rupture; if fetal bradycardia, examine for prolapsed cord; immediate Trendelenburg's position and delivery
 4. Abnormalities of the cord—absence of umbilical artery common in fetuses with defects, velamentous (veillike) insertion, and variations in cord length

C. Problems of the amniotic fluid and bleeding
 1. Hydramnios
   a. Description—more than 2,000 ml amniotic fluid; common with fetal defects; leads to premature delivery, cord prolapse, malpresentation, abruptio placentae, postpartum hemorrhage
   b. Assessment—diagnosed by sonography
   c. Interventions—transabdominal or vaginal amniocentesis
 2. Amniotic fluid embolism
   a. Description—amniotic fluid accidentally enters mother's blood through placental attachment defects; particles become emboli, stimulate DIC; mortality rate high
   b. Assessment and interventions—sudden acute respiratory distress of mother; give emergency CPR, save fetus, support family
 3. Disseminated intravascular coagulation (DIC)
   a. Description—abnormal stimulation of coagulation process, widespread thrombi formation, bleeding
   b. Intervention—intensive care unit
 4. Third-stage and fourth-stage hemorrhage—loss of more than 500 ml of blood in first 24 hours
   a. Causes—uterine atony, lacerations of cervix or vagina, retained placenta, retained placental fragments, placenta accreta
   b. Interventions—oxytocics, bimanual intrauterine compression or manual removal of placenta by physician; nurses assess blood loss, vital signs and give information and support

V. Operative obstetrics
 A. Induction of labor—use of physical or chemical stimulants to initiate or intensify contractions; cervical readiness and fetal maturity assessed beforehand
  1. Amniotomy
    a. Description—cutting of amniotic membranes; painless, 80% effective, allows assessment of amniotic fluid
    b. Interventions—auscultate FHR before, check for prolapsed cord
  2. Ocytocin infusion
    a. Description—dosage gradually in-

creased; goal: contractions every 2-3 minutes; danger of uterine rupture, water intoxication

b. Assessment and interventions—baseline assessment data, monitor every 15 minutes: mother's vital signs, contractions, dilation, effacement, station, urinary output, FHR

3. Prostaglandin administration

a. Description—IV infusion or intravaginal gel; noninvasive, free of side effects, effective

b. Assessment and interventions—baseline assessment data, monitor as for ocytocin infusion

B. Episiotomy

1. Description—surgical incision of vaginal opening made as presenting part crowns; done to reduce tissue stretching; midline or mediolateral

2. Assessment—look for hematoma, signs of infection

3. Interventions—ice during first 8 hours, then heat

C. Version

1. Description—turning of fetus within uterus by physician to facilitate delivery (external, internal, combined); external done at 37 weeks to avoid cesarean birth; internal and combined: done at delivery as emergency measure

2. Interventions—external: monitor fetus continuously, mother's vital signs every 5 minutes; internal: assess for signs of hemorrhage

D. Use of forceps

1. Description—double-bladed instruments to grasp fetal head, assist birth; types: outlet, midforceps; requires completely dilated cervix, ruptured membranes

2. Interventions—inform mother: follow breathing technique, when to push; monitor FHR; explain scalp bruises; assess neonate for Erb's palsy, cerebral trauma

E. Cesarean birth

1. Description—delivery of baby through abdominal and uterine incision; performed for one of every six deliveries; for fetal distress, breech, dystocia, and prior cesarean surgery; vaginal birth after cesarean: 74.2% successful

2. Interventions

a. Preparation for childbirth classes—information reduces fears

b. Preparation for emergency cesarean birth—explain procedures: why and what to expect; follow standard preoperative measures

c. Delivery—fathers included; general or conduction anesthesia; baby shown to mother when awake

d. Postpartum recovery period—both postoperative and postpartum care

e. Nursing care plan for cesarean birth—interventions for problems: powerlessness, recovery from surgery, fluids and nutrition, bladder drainage, hemorrhage and blood loss, pain, nausea and vomiting, incisional healing, bowel function, pulmonary status, bonding, information about self-care and infant care

f. Nursing care evaluation—good physical and emotional state, involution, bonding, understanding of self-care and infant care

● **STUDY QUESTIONS AND LEARNING ACTIVITIES**

1. What are the two most unpleasant factors of labor? What nursing measures can be taken to reduce their effects?

2. What two labor patterns result in dysfunctional labor? What nursing measures are needed for prolonged labor?

3. Preterm labor is an obstetrical emergency. Why? What factors contribute to its occurrence? What is inhibition therapy, and when is it *not* used?

4. What is the purpose of a trial labor when there is possible cephalopelvic disproportion (CPD)? How would you explain it to the woman?

5. What are the first signs of fetal distress? What nursing measure is taken immediately?

6. What are the complications of a multiple pregnancy during the pregnancy and labor?

7. How would you explain the back pain and longer labor of a woman whose fetus is in the occiput posterior position?

8. Why is labor induced when there is intrauterine fetal death (IUFD)? Why are the parents consulted about the delivery of the fetus?

9. In a group discussion, consider the stages of grieving and the purpose of grief work.

10. If you see a loop of cord on the perineum of a laboring woman, what emergency measures should you take?

11. Why is amniotic fluid embolism so dangerous? Why does the accident lead to disseminated intravascular coagulation (DIC)?

12. Explain the purpose and potential dangers of an amniotomy to a laboring mother.

13. When is an episiotomy performed? Why? Where? What measures help reduce its discomfort and enhance healing?

14. What problems should nurses address in planning postpartum care after a cesarean birth? What interventions?

REFERENCES

Affonso, DD, and Stichler, JF: Cesarean birth: women's reactions, Am J Nurs 80:468, 1980.

Bobak, IM, and Jensen, MD: Essentials of maternity nursing: the nurse and the childbearing family, ed 2, St Louis, 1987, The CV Mosby Co.

Butane, P, and others: Mothers' perceptions of their labor experiences, Matern Child Nurs J 9:73, 1973.

Genest, M: Preparation for childbirth—evidence for efficacy, a review, J Obstet Gynecol Neonat Nurs 10:82, 1982.

Lavin, JP, and others: Vaginal delivery in patients with prior cesarean section, Obstet Gynecol 59:135, 1982.

Olds, SB, London, ML, and Ladewig, PA: Maternal-newborn nursing: a family-centered approach, ed 3, Menlo Park, Calif, 1988, Addison-Wesley Publishing.

UNIT FOUR
The Newborn Baby

CHAPTER 11

Nursing Care of the Normal Newborn

VOCABULARY

Cord blood
Epstein's pearls
Erythema toxicum
Icterus neonatorum
Milia
Neutral thermal environment
Phenylketonuria (PKU)
Phimosis
Physiological resilience

LEARNING OBJECTIVES

- Compare the immediate, transitional, and periodic assessment of neonates.

- Discuss resuscitation measures used to clear the airway, provide oxygenation, and stimulate respirations.

- Describe measures used to provide a neutral thermal environment for newborn infants.

- Discuss identification measures, prophylaxis, and recording of important data about the infant.

- Discuss nursing care of neonates in the nursery.

- Discuss gestational age, including the terms used and criteria for determining gestational age.

- Describe general and specific characteristics of neonates.

- Discuss principles of newborn care and their application.

- Discuss infant feeding: breast and bottle.

- Describe parent teaching, medical supervision of the infant, and newborn screening tests.

Up to the moment of birth, fetal care is part of maternal care. As the fetus passes out of the birth canal, however, the baby becomes an independent person, requiring individual attention and supervision.

BIRTH
Time

The time of complete birth is the instant when the entire baby is separated from the mother. The cord and placenta are not regarded as part of the baby's body, so their position does not affect the birth time.

Experience

At the time of birth, many dramatic changes occur within the baby's body as it changes from dependence on to independence from the mother. From the baby's point of view, the process of birth is a traumatic experience. The fetus has been floating comfortably within the mother's uterus for 9 months. The fetus has been warm, protected, free from pain and want, and relatively unrestrained. Then labor begins, and the fetus is pushed, pounded, squeezed, and twisted through the narrow birth canal. Finally, the fetus is free. That freedom, however, is full of pain, cold, and shock. Only recently have medical personnel recognized the need to lessen the shock and stress of the birth experience as they strive to ensure the life and safety of the newborn infant.

IMMEDIATE CARE
In the delivery room
Airway

The first and most important care given to the neonate after birth is to clear the nose and mouth of mucus and amniotic fluid so the airway is open. This step is usually done by the physician or midwife moments after the baby is born. A rubber bulb syringe or soft rubber catheter with electric suction may be used. The baby's head should be placed below its body and turned to one side so any regurgitated amniotic fluid will not enter the lungs. If breathing is not satisfactory, more extensive resuscitation measures are begun at once.

Umbilical cord

The baby remains attached to the umbilical cord until the cord is severed (Fig. 11-1). Under certain circumstances clamping the cord may be delayed and the infant lowered to permit additional placental blood to flow into the baby. Such placental transfusion can increase the baby's blood volume by one half. The baby may then be placed on the mother's abdomen, in a pan of warm water, or on the back table while a cord clamp or tie is fastened securely around the cord near the baby's abdomen.

Some midwives and physicians give the scissors to the father to cut the cord. This gesture symbolizes freeing the infant and taking parental responsibility for the child's welfare.

A variety of cord-clamping devices are in current use. They all must be fastened securely to prevent fatal blood loss. A cord blood specimen is obtained from all newly delivered babies to test for such conditions as syphilis, acquired immunodeficiency syndrome (AIDS), or the presence of Rh antibodies. The cord blood is allowed to flow from the placenta into a waiting test tube before it begins to clot.

Assessment

Assessment following birth occurs in three phases:
1. Immediate, using the Apgar scoring system for physical condition and the Gray scoring system for parent-baby interaction
2. Transitional, during the periods of reactivity
3. Periodic, by systematic physical assessment.

Immediate assessment. During the first minutes of the newborn infant's life, complex

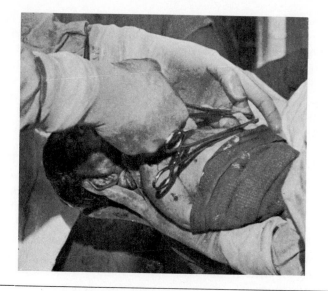

Fig. 11-1 Umbilical cord is clamped with two surgical clamps and cut between them.

physiological changes occur. One way used to assess the adjustment of the baby to extrauterine life is the Apgar scoring system, described in Chapter 9 (see Fig. 9-3). The other assessment is of parent-baby interaction, also described in Chapter 9 (see Fig. 9-4).

Transitional assessment. During the first 24 hours of life the normal infant undergoes considerable behavioral and physiological change. Assessment involves comparing an infant with the following norms:

- Period I: *reactivity* (first 30 minutes after birth). Infant is alert with open eyes, responds to stimuli, sucks vigorously, and cries. Respiratory rate to 82; heart rate to 180 per minute; bowel sounds active. *Restfulness* follows initial reactive phase and lasts 2 to 4 hours. Temperature and respiratory and heart rates fall.
- Period II: *reactivity* (lasting 2 to 5 hours). Infant awakes from deep sleep. Heart and respiratory rates rise; gag reflex active. Newborn may pass meconium stool and urine and sucks. Period ends when respiratory mucus has decreased.
- Period III: *stabilization* (12 to 24 hours after birth). Infant has vacillating periods of sleep and wakefulness. Vital signs are stable. Skin is warm and pink.

Periodic assessment. After the first 24 hours of life, the newborn infant will undergo thorough physical examinations by the attending physician and nursing personnel. Each of the body systems will be examined for structure and function.

Gray's perinatal assessment of mother-baby interaction is carried out in 2 to 3 days when possible.

Resuscitation measures

Once the umbilical cord is cut, the baby's only source of oxygen is the air. If for some reason the baby does not attempt to breathe or if the airway is blocked, oxygen cannot reach the bloodstream by way of the lungs and the baby will soon die. Even if the baby survives, sensitive brain cells may be permanently damaged from oxygen deprivation of more than 5 minutes.

Resuscitation efforts are aimed at overcoming three problems of newborn asphyxia: (1) clearing the blocked airway of mucus and fluid, (2) forcing oxygen or air into the collapsed lungs, and (3) stimulating the baby to breathe. These efforts are continued for every baby until breathing is established or the heart stops beating and the baby is pronounced dead. Usually the anesthetist, attending physician, or specially educated nurse institutes resuscitation measures at once if the baby does not breathe spontaneously.

Clearing the airway. The baby's head should be lowered, but the body does not necessarily have to be held upside down. Mucus, amniotic fluid, vernix caseosa, and meconium are removed from the mouth and trachea. This is done by putting a finger in the infant's mouth or by gently milking the trachea. A rubber bulb syringe, DeLee suction, or electric suction with a soft rubber catheter may be used. To prevent the baby from aspirating vomitus, the stomach may be emptied with suction. Great caution must be taken to prevent injury to delicate tissues. Occasionally it is necessary for the anesthetist to insert a tube into the larynx to provide an airway. This procedure is called *intubation*.

Forcing oxygen into the lungs. If the baby still does not breathe spontaneously after all obstructing mucus and fluid has been removed, it may be necessary to force air or oxygen down into the collapsed lungs. Forcing can be done by mouth-to-mouth positive pressure or by specially designed intermittent positive-pressure equipment. In either case, the lungs are filled by a positive force.

Stimulating the baby to breathe. Intermittently filling the lungs by artificial means is only a temporary measure until the baby begins to breathe independently. If the baby is sleepy because of certain drugs given to the mother during labor, the physician may prescribe stimulants. These must be chosen carefully, or an opposite effect may result. A variety of physical ways to stimulate respiration also may be used. They include rubbing or snapping the feet or spine, performing nasal suction, and stimulating the rectal sphincter. It should be remembered, however, that the body should not become chilled.

If extensive resuscitation is required, the baby usually is placed in an incubator in the neonatal intensive care nursery. In this nursery continuous observation is possible, and complete resuscitation equipment is available for emergency use.

Environment

Effects on baby. When the baby is born, the wet, warm body is exposed to the cold of the delivery room (colder by 25° to 30° F than the mother's body). This sudden chill causes the infant to gasp for breath, just as a person gasps when stepping from a warm shower into a cold room. If the infant is exposed to prolonged cold, however, the initial beneficial effect of cold to stimulate respiration is undone. Because body insulation is poor and skin surface is large, deep body temperature may drop rapidly. Although the infant does not shiver at birth, the temperature-regulating mechanism is functioning, and the body responds to cold by increasing its metabolic rate. If exposure continues, the high metabolism consumes sugar and fats with resultant acidosis and death.

To reduce this heat loss immediately after birth, various measures are used. These include giving a warm tub bath, called the Leboyer technique; placing the baby skin-to-skin against the mother's abdomen; or wrapping the infant in a warm blanket and covering the head with a stocking cap.

Neutral thermal environment. The maintenance of body heat is so important to the health of a neonate that a special term is used to describe the ideal environment for the newborn: *neutral thermal environment.*

A neutral thermal environment is one in which the infant's oxygen consumption and metabolic rate are minimal and body temperature stays within normal limits, that is, 97.7° to 98.6° F (36.5° to 37° C).

To achieve such an environment, heat loss from the baby's skin must be minimized. Heat is lost by (1) radiation, such as to cold nursery walls, (2) evaporation, such as from wet skin to dry room air, (3) conduction, such as to cold metal scales, and (4) convection, such as to cold air blown by air conditioners. Therefore nurses must seek to reduce these effects on the baby. Excessive heat is not desirable either, since it causes the neonate to increase metabolism to cool down. Thus, for minimum stress on the baby, a neutral thermal environment is ideal.

Identification

From a legal standpoint, proper identification of the newborn baby in the hospital setting is essential. The American Academy of Pediatrics recommends that "while [the infant is] still in the delivery room two identical identification bands be placed on the infant's wrists and ankles showing the mother's full name, admission number, sex (of infant), date, and time of (infant's) birth, and that the mother be fingerprinted and the infant's foot, palm, or fingers be printed" (Fig. 11-2). Many hospitals have adopted the Hollister obstetrical Ident-A-Bands, which provide three identically numbered soft plastic bands for each infant delivered, one for the mother and two for the infant (Fig. 11-3). Some hospitals also use alphabet beads to spell the baby's name, or use thumbprints and footprints in addition to the identification bands.

Prophylaxis

Ophthalmia neonatorum is a serious gonorrheal infection of the conjunctiva of the newborn baby that may be acquired as the baby passes through an infected birth canal. Because this disease may cause blindness, all states in the United States have laws that require the instillation of a bactericidal agent in the eyes of all newborn babies (Fig. 11-4). Concentrations of 1% silver nitrate in drops (Credé's prophylaxis) are effective against *Neisseria gonorrhoeae* but may cause severe irritation and even damage.

The strength and freshness of the silver nitrate should be checked before instilling it in the baby's eyes. Antibiotic ointments such as erythromycin are becoming the agents of choice, replacing silver nitrate. Erythromycin has the added advantage of being effective against *Chlamydia trachomatis.*

Recording

The newborn baby's chart usually originates in the delivery room and may include a copy of the mother's labor record. Although each hospital uses its own forms, the record should include accurate and significant information about the infant, including:

Time and type of birth
Sex
Apgar and bonding evaluation scores
Color
Cry
General condition
Obvious abnormalities or birth injuries
Medications such as erythromycin eye ointment
Ident-A-Band number if used
Oxygen
Resuscitation measures and weight if done
How the baby is to be fed (breast or bottle)
When, how, and in what condition the infant leaves the delivery room

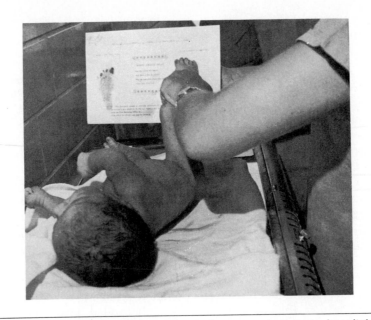

Fig. 11-2 Footprints of the newborn baby are made in some hospitals.

The chart usually goes with the newborn to the nursery. The baby, as any other patient in a hospital, must be under medical supervision. It is important, therefore, that the name of the responsible physician be indicated on the baby's record.

In the newborn nursery

In some hospitals the newborn infant is transferred from delivery to transitional nursery for intensive observation during the critical transitional period. When stabilized, the infant is admitted to a regular nursery or to the mother's room for rooming-in. Infants designated as *high risk* are admitted to an intensive care unit.

The immediate care of the newborn infant after arrival in the nursery from the delivery room includes initial cleansing and observation, weighing, measuring, estimation of gestational age, cord care, and clothing. In addition, the baby is protected from harm and observed closely and continuously.

Cleansing and assessment

The newborn baby's hair is frequently matted with dried blood from passage through the birth canal. The body may have areas where there are heavy deposits of vernix caseosa. It is not considered necessary or even wise to remove all this sebaceous gland secretion, just the excess. Most nurseries dispense with water bathing and simply wipe off the excess vernix and sponge away the dried blood. This so-called *dry skin care* reduces heat loss and potential damage to the infant's delicate skin.

Regardless of the material used, this initial cleansing is an excellent time to observe the baby closely. Axillary temperature, pulse, and respiration are measured at this time. The nurse must work quickly to avoid unnecessary chilling of the baby's body.

Weighing and measuring

Although some delivery rooms are equipped with scales, many are not, and the newborn baby is first weighed after arriving in the nurs-

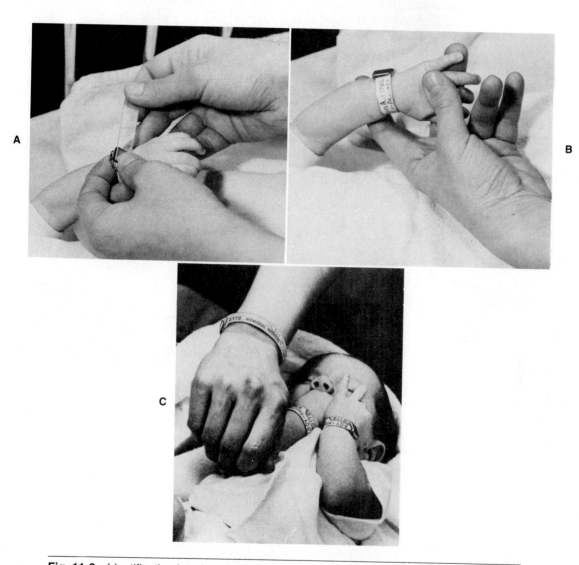

Fig. 11-3 Identification bands are attached in the delivery room. **A,** Ident-A-Band bracelet is locked in place with thumb pressure. **B,** Each band shows the mother's name and admission number, date, time of birth, and baby's sex. **C,** Bands are placed on the infant's wrists and that of the mother. *(Courtesy Hollister, Inc, Chicago, Ill; from Hamilton, PH: Basic pediatric nursing, ed 5, St Louis, 1987, The CV Mosby Co.)*

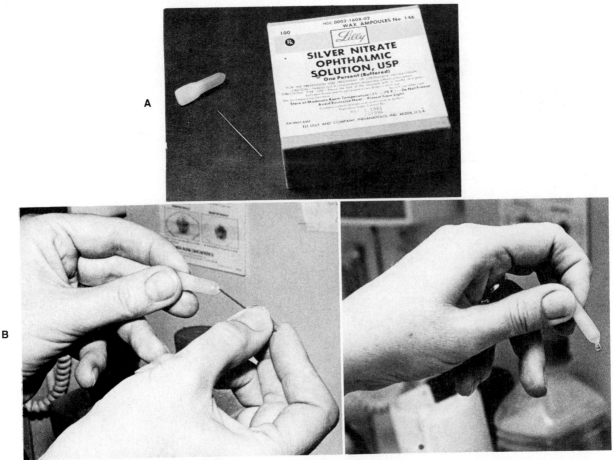

Fig. 11-4 Silver nitrate for Credé's prophylaxis. **A,** Wax ampules containing 1% silver nitrate ophthalmic solution. **B,** Puncturing wax ampule with pin. **C,** Squeezing out one drop to instill in each conjunctival sac of the newborn. *(From Phillips CR: Family-centered maternity/ newborn care, ed 2, St Louis, 1987, The CV Mosby Co.)*

ery (Fig. 11-5). The scales are balanced with a protective cloth or paper, on which the naked infant is placed. Great care is taken to protect the infant from falling off the scales. Accuracy is vital. Birth weight is important to the family and as part of the baseline data. A weight loss of 5% to 10% of birth weight is normal. This loss is caused by use of calories, loss of body

fluid, and passage of meconium. After 3 to 5 days the baby begins to gain weight. Most babies reach their birth weight after about 2 weeks.

Measurement of the head and chest circumference and length (heel to crown of the head) of the newborn baby are made at this time (Fig. 11-6). These measurements are made to

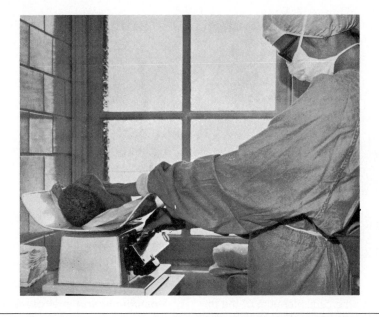

Fig. 11-5 Weighing the newborn baby. Nurse's protective hand is lifted while the scales are read.

evaluate physical maturity and to serve a standard from which future comparisons can be made. For instance, a rapidly enlarging head may indicate hydrocephalus. Unusual growth in length or size may indicate excessive anterior pituitary gland secretion.

Estimation of gestational age

The maturity of an infant affects his or her ability to survive. For example, a large for gestational age, preterm infant may weigh about the same as a small for gestational age, preterm infant, but the less mature baby is at higher risk. Accurate assessment of gestational age is vital to effective care planning.

Gestational age is determined by standardized measurements of neuromuscular maturity and physical growth (described in more detail in Chapter 12) as follows:

I. Preterm (less than 38 weeks)
   A. Small for gestational age (SGA)
   B. Appropriate for gestational age (AGA)
   C. Large for gestational age (LGA)
II. Term (38 to 42 weeks)
   A. SGA
   B. AGA
   C. LGA
III. Postterm (42 or more weeks)
   A. SGA
   B. AGA
   C. LGA

Assessment data are plotted on standardized forms, such as the one shown in Fig. 11-7.

Cord care

When the newborn baby first arrives in the nursery, about 2 inches (5 cm) of umbilical cord usually is extending from the abdomen

241

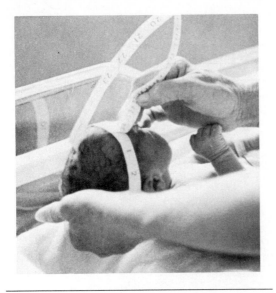

Fig. 11-6 Measuring the circumference of the infant's head. Body length from crown to heel and chest circumference are also measured.

with some type of clamp, pin, or tie fastener. In a few days the cord shrinks and darkens. In a week or so it falls off, leaving a small granulation area that eventually heals. A small, contracted scar called the *umbilicus* or *navel* remains.

Immediately after birth the umbilical vessels can still allow fatal hemorrhage if the clamp or tie becomes loose. For this reason the cord is checked initially and at frequent intervals for the first 24 hours after birth. If bleeding occurs, a second tie or clamp is applied at once and the baby watched closely.

Occasionally bacteria invade the area before healing occurs. As a precaution against such an infection, the area around the umbilical stump is scrubbed, and triple dye or 70% alcohol may be applied (Fig. 11-8).

A small, dry sterile gauze strip may be placed around the cord initially to protect the abdominal skin from the wet cord. However, belly bands and dressings are no longer used

because it was found that they harbored bacteria and kept the stump moist, thus hindering healing. The metal clamp or pin may be removed on the second or third day. By this time the umbilical vessels are sealed off, and there is no longer a danger of hemorrhage.

Clothing and cover

Although newborn infants must be kept warm, it is not desirable to constrict their movement with heavy clothes or blankets (Fig. 11-9). They are dressed in a diaper and shirt or a gown, placed in the crib, and covered by a blanket but not restricted by too much weight. Every piece of clothing and linen is washable and is often sterilized before use in the newborn nursery.

Positioning and environment

When all initial care has been given and the newborn is clothed, the baby is placed in a preheated crib or incubator, usually on the side with the head slightly lower than the rest of the body. This helps drain any remaining amniotic fluid or mucus from the stomach and nasopharynx. Extra oxygen is not administered routinely unless there is definite anoxia, as indicated by cyanosis and respiratory difficulty. Even then oxygen rarely is given in concentrations greater than 40%. *Retrolental fibroplasia*, a condition producing blindness, may result from excessively high oxygen concentrations.

After a few hours the baby of normal size and development does not need extra heat. The infant is warm enough in a regular bassinet in the warm air of the newborn nursery.

Feeding and rest

The newborn does not need food or fluids immediately after birth. The primary need is for rest. For this reason nothing is given by mouth for 12 to 16 hours after birth. (See later section on infant feeding.)

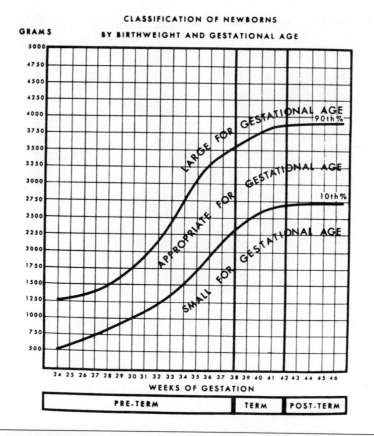

CLASSIFICATION OF NEWBORNS BY BIRTHWEIGHT AND GESTATIONAL AGE

Fig. 11-7 Intrauterine growth status for gestational ages, according to appropriateness of growth. (From Battaglia, FC and Lubchenco, LO: A practical classification of newborn infants by weight and gestational age, J Pediatr 71:159-163, 1967.)

Recording and identifying

All the observations, measurements, and care given to the newborn after first arriving in the nursery should be carefully recorded on the chart. Because each baby's crib is kept separate from all the others, it is important to label it with a clearly marked card. The crib card should have the mother's name and her room number, the baby's sex, birth time and date, and the physician's name. The crib card usually is made at the time initial care is given. It is customary to give the card to the mother when she takes her baby home.

CHARACTERISTICS OF THE NEWBORN
Terminology

According to generally accepted standards, the following terms are used for the baby:

fetus From 6 weeks' gestation to birth.
neonate or **newborn** From birth to 1 month of age.
infant From 1 month until walking alone.

The *neonatal* or *newborn period* is the first month of life. During the neonatal period the infant undergoes amazing growth and change.

243

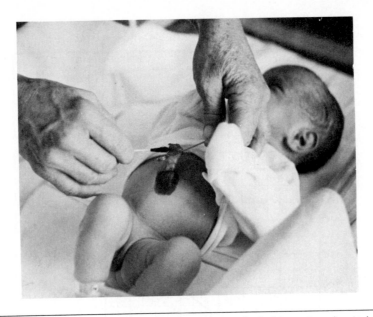

Fig. 11-8   Umbilical cord is painted with triple dye or alcohol to reduce bacterial growth.

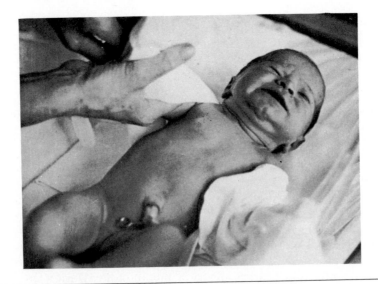

Fig. 11-9   Newborn baby is dressed to conserve body heat.

General characteristics
Body shape and measurements

The newborn baby seems to be all head and abdomen, with small, bowed legs and little hips. The neck is short and creased, the nose flat, and the baby appears to be chinless. The tiny feet look inept and flat because of the pad of fat on the sole. The genitalia, although small, seem swollen and out of proportion. The little arms are dwarfed by the large protruding abdomen (Fig. 11-10).

As a general rule, boys tend to be longer and to weigh more than girls. The first-born child is likely to be smaller than siblings, and small parents tend to produce small children. The normal ranges of body measurements at birth are as follows:

Head circumference	12½ 14 inches (31 to 35.5 cm)
Chest Circumference	12 to 13 inches (30.5 to 33 cm)
Length (crown to heel)	19 to 21 inches (48 to 53 cm)
Weight	6 to 9 pounds (2,700 to 4,000 gm)

Awareness

Six states of awareness have been identified in the newborn infant. These states do not follow any specific sequence but occur in all normal infants. They are as follows:
1. Crying
2. Quiet sleep
3. Rapid eye movement (REM) sleep
4. Active-alert
5. Quiet-alert
6. Transitional

Crying state. The infant exhibits diffuse motor activity and active crying. Crying is caused by fatigue, colic, general discomfort, hunger, and loneliness. The normal cry is lusty and loud, not weak or high pitched. The tone and pattern of crying depend on the cause and become a kind of language that parents come to understand.

Contrary to the myth that picking up a crying newborn "spoils" a baby, researchers at Johns Hopkins Medical School found that babies whose mothers responded promptly cried less by the time they were 1 year of age. The research seems to indicate that responding to

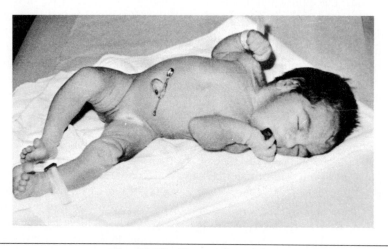

Fig. 11-10 The newborn infant.

a baby's cry helps establish trust and reduce impatience.

Quiet sleep state. The infant rarely moves, and respirations are slow and regular.

Rapid eye movement (REM) sleep state. The infant breathes irregularly and grimaces or makes other facial expressions. Rapid eye movements can be seen through the eyelids.

Active-alert state. The baby exhibits active, diffuse body movement with a quiet expression or grimace on the face.

Quiet-alert state. The infant is alert but relaxed. The eyes are open and focusing, and the baby may mimic facial expressions.

Transitional state. The infant is moving from one awareness state to another.

Physiological resilience

All normal newborn infants possess a certain physiological resilience, which is a kind of passiveness to both internal and external stressors. This resilience protects the infant during the first hours and days after birth from reacting too greatly to the new and hostile world outside and to the physiological revolution taking place inside the body. Because of this resilience, newborn infants can survive extremes of cold and heat, abnormal levels of substances in the blood, and a lack of food and water. There are, however, limits to their reserve that should not be risked. The premature infant does not have this resilience so must be protected from as many stressors as possible.

A week or so after birth, when the regulating mechanism and the body systems of the infant begin to function in their intended way, this special physiological resilience is no longer needed and disappears. Then the baby reacts more acutely to cold and heat and imbalances of body chemistry.

Immunity

If the mother has antibodies to certain infectious diseases, they pass through the placenta to the infant. Among these may be antibodies to mumps, diphtheria, and measles. This passive immunity lasts from a few weeks to several months. Few if any antibodies are passed on for pertussis and chickenpox (varicella), so infants may fall easy prey to these diseases. At 2 to 3 months of age they can be immunized against pertussis, but at present no commercial serum against chickenpox is available.

Vital signs

Temperature, pulse, and respirations of the newborn infant vary in response to the environment.

Temperature. At birth the infant's temperature is about the same as the mother's. However, the infant has little fat insulation, a large body surface, and relatively poor circulation and does not yet sweat or shiver. Thus the infant's ability to regulate body temperature is poor. In addition, excessive cold may overload the heart, and excessive warmth can cause "prickly heat," a pinpoint rash called *miliaria*. Therefore the nurse must regulate the environment to provide constant body temperature of 97.7° to 99° F (36.5° to 37.2° C), that is, a neutral thermal environment.

Pulse. The pulse rate of a newborn baby is 120 to 150 per minute, depending on activity. Pulse may become irregular from any one of several physical and emotional stimuli, such as being startled, crying, or undergoing a sudden temperature change. The apical cardiac pulse is counted for a full minute to ensure accuracy.

Respirations. The respirations of a newborn infant are irregular in depth, rate, and rhythm and vary from 30 to 60 per minute. As with the pulse rate, respirations are affected by such things as crying. Normally respirations are gentle, quiet, rapid, and shallow. They are most easily observed by watching abdominal movements because newborn respiration is accomplished mainly by the diaphragm and abdominal muscles.

Blood pressure. Blood pressure of the new-born infant is characteristically low and difficult to measure accurately with conventional sphygmomanometers. When a cuff 1 inch (2.5 cm) wide is used, average systolic pressure is 80 to 60/45 to 40 mm Hg at birth and 100/50 mm Hg by the tenth day of life. As the child grows older, blood pressure gradually rises and pulse and respiration rates drop.

Basic needs

All humans are born with basic needs that, according to Maslow, are essential for health. These needs are for survival, safety and security, belongingness and affection, respect and self-respect, and self-actualization. Some persons believe that the basic needs are fulfilled sequentially over time. Others believe that the basic needs may be filled at all ages in different ways. There is no debate, however, that the newborn infant must have the first three: survival, safety and security, and belongingness and affection. Nor is there any question that the baby depends on others to supply those needs. For this reason great care is taken to meet the physical needs of the baby, to provide a safe environment, and to hold and cuddle the infant, particularly during feedings.

Specific characteristics
Head

The neonate's head is proportionately much larger than it will be in adulthood. It represents one-fourth the infant's total body length, whereas an adult's head is only one-eighth the total height. The circumference of the baby's head ranges from 12½ to 14 inches (31 to 35.5 cm) and equals or exceeds that of the chest. During delivery, for the large head to pass through the small birth canal, the skull bones may actually overlap in a process called *molding*. Such molding reduces the diameter of the skull temporarily. This strange-looking elongation usually disappears a few hours after

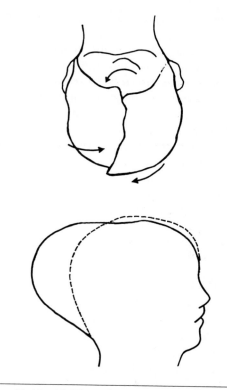

Fig. 11-11 Molding of the fetal head during the birth process is made possible by the overlapping of suture lines between skull bones.

birth as the bones assume their normal relationships (Fig. 11-11).

The six bones of the infant's skull are separated from one another along the suture lines. Where more than two bones come together, the space is called a *fontanel,* (or "little fountain") because the pulse is sometimes visible there. The anterior fontanel is the largest and is called the *bregma,* or soft spot. It normally is closed in with bone by the eighteenth month. The posterior fontanel closes in about 2 months. If closure occurs too soon, there is inadequate space for brain growth. During infancy the anterior fontanel provides valuable information about the baby's condition. A sunken fontanel indicates dehydration; a bulging fontanel indicates increased intracranial pressure.

Skin

At birth the delicate skin of the newborn infant appears dark red because it is thin, and the layers of subcutaneous fat have not yet covered the capillary beds. This redness shows through even heavily pigmented skin and becomes even more flushed when the baby cries. Some common characteristics of the skin of newborn infants follow.

Vernix caseosa. During the months of intrauterine life the fetus floats in amniotic fluid. The tender skin is protected by a cheeselike, cream-colored paste, called *vernix caseosa*, that is secreted by sebaceous glands and epithelial cells (Fig. 11-12). At birth some infants are covered thickly, whereas others may have deposits only in the body creases. Many physicians prefer that a minimum of the vernix be removed so it can continue its protective function. Others believe that it be thoroughly

removed to prevent the possibility of its harboring bacteria. In any case, the vernix usually disappears in 2 or 3 days.

Milia. Milia are tiny whitish dots typically seen on the nose, forehead, and cheeks of newborn infants. These dots are clogged sebaceous glands that have not yet begun to function. After about 2 weeks, when sweat begins to be secreted, milia gradually wash away and disappear.

Lanugo. Lanugo is soft, downy hair that covers the fetus beginning about the sixteenth week of gestation and continuing until the thirty-second week, when it begins to disappear. Thus the more premature an infant is, the more lanugo is present at birth. Lanugo is distributed over the entire body but is more dense on the shoulders, back, extremities, and temples. Lanugo tends to disappear during the first week of life.

Desquamation. Desquamation is the peeling of the skin that occurs normally during the first 2 to 4 weeks of life. This may be pro-

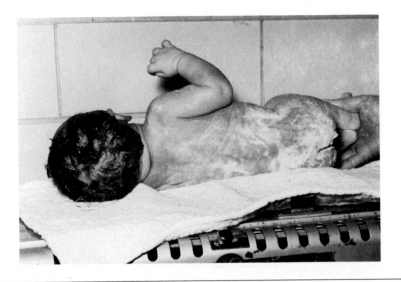

Fig. 11-12 Vernix caseosa on the back and buttocks of a newborn baby before the excess has been removed.

nounced or quite minimal and is most common in low-birth-weight infants.

Erythema toxicum. This is a type of "allergic redness" that appears as red blotches on the skin of otherwise normal infants. Erythema toxicum may appear on the day of birth and persist for many days. The red blotches may become raised and even develop blisters before they gradually disappear. There is no known cause or cure. Erythema toxicum is not contagious and most often affects healthy, vigorous babies.

Mongolian spots. Occasionally, bluish black pigmented areas occur on the buttocks or lower portion of the back of infants with yellow, brown, or black skin. Mongolian spots are of no permanent significance because they usually disappear during the first or second year of life.

Birthmarks (nevi). There are various types of birthmarks; some are temporary, some permanent, some result from birth trauma. Others result from structural abnormalities of pigment, blood vessels, hair, or other tissues. Nevi may be elevated or flat and of any size or shape. They may occur any place on the body and may even develop days or weeks after birth, as does the "strawberry mark." Cosmetic surgery, if attempted, is usually delayed for a number of years to allow for possible fading.

Jaundice. Jaundice is a yellow discoloration that may be seen in the skin or in the sclera of the eye. Jaundice is caused by excessive amounts of free bilirubin in the blood and tissue. Complex enzyme processes within the liver are responsible for the maintenance of bilirubin levels in the body. Because of the immaturity of the newborn infant's liver, there is an excessive amount of bilirubin in the blood at birth. During the first week further breakdown of hemoglobin occurs from the reduction of red blood cells. As a result, on about the second or third day, approximately 60% of all infants begin to show some jaundice. By about the seventh day it usually disappears.

This is called *physiological jaundice,* or *icterus neonatorum.*

If jaundice occurs before the third day, it indicates abnormal blood cell destruction. Such pathological jaundice may be caused by Rh factor or blood group A, B, or O incompatibility. This jaundice is discussed in greater detail in Chapter 12. Any jaundice should be reported promptly, particularly when appearing soon after birth.

Hair and nails

Infants may be born with long, thick hair or may be bald. The hair can be quite different in color, coarseness, and curliness from what it will be in later life. Eyelashes and eyebrows are normally present at birth. Fingernails may be long and sharp enough to make deep scratches. To prevent infants from injuring themselves, some nurseries use shirts with closed long sleeves. Nurses should not attempt to cut infant's fingernails; the danger of cutting the fingertips is too great.

Breasts

The breasts of both boys and girls may be enlarged at birth because of high levels of female hormone in the mother's blood. The breasts even may secrete a substance similar to colostrum, but without continued hormone stimulation the response disappears soon after birth.

Genitalia

In boys the testes normally descend during intrauterine life and are present in the scrotal sac at birth. Failure to do so is called *cryptorchidism* (hidden testes). Surgery may be required in later years, before puberty, if descent does not occur spontaneously.

Hydrocele, an accumulation of fluid around one or both of the testes, may occur and in most cases is absorbed in a few months. A condition called *phimosis,* in which the foreskin or prepuce cannot be retracted to expose the glans penis, also may occur and usually is self-corrected by growth during the first year.

Tiny glands located under the prepuce secrete a cheeselike matter called *smegma.* To promote cleanliness, prevent continued phimosis, or fulfill a religious rite, the foreskin may be cut or removed in whole or in part. This surgical procedure, called *circumcision,* is most frequently performed during the first week of life and sometimes immediately after birth.

In girls the labia minora and clitoris may be swollen at birth as a result of the high female hormone levels in the mother's body. A white mucoid discharge may fill the vagina. Occasionally this discharge is tinged with blood because of the sudden withdrawal of female hormones from the mother, called *withdrawal bleeding.*

Urinary system

At birth the kidneys function at 30% to 50% of adult capacity and are not yet mature enough to concentrate urine. A dilute urine, however, is collected in the bladder. The infant usually voids within 24 hours. It is important to record the time of first voiding. Complete anuria should be reported, since this may indicate a congenital anomaly of the urinary system.

Respiratory system

During intrauterine life the fetus does not need its lungs to obtain oxygen, since this is supplied from the mother's blood by means of placental circulation. Long before birth, however, the mechanism of respiration is established. As early as the fourth month of gestation, prerespiratory movements begin. The lungs develop, but their air sacs are in an almost total state of collapse, or *atelectasis.* At birth placental oxygen is cut off, carbon dioxide builds up in the infant's blood, and the infant suddenly is exposed to a shocking new environment. In response the baby draws a first breath, fills the lungs with air, and utters a robust cry with the first expiration.

Mucus and amniotic fluid must be removed from the air passages so the infant will not aspirate them. During the first weeks of life the respiratory rate may be irregular because of the immaturity of the respiratory center in the brain. The rate should not drop below 30 or rise above 60. Abdominal breathing is normal; sternal retraction ("chest breathing") and cyanosis are abnormal and indicate dyspnea. These signs should be reported promptly.

Circulatory system

During fetal life the blood largely bypasses the lungs and liver by means of the ductus venosus, foramen ovale, and ductus arteriosus (see Fig. 3-7). When umbilical blood stops flowing at birth, sudden pressure differences occur within the circulatory system. These differences cause the blood flowing to the lungs and liver to increase and the blood flowing through the bypass channels to decrease. Specifically, when the pressure in the left atrium exceeds that in the right side, the foramen ovale closes. Umbilical arteries and veins contract and close, and within 24 hours the ductus arteriosus closes. The ductus venosus, which bypassed the liver, and the ductus arteriosus shrivel up and are converted to fibrous ligaments within 2 to 3 months (see Fig. 3-8).

Blood

During intrauterine life and for the first few postnatal days before the lungs expand fully, a relatively high number of red blood cells and level of hemoglobin are needed to provide the fetus with adequate oxygen. During the first 2 weeks after birth, oxygenation improves and large numbers of red cells are no longer needed; thus hemolysis occurs. The red cell count and fetal hemoglobin continue to fall for the first 3 months of life, resulting in physiological anemia (Table 11-1). Fetal hemoglo-

Table 11-1 Hemoglobin content in blood according to age

Age of child	Grams of hemoglobin per 100 ml of whole blood
At birth	17 to 20
3 months	10.5 to 12 (physiological anemia)
1 year	11 to 12.5
5 years	12 to 13
10 years	13 to 14
Adult	14 to 16

bin differs chemically from adult hemoglobin. Gradually new red blood cells with adult-type hemoglobin replace the hemolyzed cells.

As mentioned earlier with signs of jaundice, bilirubin levels in the newborn infant's blood are high at birth and rise still higher, to 18 to 20 mg per 100 ml of serum. When the liver matures sufficiently, this level drops to the normal level (1 mg per 100 ml). Continuing high levels beyond the first 2 weeks indicate a pathological condition such as obstruction, abnormal blood destruction, or serious infection.

During the first few days of life, the prothrombin level decreases and clotting time in all infants is prolonged. This process is most acute between the second and fifth postnatal days. It can be prevented to a large extent by giving vitamin K to the infant after birth. With the ingestion of food, establishment of digestion, and maturation of the liver, vitamin K is manufactured by the baby, and clotting time stabilizes within a week to 10 days.

Digestive system

Mouth. The newborn infant's lips should be pink and the tongue smooth and symmetrical. The tongue should not extend or protrude between the lips. The connective tissue attached to the underside of the tongue (frenulum) should not restrict the mobility of the tip of the tongue. An existing restriction is called

tongue-tie (*ankyloglossia*), and the physician may cut the constrictive tissue.

The gums may have tooth ridges along them, and rarely a tooth or two may have erupted before birth. The roof of the mouth (hard palate) should be closed, and the uvula (soft palate) should be present. Sometimes there are white glistening spots along the hard palate, called *Epstein's pearls,* where the two halves of the hard palate fused. They will disappear in time.

Stomach. At birth the capacity of the infant's stomach is about 1 to 2 ounces (30 to 60 ml) and increases rapidly. The infant is fed formula from a bottle or milk at the mother's breast. As the infant sucks the nipple, air as well as milk may be swallowed. This creates a false feeling of satisfaction from a full stomach. If the baby is not lifted to a head-up position so that the air can escape by rising (burping), air will remain in the stomach for some time. When air does escape, it may force the milk out with it (regurgitation). After being burped, the baby can then take more milk.

As the feeding continues, milk leaves the stomach almost immediately, passing through the pyloric sphincter into the small intestine. Occasionally this valve is stenosed (too tight) and the milk, instead of passing through, is vomited with great force immediately after the feeding. Such projectile vomiting should be reported promptly, since it may indicate a pathological condition called *pyloric stenosis* that may require surgical intervention.

Intestine. The baby's first stool is a blackish-green, odorless, sticky substance called *meconium.* It consists of amniotic fluid, vernix, digestive tract secretions, bile, lanugo, and waste products from the body tissues. As soon as the baby begins to take milk, the stool begins to change to what is known as *transitional stool,* then typical milk curd stools follow. Stool of the breast-fed infant is golden yellow, watery, and acid in reaction. As a result, the baby's buttocks may become excoriated. The stool of a formula-fed infant is usually bright yellow, formed, less frequent, and neutral to slightly alkaline.

Normally there is some type of defecation within the first 24 hours after birth. The absence of any stools during this period may indicate a congenital defect and should be reported.

Skeletal system

The bones of the neonate are soft because they are composed chiefly of cartilage, which contains only a small amount of calcium. The skeleton is flexible and the joints are elastic to ensure a safe passage through the birth canal.

The infant's back is normally flat and straight. The spinal curves develop later when the infant sits up and begins to stand. The legs are small, short, and bowed. The hands are plump and the fingers relatively short.

The hands may open completely when relaxed, but they close reflexly when the palm is touched; this is called the *grasp reflex*. The feet appear flat and the legs bowed. True deformity of the hips, legs, or feet must be diagnosed by an experienced physician.

Neuromuscular system

At birth the infant's muscles are firm and resilient. They have tonus, the ability to contract when stimulated, but the infant lacks the ability to control them. The infant wriggles and stretches, but movements are uncoordinated. When picking the baby up, the nurse must support the heavy head because as yet the neonate lacks the strength to hold up the head. Normally the infant is not limp in the nurse's hands, and the muscles do not twitch or jerk. Instead, a certain normal resistance to gravity makes the baby "hold together." Any lack of this may indicate brain damage or narcosis from drugs given to the mother during labor. Muscular development of the infant

awaits further development of nervous control.

The nervous system of the newborn is sufficiently developed to sustain life but is incompletely integrated. Bodily functions and responses are mainly carried on by the lower centers of the brain and reflexes in the spinal cord. Nervous control from the higher centers gradually develops, making possible more complex and purposeful behavior.

Reflexes and special senses

Reflexes are responses to stimuli that do not have to be consciously directed by the brain. The infant is born with a number of life-preserving reflexes. Some of these will disappear during development and will no longer be needed; others remain throughout adult life (Fig. 11-13).

The special senses have not had an opportunity to mature in infants, who have not developed the capability to interpret the input of all these senses. Newborns feel pain, temperature change, and pressure and they respond in appropriate ways (Table 11-2).

CONTINUING HOSPITAL NURSING CARE

The goal of continuing nursing interventions for newborn infants and their mothers is to promote healthy adaptation. Nursing procedures are geared toward aseptic, individualized care.

Principles and practice

Procedures are ways of putting principles into action. Each newborn nursery develops its own procedures, but the principles of newborn care are quite universal because they are based on scientific facts. For example, it is known that infection occurs because pathogenic organisms invade the body. If the body could be separated from such organisms, infection would be prevented. Thus a principle of newborn care is that newborns should be

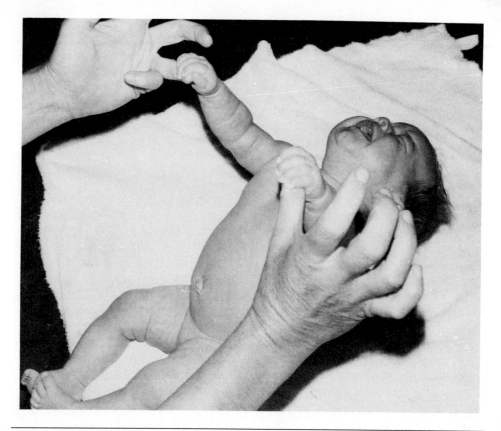

Fig. 11-13 The grasp reflex, one of the protective reflexes, causes the infant to hold so tightly to any object placed in the hands that the whole body can be lifted up.

isolated from pathogenic organisms.

To implement this principle, the following practices have become almost standard in hospitals across the United States:

1. Any person with an infectious disease is barred from the nursery area, including visitors, nurses, physicians, and auxiliary persons.
2. All supplies, especially linens, that are to be used in the newborn nursery are handled separately and sometimes sterilized.
3. Any infant suspected of infection, including those infants born out of asepsis, is removed from the regular nursery. No infant is returned to the regular nursery

after having had a diagnosed infection.
4. Newborns are separated from each other by the practice of barrier technique. The nurses wash their hands between care of babies and mothers.
5. Personal cleanliness is required of all personnel. Clean clothing is worn; gowns are placed over nursery clothing when nurses leave the nursery; and scrupulous handwashing technique is observed before touching each baby.
6. The air, all cribs, the walls, and all equipment are made as free of bacteria as possible by every means available, including disinfectant lamps and chemicals.

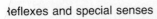

Reflexes and special senses

	Description	Presence and duration
VE REFLEXES		
oro's)	Sudden stimulus causes arms to fly out and up, tremble, and slowly relax	At birth; fades at about 2 months of age
Tonic neck	Postural "fencing" response; head, arm, and leg turn to one side, slowly relax	At birth; fades at about 2 to 3 months of age
Grasp	Infants grasp any object put in their hands firmly enough to hold their body weight, relax	At birth; fades at about 2 months of age
Eye blinking	Eyelids close and open when stimulated by touch or light	At birth; lifelong
Crying	Sudden pain, cold, hunger cause air to pass through vocal cords	At birth; lifelong
FEEDING REFLEXES		
Sucking	Lips pucker, tongue rolls, inward pull or sucking caused by hunger, lip stimulation	At birth; 6 to 8 months of age (as a reflex movement)
Rooting	Touch of cheek or lips causes head to turn toward touch	At birth; 6 months
Swallowing	Throat muscles close trachea and open esophagus when food is in mouth	At birth; lifelong
Gag	At stimulation of uvula, esophagus opens; reverse peristalsis occurs	At birth; lifelong
BREATHING REFLEXES		
Respiratory motion	Chest and abdominal muscles cause inspiratory and expiratory muscle movement	At birth; lifelong
Sneeze	Violent reverse flow of air from nose and throat	At birth; lifelong
Cough	Violent reverse flow of air from throat and lungs	1 year; lifelong
SPECIAL SENSES		
Touch, pain, pressure	Infant's lips most sensitive	At birth; lifelong
Smell	Odor perception	At birth; lifelong
Taste	Sweet and sour; flavors learned later	At birth; lifelong
Hearing	Loud noise perception	2 to 3 days when eustachian tubes clear
	Voice recognition	6 months
Sight	Light sensitive	At birth; lifelong
	Perceives light and follows it	At birth; lifelong
	Focus and tear formation	At birth; lifelong

Another principle of newborn care grows out of the knowledge that the infant is weak and helpless, needs extra body heat, and is in a dangerous period of life. The resulting principle is that the newborn should have a protected, regulated environment under constant observation. To implement this principle, the following practices are followed:

1. The newborn nursery is never left unattended.
2. All newborns are kept in unobstructed sight of the nurse.
3. Humidity and heat are carefully controlled (humidity of 50% and a temperature of 74° to 76° F).
4. A baby is never left unattended on a table or on the scales.
5. Babies are held for every feeding, never left with propped bottles.

Daily care

Every day each newborn is examined, cleansed, and weighed and the temperature taken. All this information is then recorded. This provides the physician with valuable facts about the infant's progress.

Nurses must handle infants gently, avoiding unnecessary exposure, and check general appearance, nose, eyes, mouth, ears, skin, cord, genitalia, and the character of stools. This is done before morning feeding so that movement will not cause newly ingested milk to be regurgitated.

Nurses should care for only one infant at a time and wash their hands after each baby is handled. Each baby is kept completely separate from the others. An individual thermometer, hairbrush or comb, and linen pack is needed for each baby. A typical procedure is as follows:

1. Cleanse the eyelids with water, wiping from the inner canthus outward.
2. Inspect the nostrils; if there is mucus or milk curd in them, remove it with a small, moist piece of twisted cotton.
3. Wipe the face.
4. Use a mild soap if washing the hair.
5. Remove the shirt; inspect and wash the hands, arms, and axillae.
6. Take axillary temperature.
7. Inspect the cord and cleanse the base with 70% alcohol.
8. Remove the diaper; cleanse and inspect the feet, legs, groin, genitalia, and buttocks.
9. Turn the infant, and cleanse and inspect the back.
10. Place a clean paper or cloth on the scales, balance them, and weigh the infant.
11. Dress the infant in a shirt and diaper.
12. Place the infant on the bassinet tray and change the linen.
13. Replace the infant in the bassinet, and cover with a top cover.
14. Wash hands and record nursing observations in the baby's record.

Infant feeding

At delivery the mother indicates whether she wishes to breast-feed or bottle-feed her infant. Because this is a highly personal decision and because neither breast nor bottle can be called better in all cases, nurses support mother's choice without passing judgment.

Usually newborn babies are given nothing by mouth (NPO) for the first 12 hours of life. This allows time for the mucus and amniotic fluid to leave the oral passages and for the baby to rest. Practice varies, but in some hospitals all babies receive glucose water after they are 12 hours old and milk formula or breast-feedings after 24 hours.

Breast-feeding

The mother who indicates her intention to breast-feed should be given special instructions on the care of her nipples and breasts.

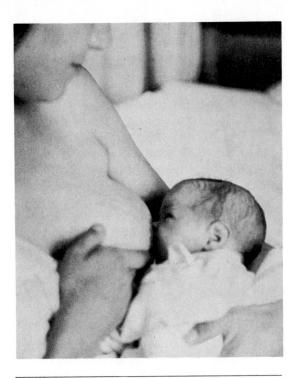

Fig. 11-14   Baby at breast. Nipple extends well into the baby's mouth.

The first time the baby goes to breast, an experienced nurse brings the baby to the mother to provide her with assistance and encouragement. The following instructions are given to ensure the mother and infant safety and success in the nursing experience.

1. The mother showers or bathes daily to provide general cleanliness.

2. Before touching her breasts or the baby, the mother washes her hands thoroughly with soap.

3. The mother needs to find a comfortable position, either sitting or lying down, using pillows for support.

4. The baby is held in a natural position with the nipple extending well into the mouth (Fig. 11-14).

5. At first both breasts should be nursed at each feeding for as long as the baby will feed. The mother should switch breasts when the baby becomes agitated and end the feeding when the baby falls asleep or detaches from the breast.

6. Babies are fed "on demand" or every 2 to 3 hours. The more the baby sucks, the more milk is produced. Sucking causes the pituitary gland to release two hormones: oxytocin and prolactin. *Oxytocin* causes contractions within the breast that squeeze milk out to make feeding easier for the baby. This is called the "let-down" reflex. *Prolactin* stimulates the cells to produce milk. The more the baby sucks, the more prolactin is produced. Nursing helps the mother's body adjust the milk supply to the baby's need.

Bottle-feeding

Babies who are not breast-fed are given formula in a nursing bottle. A great variety of nursing devices have been invented, each seeking to duplicate the human breast as closely as possible and still be safe, economical, and easy to use. Generally the breast-fed infant must suck harder and longer to obtain the same amount of milk as the bottle-fed infant.

A formula is an infinitely variable recipe that can be made to precise specifications as to caloric, carbohydrate, protein, fat, mineral, vitamin, and water content. The amount may also be adjusted and measured exactly and the temperature varied.

All formulas, regardless of their content, must be sterile, fresh, and clearly labeled. Formula prepared for the newborn nursery is usually put in 4-ounce bottles, because few newborn babies can tolerate more than that amount at one time. Any unused portion of an opened bottle should be discarded.

Bottle-fed babies are usually started on a dilute formula by the time they are 16 hours

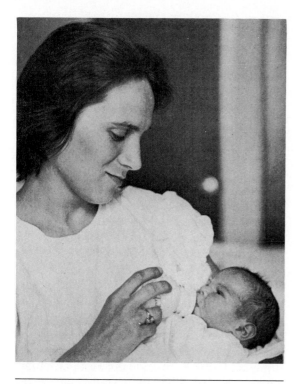

Fig. 11-15 Baby in the mother's arms for bottle-feeding. Nipple should be at the same angle as the baby's tongue.

old. Four ounces of this formula is offered every 4 hours until the baby is 3 days old. The concentration of the formula is usually increased at that time. As the infant grows and nutritional needs increase, the formula will be altered and solid foods added to the diet.

The mother of the bottle-fed infant is encouraged to hold her baby for every feeding, just as a breast-fed infant is held (Fig. 11-15).

Before feeding her infant, the mother should wash her hands and find a comfortable position. The baby is held in the crook of one arm and the bottle held in the other hand. The nipple should be placed in the infant's mouth at the angle of the tongue. After the baby has

taken an ounce, the baby should be burped to allow swallowed air to escape from the stomach. Then a second ounce may be given, followed again by burping. Two ounces are usually enough at the beginning. Overfeeding may cause hiccups or regurgitation and should be avoided. Most babies stop sucking and go to sleep when they have had enough.

Parent teaching

It is the privilege and obligation of the maternal-child care team to teach the mother and father how to care for their new baby. Classes are taught by hospital and school personnel on such subjects as parenting and care of the infant. Numerous books, pamphlets, and magazines are available to new parents.

Perhaps the most valuable teaching is done by the staff in the maternity unit as they instruct and demonstrate to the parents. Some hospitals provide a checklist of subjects to be taught parents by the staff, including changing diapers, giving cord care, and using a bulb syringe for gentle nasal suction. When the mother and baby are discharged, these items are reviewed and discussed with the parents.

Medical supervision

Every infant born in a hospital must have a physician who is responsible for medical supervision. Within a few hours after birth, the physician examines the baby thoroughly and then prescribes specifics for the infant's care, including feeding, medications, treatments, and special laboratory tests. Thereafter, medical supervision includes a regular check of the infant's weight gain or loss, vital signs, feeding, elimination, color, and general condition. Unless there is some contraindication, the baby is discharged at the same time as the mother.

Birth registration

Each of the 50 states of the United States has a department or division of vital statistics in which all births, deaths, marriages, divorces, and so on are registered. It is the legal responsibility of the one who attends a birth to see that it is properly registered. Often registration is channeled through a local county seat or township and then to the state office. When a baby is born in a hospital, the form usually is made out by the medical records department, then signed by the mother and her physician.

Information included on a typical birth certificate includes the mother's name and address, a description of her pregnancy and delivery, the baby's name, information about the birth, the father's name and address, and birth attendant.

A clerk from the medical records department of the hospital may come to the obstetrical ward to obtain information for the birth certificate. When the clerk has prepared the original form, it is signed by the mother. She is not given a copy of the legal birth certificate at that time, but sends to the state department of vital statistics for a photostatic copy after it has been registered with the department. This official document is not to be confused with the "hospital birth certificate" sometimes given as a memento to the mother.

Newborn screening tests

Before the baby and mother are discharged from the hospital, parents are told about standard screening tests for newborn infants and when to return to have these tests completed. Screening tests detect disorders that cause mental retardation, physical handicaps, and death if left undiscovered. Conditions that can be identified from a drop of blood from a heel stick on the second or third day are phenylketonuria (PKU), galactosemia, hypothyroidism, maple syrup urine disease, and homocystinuria. If tests results are positive, more definitive tests are performed. If the diagnosis is confirmed, treatment is begun at once.

Discharge

An infant in normal health is discharged from the hospital at the same time as the mother. The physician examines the baby and writes discharge prescriptions, including a date on which the parents should bring the baby for an office visit. Frequently physicians spends time with the parents, establishing rapport and answering questions. They may recommend a visit of a community health nurse.

When the mother is ready to go home, the nursery is notified and the infant prepared for discharge. The nurse takes the baby to the mother's bedside. The mother watches the nurse cut off one of the baby's identification bands, and together they check the number against the mother's band. If the numbers are identical, the mother knows that this is indeed the baby she delivered. She signs a form to that effect, and the band that was removed is attached to the form and kept as a permanent hospital record. The other band is left on the infant.

The infant is then dressed in clothes provided by the parents. The nurse can take advantage of this time for last-minute instructions about infant care, as follows:

1. Cord care: paint the base with 70% alcohol twice a day until it drops off and heals in about 2 weeks. Do not use binders and keep dry.
2. Bathing: give sponge baths until the naval is healed.
3. Diapering: change diapers when wet. Wash and dry buttocks at each change. Expose to air or apply antiammonia salve if buttocks become excoriated.

The mother and father are encouraged to ask questions and participate in the discussion. The plan for continued nursing or medical supervision, such as a number to call or appointment to keep, is reviewed.

The crib card may be given to the mother as well as photographs, certificates, and other mementos provided by the hospital. If the baby is receiving formula, some hospitals provide courtesy feedings. In addition, many large baby-supply companies give courtesy packs of baby care products including diapers, lotion, and so on.

When all is in readiness, the mother is seated in a wheelchair, the baby is placed in her arms, and they are wheeled to the automobile exit. The mother should never attempt to walk from the maternity ward with the baby in her arms; a fall would be disastrous, and the risk is unnecessary. At the exit the discharging nurse or attendant should hold the baby while the mother gets into the automobile and then place the baby in her arms when she is ready.

▶ **KEY CONCEPTS**

1. Making sure that the neonate's airway is open is the primary concern in the delivery room.
2. Three phases of assessment of the newborn are immediate, transitional, and periodic.
3. A neutral thermal environment is one in which the infant's oxygen consumption and metabolic rate are minimal.
4. The infant is identified with two identical name bands in the delivery room.
5. Prophylactic treatment of the infant's eyes after birth is done to protect the infant from gonorrheal and chlamydial infections.
6. Data about weight, height, and head size are collected immediately after birth to provide a baseline for comparison with future measurements.
7. SGA, AGA, and LGA are terms used to describe intrauterine growth when age and weight are compared.
8. The six states of awareness of neonates are crying, quiet sleep, rapid eye movement, active and alert, quiet and alert, and transitional.
9. Physiological resilience is a mechanism that protects neonates against stressors until body systems begin to function fully.

10. Common characteristics of the skin of newborns include vernix caseosa (cheeselike paste), milia (facial whiteheads), lanugo (fine hair over body), desquamation (peeling), erythema toxicum (nonserious allergic rash), mongolian spots (bluish black pigment), and jaundice (yellowness).
11. Cryptorchidism (failure of testes to descend into the scrotal sac) and phimosis (a foreskin that does not retract) are common defects of the male genitalia; anuria for more than 24 hours should be reported.
12. The newborn's respiratory rate is irregular at first because of immaturity of the respiratory center in the brain.
13. Special ducts of fetal circulation convert to fibrous ligaments within 2 to 3 months after birth.
14. Physiological anemia typically occurs for the first 3 months, then disappears.
15. Tongue-tie is caused by excessive frenulum; Epstein's pearls are found along hard palate; meconium is a black, sticky substance found in bowel at birth; transitional stool is part meconium, part milk curds.
16. Many protective, feeding, and breathing reflexes are present in the newborn at birth; all special senses except hearing are present at birth.
17. Principles of asepsis are put into practice in the nursery.
18. Breast feeding "on demand" helps establish milk supply; "let-down" reflex results from oxytocin stimulation; prolactin stimulates milk-producing cells.
19. Parent teaching is a nursing function.
20. Birth registration is the responsibility of the birth attendant.
21. Newborn screening tests for phenylketonuria, galactosemia, hypothyroidism, maple syrup urine disease, and homocystinuria are done from a drop of newborn blood.

■ **ANNOTATED SUMMARY**

I. Birth
   A. Time—when entire baby is separated from mother

B. Experience—shocking and stressful to infant

II. Immediate care
  A. In the delivery room
    1. Airway—clearing airway is most important care
    2. Umbilical cord—cut by midwife, physician, or father and clamped or tied
    3. Assessment
      a. Immediate
      b. Transitional
      c. Periodic
    4. Resuscitation measures
      a. Clearing the airway—suctioning
      b. Forcing oxygen into the lungs—mouth-to-mouth or intermittent positive-pressure breathing
      c. Stimulating the baby to breathe—physical methods
    5. Environment
      a. Effects on baby—sudden chill initially stimulating; afterward, cold has adverse effects
      b. Neutral thermal environment—ideal; maintains a constant warm body temperature
    6. Identification—three bands: one on mother, two on infant
    7. Prophylaxis—to prevent ophthalmia neonatorum and chlamydial infections, antibiotic ointment is put in baby's eyes
    8. Recording—hospital record begins in delivery room
  B. In the newborn nursery
    1. Cleansing and assessment—do not chill; use minimum of water
    2. Weighing and measuring—weight, length, and head circumference
    3. Estimation of gestational age—three categories: preterm, term, and post-term; three subgroups: SGA, AGA, and LGA
    4. Cord care—observe for hemorrhage, scrub, paint with 70% alcohol
    5. Clothing and cover—must be lightweight and sterile
    6. Positioning—on side with head down
    7. Feeding and rest—NPO for 12 to 16 hours
    8. Recording and identifying—essential data must be recorded; card is left on crib

III. Characteristics of the newborn
  A. Terminology—fetus, 6 weeks to birth; neonate, birth to 1 month of age; infant, 1 month to walking age
  B. General characteristics
    1. Body shape and measurements—large head and abdomen
    2. Awareness—six states: crying, quiet sleep, REM, active-alert, quiet-alert, and transitional
    3. Physiological resilience—passive resistance to stressors
    4. Immunity—antibodies pass from mother through placenta; none for pertussis or chicken pox
    5. Vital signs
      a. Temperature
      b. Pulse
      c. Respirations
      d. Blood pressure
    6. Basic needs—survival, safety and security, belongingness and affection, respect and self-respect, and self-actualization
  B. Specific characteristics
    1. Head—bones overlap at birth, then return to position
    2. Skin
      a. Vernix caseosa—cheeselike paste
      b. Milia—white dots on face
      c. Lanugo—downy hair over body
      d. Desquamation—peeling-off of skin
      e. Erythema toxicum—allergic redness
      f. Mongolian spots—pigmented areas
      g. Birthmarks (nevi)
      h. Jaundice—yellowness caused by hyperbilirubinemia
    3. Hair and nails—variable
    4. Breasts—may be enlarged from mother's hormones
    5. Genitalia—infant examined for defects
    6. Urinary system—first voiding usually in 24 hours
    7. Respiratory system—atelectasis until first breath
    8. Circulatory system—fetal bypass structures close soon after birth

9. Blood
   a. Hemoglobin—high at birth, then drops
   b. Vitamin K—necessary for clotting; ordered for some babies
10. Digestive system
    a. Mouth—Epstein's pearls, tongue-tie
    b. Stomach—pyloric stenosis
    c. Intestine—meconium precedes normal stool
11. Skeletal system—bones soft in neonate
12. Neuromuscular system—infant should not be flaccid
13. Reflexes and special senses—protective, feeding, and breathing reflexes
IV. Continuing hospital nursing care
    A. Principles and practice
    B. Daily care—examined, weighed, temperature taken, cleansed, and held and fed
    C. Infant feeding—mother's decision is valid
       1. Breast-feeding—nipple care; mother needs assistance
       2. Bottle-feeding—various formulas
    D. Parent teaching—responsibility of staff; checklist of subjects for parents
    E. Medical supervision—necessary
    F. Birth registration—required by law
    G. Newborn screening tests—to detect potential disorders
    H. Discharge—infant identification is vital

● STUDY QUESTIONS AND LEARNING ACTIVITIES

1. Resuscitation efforts are aimed at overcoming three problems of asphyxia. Name them and discuss measures to overcome each one.
2. Why is ophthalmia neonatorum a serious condition? What measures are used to prevent the infection?
3. Why is the measurement of the newborn infant's head circumference important?
4. Define the following conditions of the skin: milia, mongolian spots, vernix caseosa, and desquamation.
5. What information about the infant's condition can be obtained from the bregma?
6. What is the normal range for newborn infants for each of the following vital signs: pulse, respiration, and blood pressure?
7. Discuss the ways in which the principle that the infant should be isolated from as many pathogenic organisms as possible is implemented in your hospital.
8. List three laboratory tests made on newborn infants and the reasons they are performed.
9. Describe discharge procedures at your hospital.

REFERENCES

American Academy of Pediatrics: Hospital care of newborn infants, Evanston, Ill, 1971, The Academy.

Battaglia FC, and Lubchenco LO: A practical classification of new born infants by weight and gestational age, 71:159-163, 1967.

Bobak IM, and Jensen MD: Essentials of maternity nursing: the nurse and the childbearing family, ed 2, St. Louis, 1987, The CV Mosby Co.

Bower TGR: The perceptual world of the child, Cambridge, Mass, 1977, Harvard University Press.

Hamilton PM: Basic pediatric nursing, ed 5, St. Louis, 1987, The CV Mosby Co.

Klaus M, and Kennel J: Parent-infant bonding, ed 2, St. Louis, 1982, The CV Mosby Co.

Korones SB: High-risk newborn infants: the basis for intensive nursing care, ed 4, St. Louis, 1986, The CV Mosby Co.

Meltzoff A, and Moore M: Imitation of facial and manual gestures by human neonates, Science 198:75, 1975.

Olds SB, London ML, and Ladewig PA: Maternal-newborn nursing: a family-centered approach, ed 3, Menlo Park, Calif, 1988, Addison-Wesley Publishing.

Tsikouris C: Increasing your milk, informational sheet #85, Franklin Park, Ill, 1982, LaLeche League International.

Whaley LF, and Wong DL: Essentials of pediatric nursing, ed 2, St. Louis, 1985, The CV Mosby Co.

Williams JK, and Lancaster J: Thermoregulation of the newborn, M.C.N. 1(6):355, 1976.

CHAPTER 12

Newborns with Special Needs

VOCABULARY

Ectromelia
Fistula
Gestational age
Hyperplasia
Orchiopexy
Prophylactic
Relinquishment
Subluxation
Talipes

LEARNING OBJECTIVES

- Define the terms used to describe infants' gestational age and growth.

- Discuss signs of physiological distress one might observe in high-risk infants.

- Describe typical preterm and postterm infants, stating handicaps, special needs, and appropriate nursing interventions.

- Discuss oxygen needs, conservation of energy, safety, body temperature maintenance, and nutritional needs of preterm infants.

- Describe some common perinatal injuries, and discuss assessment and nursing interventions for each.

- Describe congenital defects typically found in neonates, and discuss assessment and nursing interventions for each.

- Discuss common disorders that affect neonates, including diarrhea, jaundice, vomiting, and convulsions.

- Describe retrolental fibroplasia, respiratory distress syndrome, phenylketonuria, and omphalitis, and discuss assessment and nursing interventions for each.

- Discuss sexually transmitted diseases, their effects on the fetus and neonate, and nursing interventions.

scuss complications and nursing interven-
uuns for infants of diabetic mothers.

- Discuss the effects of alcohol on the developing fetus and the care of infants with fetal
alcohol syndrome.

- Discuss assessment of infants of drug-
dependent mothers and the goal of care.

- Discuss the needs of parents whose children
are at risk and appropriate nursing interventions.

- Describe circumcision surgery, its indications, and nursing interventions.

- Discuss religious rites maternity nurses
might need to understand, and describe the
adoption process.

Most babies are mature, healthy, and perfectly formed at birth. A small percentage are
not. For those few who are not, early detection
and treatment of problems are vital. Nurses
must be able to assess deviations from normal
and know what action to take. They must also
know of special situations not common to
every baby, such as circumcision, religous
rites, and adoption.

HIGH-RISK INFANTS
Terminology

Once all underdeveloped infants were called
"premature." Then it was recognized that both
gestational age and growth, as measured by
weight, were important indicators of the degree to which infants were at risk. For example, in Fig. 12-1, the three infants are all
the same age, but note the difference between
them. Gradually a more precise system of ter-
mology evolved, as follows:

Infant	Description
Preterm; premature	Before 38 weeks of gestation regardless of birth weight
Term; full-term	38 to 42 weeks of gestation
Postterm; postmature	42 weeks of gestation or more, regardless of birth weight
Low birth weight (LBW)	Weighs less than 2,500 gm regardless of age
Small for gestational age (SGA); small for date (SFD)	Weighs below the 10th percentile on intrauterine growth curve
Appropriate for gestational age (AGA)	Weighs between the 10th and 90th percentiles of neonates of a given gestational age
Large for gestational age (LGA)	Weighs above the 90th percentile on intrauterine growth curve
Intrauterine growth retardation (IUGR) or acceleration (IUGA)	Fetal undergrowth or overgrowth for any reason
Infants at risk	Likelihood of mortality higher than 10%
Fetal death	Death of fetus after 20 weeks of gestation and before delivery, regardless of gestational age, with no signs of life following birth

Assessment of neonates

Generally speaking, preterm infants and
those of low birth weight have a significantly
higher mortality than full-term babies of appropriate weight. Those babies with problems
related to growth are subject to respiratory,
neurological, and thermal disorders.

Scoring systems

Assessment scoring systems have been devised by a number of researchers. Although
the systems are not identical, they all use
growth and maturity criteria as indicated by
weight and neuromuscular signs.

The most common scoring system is the Apgar system. (see Table 9-2), used to evaluate
infants at birth.

Other, more detailed systems are used fol-

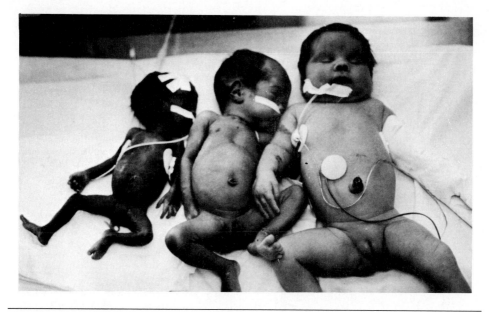

Fig. 12-1 Three babies of the same gestational age. They weigh 600, 1,400, and 2,750 gm, respectively, from left to right. *(From Korones SB: High-risk newborn infants: the basis for intensive nursing care, ed 4, St Louis, 1986, The CV Mosby Co.)*

lowing the initial assessment to evaluate certain critical characteristics, such as the growth of ear cartilage. Examples of such systems are given in Figs. 12-2 and 12-3. Using a chart, the examiner assigns a score for each characteristic. The higher the score, the more mature the baby.

Physical examination

Each body system is examined to identify any disease, injury, or defect with which the child may have been born or that may develop. The assessment is made by the following means:

auscultation Use of hearing to identify typical sounds such as breath or bowel sounds.

inspection Use of sight to identify deviations from normal, such as birthmarks.

palpation Use of touch to identify variations between soft and firm or hot and cold.

percussion Striking a portion of the baby's body to evaluate the condition of the underlying structures or to elicit responses.

Signs of physiological distress

Important symptoms to be noted include:

abdominal distention Especially if it occurs suddenly, may be caused by defects or disease of the gastrointestinal system.

anuria May indicate urinary system defect if lasts more than 24 hours.

bulging or sunken fontanels of skull Indicate increased or decreased intracranial pressure.

convulsions, muscle twitching, facial grimacing Caused by irritations of the central nervous system.

cyanosis of skin Blueness, especially a single, sud-

265

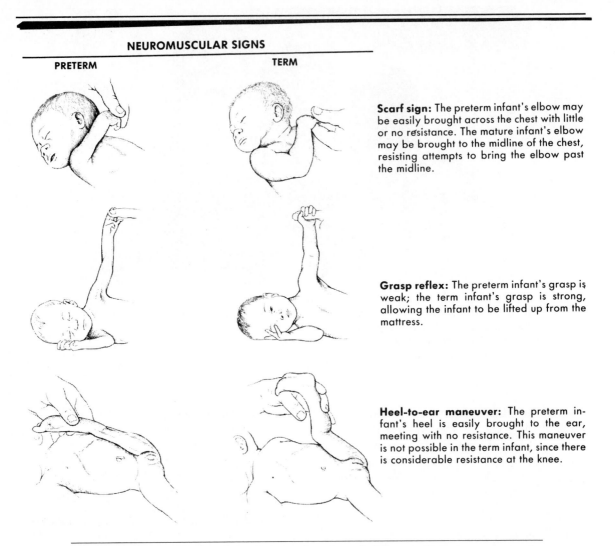

NEUROMUSCULAR SIGNS

PRETERM   TERM

Scarf sign: The preterm infant's elbow may be easily brought across the chest with little or no resistance. The mature infant's elbow may be brought to the midline of the chest, resisting attempts to bring the elbow past the midline.

Grasp reflex: The preterm infant's grasp is weak; the term infant's grasp is strong, allowing the infant to be lifted up from the mattress.

Heel-to-ear maneuver: The preterm infant's heel is easily brought to the ear, meeting with no resistance. This maneuver is not possible in the term infant, since there is considerable resistance at the knee.

Fig. 12-2 Estimation of gestational age using characteristic growth and neuromuscular signs. (From Pierog, SH, and Ferrara, A: Medical care of the sick newborn, ed. 2, St. Louis, 1976, The C.V. Mosby Co.)

den episode, caused by anoxia, may result from defects or disease of the circulatory, respiratory, or nervous systems.

discharge or redness of umbilicus or eyes May result from infection.

dyspnea Rapid or labored respirations, may be caused by defects or disease of circulatory or respiratory systems.

excessive salivation May be caused by gastrointestinal system defect.

jaundice of skin Yellowness caused by bilirubin, a product of blood destruction, may be normal or may be caused by disease.

no stools Beyond first 24 hours or **watery stools** may be caused by infection or defects of gastrointestinal system.

GROWTH

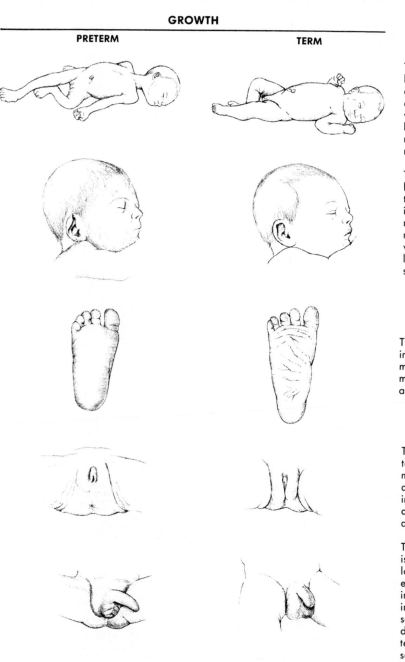

PRETERM   TERM

The preterm infant lies in a "re-laxed attitude," limbs more extended; his body size is small, and his head may appear some-what larger in proportion to the body size. The term infant has more subcutaneous fat tissue and rests in a more flexed attitude.

The preterm infant's ear carti-lages are poorly developed, and the ear may fold easily; the hair is fine and feathery, and lanugo may cover the back and face. The mature infant's ear cartilages are well formed, and the hair is more likely to form firm separate strands.

The sole of the foot of the preterm infant appears more turgid and may have only fine wrinkles. The mature infant's sole (foot) is well and deeply creased.

The preterm female infant's cli-toris is prominent, and labia majora are poorly developed and gaping. The mature female infant's labia majora are fully developed, and the clitoris is not as prominent.

The preterm male infant's scrotum is undeveloped and not pendu-lous; minimal rugae are pres-ent, and the testes may be in the inguinal canals or in the abdom-inal cavity. The term male infant's scrotum is well developed, pen-dulous, and rugated, and the testes are well down in the scrotal sac.

Fig. 12-2 For legend see opposite page.

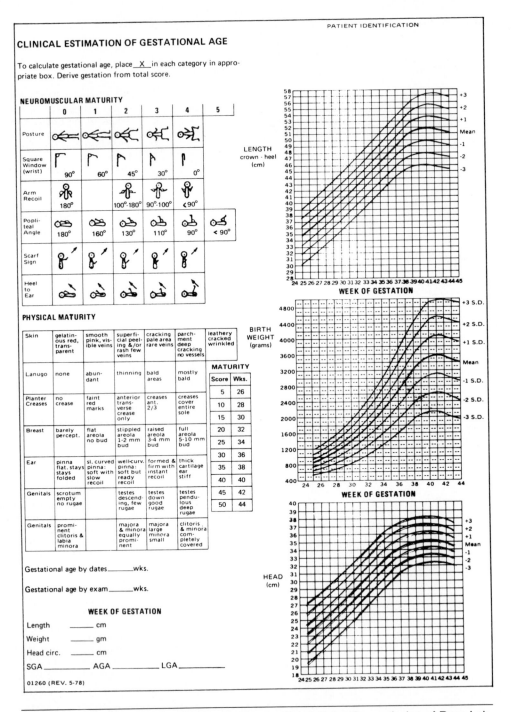

Fig. 12-3 Clinical estimation of gestational age. (Reprinted with permission of Ross Laboratories, Columbus, Ohio, 43216. Rev. May, 1978.)

shrill or weak cry May be caused by defects or disease of the nervous system.

tachycardia (rapid pulse) or **bradycardia** (slow pulse) May result from defects or disease of circulatory or respiratory systems or from high or low body temperature.

vomiting Not just spitting up small amounts of milk; is forceful, is continuous, or occurs with every feeding; may result from defects of the gastrointestinal or nervous systems.

weak or absent sucking effort May result from immaturity, defects, or disease of the nervous system.

Common measures of function include vital signs, height, weight, head circumference, and the presence of absence of necessary bodily functions such as the ability to take food, to pass stool, and to void.

Various laboratory tests are also performed, including hematocrit, thyroid function, galactose enzyme, phenylalanine for phenylketonuria (PKU), blood glucose, Veneral Disease Research Laboratory (VDRL) for syphilis, and others as indicated.

Assessment is folllowed by a medical treatment plan and a nursing care plan. These plans include various interventions that are evaluated as to their effectiveness and then adjusted.

Description

Preterm infants

Infants who are born before term are deprived of the benefits of intrauterine life for varying periods. They must breathe, eat, and carry on the functions of mature babies while they are still immature. As a result, it takes them longer to catch up with babies who remained in the ideal environment of the uterus until they were fully mature. A standardized growth chart has been developed for premature infants (Fig. 12-4).

The preterm infant resembles a little old man. The features are sharp and the bones pronounced and unsoftened by subcutaneous fat. Through the transparent skin, exposed capillary beds give a dark red hue. The fontanels and suture lines of the too-large skull are prominent. Fine lanugo hair may cover the entire body in a downy coat, while the pasty, lubricating vernix caseosa, so conspicuous on a full-term baby, is absent. The infant's cry is weak and pitiful, matching the frail appearance (Fig. 12-5).

Handicaps. The preterm infant has numerous handicaps:

1. Reduced respiratory function caused by the incomplete development of the air sacs, thoracic muscles, blood supply, and nervous reflexes of the respiratory system.
2. Inadequate regulation of the body temperature caused by feeble muscle activity, immature sweat glands, a surface area that is too large in proportion to the infant's weight, and a lack of subcutaneous fat.
3. Inadequate development of the mouth, stomach, and reflexes of sucking and swallowing, making it difficult to supply nutritional needs.
4. Inefficient elimination of body wastes by immature kidneys and skin.
5. Reduced resistance to disease caused by incomplete development of the enzyme system, of body chemistry balance, and of antibody production. Reduced disease resistance also caused by not receiving sufficient immune substances, hormones, and nutrients from the mother.
6. Reduced storage of body nutrients and production of blood-clotting elements resulting from immature liver function.
7. Defective hemopoiesis (blood cell production) and increased capillary fragility, making even a small blood loss dangerous.
8. Increased possibility of brain damage during the birth process caused by fragility of capillaries and by a tendency to bleed.

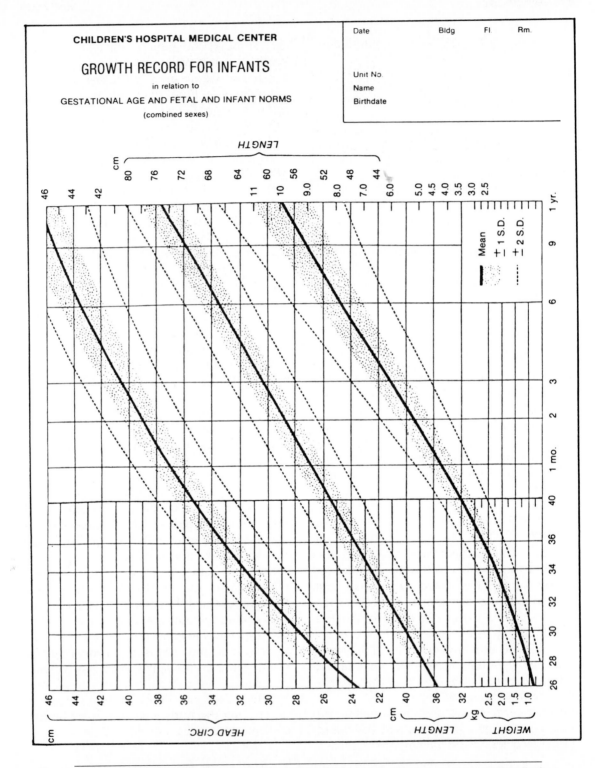

Fig. 12-4 Growth chart for premature infants. (Courtesy Childrens's Hospital Medical Center, Oakland, Calif.)

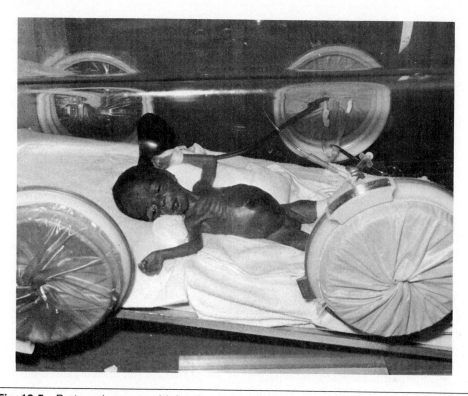

Fig. 12-5 Preterm (premature) infant in incubator. Baby was less than 27 weeks' gestation and weighed less than 2 pounds (about 900 gm) at birth. Immediate surgery was performed for herniation of the abdominal contents of the umbilicus, called an *omphalocele*.

9. Lack of adequate amounts of surface-active material (surfactant) needed to reduce surface tension in air sacs of the lungs. This lack of surfactant leads to two common complications associated with prematurity—hyaline membrane disease and retrolental fibroplasia.

Postterm infants

Most babies are born after 38 to 40 weeks of gestation. About one in 20, however, stays in the uterus beyond 42 weeks. Surprisingly, postterm infants are not better off for having remained in their watery prison. They lose weight and grow long fingernails and hair. Their skin becomes waterlogged because it is no longer protected by vernix caseosa. Meconium from the bowel stains their nails and may be found in the lungs.

Generally, postterm infants are at risk. Their mortality rate is two or three times higher than that of full-term infants. Their poor condition and apparent malnutrition are caused by placental aging. As gestational weeks pass, the placenta becomes less and less efficient in providing infants with needed nutrients and oxygen. As a result, they suffer varying degrees of malnutrition and hypoxia.

When mothers are sure of the date of conception so that the calculated length of the pregnancy is known, physicians may recommend induction of labor or cesarean birth to reduce risk for postterm infants.

Assessment of needs and Interventions

Every effort is made to prevent labor and delivery before term. If preterm delivery is inevitable, however, preparations for the infant are made. These same special preparations are made for the labor of a woman who has been pregnant more than 42 weeks. The nursery is alerted, and a person knowledgeable in resuscitation stands by at the delivery. Essential equipment includes a preheated incubator and ready-to-use resuscitation devices. At the birth the physician evaluates the baby's condition, and energency care is given as needed. The cord is clamped, and the naked baby is placed in an incubator. After proper identification and eye care, the baby is transferred to the neonatal nursery. Weighing, measuring, and other care are secondary to life-maintaining measures. Sometimes it is several days before the baby is strong enough to be weighed.

The preterm or postterm infant may be cared for in the regular newborn nursery. The infant also may be transferred to a neonatal intensive care unit, where specially prepared personnel care for babies at risk, using the most advanced equipment and techniques.

Objectives of care include the following:

1. Maintenance of the airway and adequate oxygen
2. Conservation of the infant's energy
3. Maintenance of body temperature
4. Safety and prevention of infection
5. Provision of nutritional needs

Airway and oxygen. Oxygen is essential for life. Preterm infants are often not able to obtain enough oxygen from the atmosphere to survive. Airways are blocked with mucus, and the 21% concentration of oxygen that is present at atmospheric pressure is insufficient to penetrate mucus in the lung. To compensate for this problem, high concentrations of oxygen may be administered directly into the lung, or the infant may be placed in an oxygen-rich environment.

Concentrations of oxygen administered, or present in the environment, do not accurately reflect levels of oxygen within the baby's circulation. Only by measuring blood concentrations can the actual amounts be known. These are monitored with devices such as transcutaneous oxygen monitors ($tcPO_2$) or pulsoximeters, or they are measured by direct sampling of arterial blood. Ideal arterial oxygen tension or pressure (PaO_2) is 60 to 80 mm Hg. Less than this causes cell death. However, prolonged use of pure oxygen has been found to produce the following adverse effects[*]:

1. Vasoconstriction occurs in the retina and progresses to obliteration; new vessels subsequently proliferate through the retina. Hemorrhages may occur, followed by traction on the retina, which may cause detachment and blindness. This condition, called *retrolental fibroplasia*, is discussed later in this chapter.

2. Progressive respiratory distress occurs in the lungs with pulmonary edema, atelectasis, irritation of the bronchial glands causing hypersecretion of mucus, thickening of alveolar basement membranes, proliferation of capillary tufts, and fibrosis.

3. In animal studies, high concentrations of oxygen appear to cause a change in the vascularization of the brain.

To prevent such tragic occurrences, oxygen is administered only when it is definitely needed. To enhance oxygen absorption by the lungs, and thereby reduce the amount of oxygen needed, steroids and other drugs may be given to preterm infants.

Conservation of energy. The premature infant is handled as little as possible to conserve his or her energy. Usual bath procedures are

---

[*]Adapted from Pierog SH, and Ferrara A: Medical care of the sick newborn, St Louis, 1976, The CV Mosby Co.

reduced to absolute essentials. Because the environment is warm and moist and there is no need for clothing, the infant is placed on a diaper. Thus the extra handling required for dressing is avoided, and absence of clothing makes close observation of the infant possible. Monitors attached to the skin give continuous data about vital functions, thus eliminating the handling that would otherwise be necessary for periodic assessment.

The delicate skin tends to become dry and the buttocks excoriated. Gentle cleansing, exposure to the air, or application of protective ointments may enhance healing.

Waterbeds and foam-rubber and oscillating mattresses are used in some nurseries to provide soft, stimulating support. Preterm infants may be too weak to turn themselves. They must be turned from side to side at least every 1 to 2 hours. They may be placed with the head down and to the side to help drain mucus. Because these babies are totally dependent on others for life, intensive care nurseries are usually staffed with a nurse for each baby.

Maintenance of body temperature. The maintenance of a constant neutral thermal environment, discussed in Chapter 11, is necessary for survival of the premature infant. To provide such an environment, specialized equipment is used, including Isolette incubators, radiant cribs, and other warming systems, as well as oxygen delivery devices, fluid-administration equipment, and various monitoring devices (Fig. 12-6). Nurses must know how each of these devices works, and what to do if any piece of equipment ceases to function properly.

Safety and prevention of infection. Because of the untimely birth of preterm infants, their defenses are underdeveloped. They are easy prey to every variety of infectious disease. Nurses in the intensive care unit therefore must maintain meticulous cleanliness in every aspect of care, including hand washing, sterilization of supplies and equipment,

maintenance of barrier technique, and isolation of the infant from all sources of infection.

Provision of nutritional needs. Nutrition plays an important part in the maintenance and growth of preterm infants. Fluids and nutrients were once withheld for the first 1 to 3 days of life but now are given within a few hours after birth. Thereafter the infant's needs are calculated every 12 to 24 hours on the basis of clinical information (such as intake, output, and weight) and blood chemistry.

When human milk is prescribed, the mother will express it manually and provide a supply to the nursery until the infant is strong enough to nurse at the breast. The method of feeding and the amount given depend on the baby's development, size, and strength. Most preterm infants are bottle-fed, but particularly small ones may be fed by nasogastric or nasojejunal tube until they are able to suck and to swallow enough nourishment to meet their needs. If necessary, intravenous feedings may be prescribed.

Intravenous feedings. Total parenteral nutrition (TPN), or *hyperalimentation,* is the administration of a nutrient solution that provides total nourishment for the infant. It is administered by an intravenous catheter inserted into a central vein such as the internal or external jugular vein. Frequent clinical monitoring of the infant's metabolic status is necessary.

Oral feedings. Oral feedings are given by a variety of means, including medicine droppers with rubber tips and bottles with nipples that are small and very soft. Sometimes it is necessary to insert a tiny nasogastric tube into the stomach. Because of the danger of damaging the delicate tissue or of inserting the tube into the lungs, only nurses who have received special instruction should undertake this procedure. Even when the tube is left in place between feedings, its placement must be checked before each feeding.

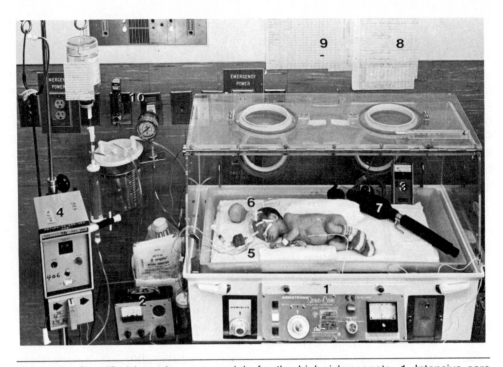

Fig. 12-6 Simplified intensive care module for the high-risk neonate. *1,* Intensive care incubator to regulate automatically environmental temperature to maintain the infant's temperature at a preset level by means of a skin sensor attached to the infant's abdominal skin (Ohio Armstrong); *2,* battery-powered heart rate monitor with audible and visual beat and a low alarm signal; monitor cable attached to the skin with Grass' needle electrodes (Parks Electronics, Grass Intruments Co.); *3,* oxygen continuous analyzer (BMI); *4,* infusion pump to regulate parenteral fluid administration (IVAC); *5,* Millipore filter to screen out bacteria and particulate matter from parenteral solution (Millipore); *6,* suction bulb and DeLee trap; *7,* bag and mask used for resuscitation (Penlon); *8,* graphic record to portray the longitudinal physiological state of an infant; *9,* flow sheet for recording of sequential blood gas and other laboratory data of an infant; *10,* utilities providing outlets for electricity, oxygen, air, and vacuum. *(From Pernoll ML, Benda GI, and Babson SG: Diagnosis and management of the fetus and neonate at risk: a guide for team care, ed 5, St Louis, 1986, The CV Mosby Co.)*

Feeding techniques. Preterm infants must be fed with great care. They are given small amounts slowly, with frequent rest periods and burpings, at 1- to 3-hour intervals. Overfeeding is dangerous, since it may cause regurgitation. The gag reflex is weak, and they may aspirate the regurgitated milk into the lungs.

To help prevent regurgitation, preterm infants are positioned with the head elevated for several minutes after each feeding.

An accurate record of the exact amount of formula taken at each feeding and of the infant's response is important in evaluating the infant's progress.

Perinatal injuries

Although modern obstetrics places much emphasis on prevention, injuries sometimes occur as a result of the birth process. Some of the most common ones are described briefly here.

Forceps marks

Forceps marks are bruises made by the pressure of forceps on the infant's head. They disappear in a few days with no scarring or aftereffects.

Caput succedaneum

Description. Caput succedaneum is a swelling over the area of the scalp that presents in a vertex delivery. It is caused by an effusion of serum and blood into the tissue as a result of pressure on the head during labor.

Assessment and interventions. The swelling is obvious at birth and can be felt as a soft mass. The size and location are noted, and the area is monitored until swelling subsides, usually about 3 days. No treatment is required, but parents may need to be assured that the condition is relatively common and temporary.

Cephalohematoma

Description. Cephalohematoma is an accumulation of blood between one of the skull bones and its membranous covering, the periosteum. Because it is limited by the attachment of the peristeum to the bone affected, margins are well defined.

Assessment and interventions. A cephalohematoma is a soft, movable mass that may not be evident the first day after birth because of the presence of a large caput succedaneum. It may then increase in size for about 2 to 3 days. The size, shape, and location are noted and monitored until swelling subsides.

A cephalohematoma is not aspirated because the needle might carry infectious organisms into the area, causing a dangerous infection. Gradually the blood is absorbed. Although not life threatening, cephalohematoma may be distressing to parents, who need information and reassurance.

Intracranial hemorrhage

Description and assessment. Intracranial hemorrhage is a serious birth injury that is seen most often in infants with bleeding tendencies and infants born of difficult deliveries. Rupture of blood vessels causes bleeding into the brain tissue, producing symptoms of increased intracranial pressure that appear at birth or after several hours. The infant becomes irritable or lethargic and may twitch, convulse, vomit, or become feverish and cyanotic. The baby may have a shrill cry, bulging fontanel, and difficulty sucking or breathing. Sometimes the bleeding stops of itself before serious complications develop, and there are no permanent effects. More severe hemorrhages may cause immediate death or residual damage, such as hydrocephalus, mental retardation, and cerebral palsy.

Interventions. Nurses monitor vital signs and neurological status and assist with various medical and surgical treatments. They elevate the baby's head to about 30 degrees.

Parents are kept informed of the child's status, and tests and treatments are explained. Nurses are available to help the family cope with their fears and grief.

Subdural hematoma

Subdural hematoma is a collection of blood below the dura mater, the outermost membrane covering the brain. The acute form occurs immediately after head trauma. The chronic form occurs in infants with bleeding tendencies. Symptoms of increased intracranial pressure develop. Blood is withdrawn by needle or surgical operation to prevent compression and permanent brain damage, and the infant's condition is monitored closely.

Fractures

Fractures of the bones sometimes occur during delivery. The bones most frequently injured are the clavicle, humerus, and femur. Symptoms of fractures in the newborn infant are (1) discoloration of tissue at site, (2) deformity in alignment or swelling, (3) abnormal mobility or lack of movement, and (4) a shrill cry when the bone is moved.

If fracture is suspected, great care must be taken to immobilize the part and prevent further damage. Traction and splints may be used to immobilize the part during the healing period.

Brachial plexus palsy (Erb-Duchenne paralysis)

Description. Brachial plexus palsy is a paralysis of the upper arm caused by damage to the fifth and sixth cervical spinal nerves. The injury occurs when the infant's shoulder is pulled away from the head during delivery. The arm on the affected side lies limp alongside the body and turns inward. The hand and fingers of the arm are not affected. If paralysis is caused only by edema and hemorrhage around the nerve fibers, function will return in about 3 months. If it is caused by tearing of the nerves, permanent paralysis may result.

Assessment and interventions. Diagnosis is based on a history of a difficult delivery, weakness of the affected arm on examination, loss of the biceps reflex, and decreased Moro's reflex. Extent of injury is determined by the recovery rate.

Treatment is aimed at preventing contractures and maintaining correct placement of the humeral head within its position in the scapula. If function does not return within 3 to 6 months, surgical neuroplasty may be attempted.

Nursing interventions consist of positioning the affected arm so that it is abducted and externally rotated, maintaining range of motion, and teaching parents (Fig. 12-7).

The desired position may be maintained by pinning the shirt sleeve to the mattress. Sometimes a splint or cast is applied. The arm is put through complete passive range of motion exercises daily to maintain muscle tone and function. When dressing the infant, the nurse begins with the affected arm. When undressing the infant, the nurse begins with the unaffected arm. Parents are taught to position and exercise the affected arm and to dress and undress the infant.

Facial nerve paralysis (Bell's palsy)

Description. Injury to facial nerves occurs as a result of pressure on cranial nerve VII. It may take place in utero from fetal positioning, or it may result from pressure by the mother's sacral bone or by a uterine fibroid. Injury also may result from forceps pressure at birth. One or both sides may be affected, causing paralysis of the facial muscles so that the corner of the mouth droops, the eye does not close completely, and sucking is impaired (Fig. 12-8). Paralysis is most noticeable when the infant cries.

Prognosis depends on the extent of nerve damage. More than 90% of those affected recover completely in 6 to 12 months without treatment. If recovery does not occur, surgical neuroplasty may be attempted.

Assessment and interventions. Observation of the face for symmetry (sameness) is part of the initial assessment of neonates. When facial paralysis is present, there is an absence of wrinkling of the forehead and skin around the nose. There is also partial closure of an eye and twisting of the mouth.

No medical or surgical treatment is attempted for at least a year because most children recover completely. If paralysis continues beyond that time, neuroplasty may be

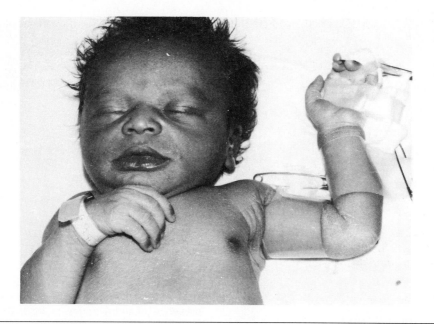

Fig. 12-7 Corrective positioning of left arm of infant with brachial plexus palsy. Note abduction and external rotation of shoulder, flexion at elbow, supination of forearm, and slight dorsiflexion at wrist. *(From Behrman RE, and Seeds AE, eds: Neonatology: diseases of the fetus and infant, ed 2, St Louis, 1977, The CV Mosby Co.)*

considered, although it is not always successful.

Nursing interventions involve helping the infant suck, because part of the mouth cannot close tightly around the nipple. A soft nipple with a large hole may help. Gavage may be necessary to prevent aspiration. Breast-feeding is difficult; the mother may need to compress the areolar area with her fingers to help the infant grasp the nipple.

The eye on the affected side must be protected from injury if the lid does not close completely. To prevent drying of the cornea, an eye patch is applied and artificial tears are instilled. Parents are taught to give eye care, and they also need information and reassurance. The infant's condition is followed closely until facial muscles regain normal movement.

Congenital defects

Sometimes babies are born with defects of body structure. Such defects may be inherited, or they may be caused by irradiation, drugs, or maternal disease. The most critical period of gestation for defects to occur is the first 12 weeks after the ovum is fertilized, as body systems are forming. If the complex process of cell differentiation is disrupted, body organs may be seriously deformed.

Despite these hazards, congenital defects are relatively rare. Those babies born with abnormalities have a greater chance for survival if they are recognized early and if appropriate treatment is begun immediately. For this reason, nurses working in the delivery room and newborn infant nursery should be alert for defects. Once diagnosis is made, treatment is usually carried out in the pediatric depart-

277

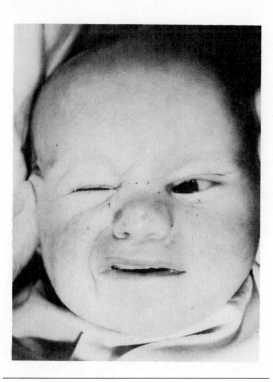

Fig. 12-8 Facial paralysis caused by birth injury of facial nerve.

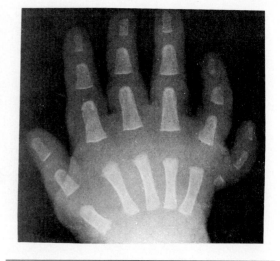

Fig. 12-9 Polydactyly. This child was born with six fingers on each hand and six toes on each foot. The presence of three bones in the extra digit is not unusual.

ment. Some of the most common defects are described here.

Developmental anomalies of the extremities

Description and causes. Congenital anomalies of the extremities vary in severity from slight defects of a finger to the complete absence of all four extremities (Figs. 12-9 and 12-10). These defects result from abnormal embryonic development, which may be caused by inherited traits, by maternal irradiation, or by ingestion during early pregnancy of teratogenic substances such as the drug thalidomide. Defects are described as follows:

adactyly Absent digits; one or more fingers or toes are missing.

amelia Absent limbs; neither arms nor legs develop.

ectromelia Abortive limbs; there is an absence of a limb or limbs (Fig. 12-10).

hemimelia Half limb; the distal portion (hands or feet) is missing.

micromelia Small limbs; the shaft of an extremity is absent, causing severe shortening.

phocomelia Seal limbs; only the distal portion of an extremity is present.

polydactyly Many digits; there are extra fingers or toes (see Fig. 12-9).

syndactyly Joined-together digits; fingers or toes grow together, may involve only skin or may involve bones.

Assessment and interventions. All these anomalies are obvious at birth. When they occur, it is likely that other deformities are present. As a result, these infants are examined carefully and observed closely for signs and symptoms of other defects.

Simple defects are treated immediately. Extra fingers or toes are amputated, or they are

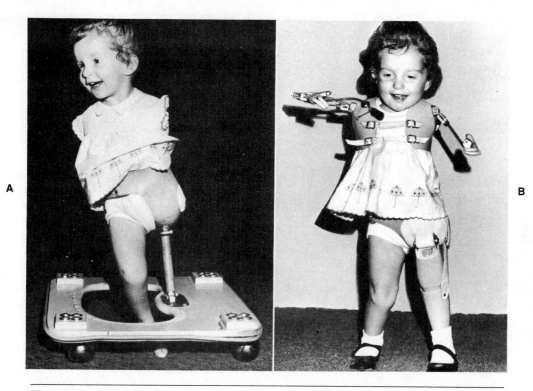

Fig. 12-10 A, Ectromelia of three limbs showing a walking platform created to permit this child to ambulate during her toddler years. **B,** Same little girl as pictured in **A** after she learned to walk with a full leg prosthesis, using her prosthetic arms for balance. (Courtesy The National Foundation—March of Dimes.)

merely tied off with a tight suture, which causes them eventually to drop off. Major defects require careful planning and cooperation of a whole medical team, including pediatrician, orthopedist, prosthetist, social worker, psychologist, occupational therapist, physiotherapist, educators, and nurses. The objective of treatment is to help the child grow to adulthood with minimum dependency and maximum physical and mental health.

Parents play an important role. Initially, the impact of a congenital limb deficiency on parents is profound. Usually the attending physician discusses the problem with them soon after birth. They are included in decisions about treatment. Because tremendous strides have been made in the fields of prosthesis, physical therapy, and occupational therapy, the future is not as bleak as it once was for these children. Public and private funds are available for special equipment and treatment.

Even with information, parents need help to accept their feelings of guilt, fear, helplessness, and sorrow. Talking about these emotions helps, as does sharing them with other parents of disabled children. Nurses also may need to talk about their own anger and feelings of helplessness.

In recent years much research has been devoted to prevention of birth defects. One of the largest private organizations devoted to this cause is the National Foundation–March of Dimes. Originally formed to fight poliomyelitis, the organization now spends millions of dollars for public information, direct services to clients, and research to fight birth defects.

Clubfoot (talipes)

Description and causes. A clubfoot is a foot that is twisted out of its normal position. Any foot deformity that involves the ankle is called *talipes*, derived from *talus*, meaning ankle, and *pes*, meaning foot (Fig. 12-11). Clubbing may involve one or both feet, may be mild or severe, and may be associated with other defects or occur alone. Boys are affected twice as often as girls.

The exact cause of clubfeet is unknown. Some believe it results from arrested embryonic development or abnormal positioning in utero. Because some families have a higher incidence than others, heredity is a factor.

Clubfoot deformities are named by the distorted position of the foot. The two primary types are equinus and calcaneus. *Equinus* means horselike with toes down and foot in plantar flexion. *Calcaneus* means heel prominent with toes elevated and foot in plantar extension. Each type may be *varus* (bent in) or *valgus* (bent out). Talipes equinovarus accounts for 95% of all clubfoot deformities. Talipes calcaneus is the next most common; other types are rare.

Without treatment, children eventually learn to ambulate on the twisted, painful clubs, much as the little girls of ancient China learned to hobble about on their wrapped, deformed feet. When treatment is begun soon after birth and conscientiously continued, prognosis is excellent.

Assessment and interventions. The deformity can be detected at birth by moving the foot to the midline position. Resistance indicates a clubfoot defect.

Once clubfoot is diagnosed, treatment begins immediately. It consists of correction of the defect, maintenance of the correction until normal muscle strength is attained, and fol-

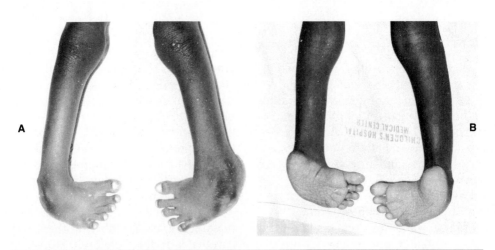

Fig. 12-11   Talipes equinovarus (horselike and bent in) is the most common type of clubbed feet. **A,** View of feet from top. **B,** View of feet from bottom.

low-up observation to prevent recurrence.

Correction consists of serial casting and recasting every 1 to 2 weeks to accommodate the infant's growth and allow for gradual manipulation of the foot to an overcorrected position. Casts extend from toes to groin, with the knees flexed to control heel position and leg rotation. Some surgeons favor manipulation several times per day for the first week or two before casting is begun.

An alternate method of treatment is use of the Denis Browne splint, a device that consists of two padded metal plates to which the infant's feet are securely fastened with adhesive tape or shoes connected to a metal crossbar.

Correction is maintained by special clubfoot shoes designed to maintain the position of the feet. If the defect is left untreated or if treatment is not maintained, surgical repair followed by casting may be necessary.

Nursing interventions consist of performing initial manipulation, when prescribed, and teaching parents to do so. Success of treatment depends on maintenance of the corrected position, which requires the cooperation of parents. Nurses need to encourage parents and teach them how to follow the treatment plan.

Hip dysplasia

Description. Hip dysplasia (underdevelopment) is the most common congenital deformity in the Western world, occurring in 1 in 750 births. It occurs seven times more often in girls than in boys. The defect is rare in the Orient, where infants are carried with their legs astride their mothers' backs, so that if the condition occurs, it is corrected in the course of normal childrearing. Both hips are affected in half the cases. The degree of underdevelopment is described as:

acetabular dysplasia or preluxation Head of femur in place, but acetabulum inadequately developed
dislocation of the hip joint Head of femur not in contact with acetabulum and displaced upward and backward, over fibrocartilaginous rim
subluxation of the hip joint Head of femur in contact with acetabulum but partially displaced, causing pressure on roof and flattening of the socket

If hip dysplasia is not treated in infancy, walking will be delayed, one leg will be shorter than the other, and treatment will be prolonged and less successful.

Assessment. Newborns are assessed for possible hip dysplasia using various maneuvers, such as Ortolani's manipulation (which produces a characteristic click) and Barlow's modification (in which the joint is felt to be unstable). These tests are performed with great care by experienced practitioners only.

Other physical signs include restricted abduction of the affected hip, shortening of the limb on the affected side (Allis's sign), asymmetrical thigh and gluteal folds, and broadening of the perineum (in bilateral dislocations). These signs are the primary means of diagnosis because the bones of infants are mostly cartilage and difficult to visualize on radiographs.

If the diagnosis is missed before a child begins to walk, the affected leg will be shorter than the other one with "piston mobility," that is, the head of the femur can be felt to move up and down in the buttocks. A waddling gait and marked lordosis (swayback) are typical signs. In older children, diagnosis is confirmed with radiography.

Interventions. The object of treatment is to place the head of the femur within the acetabulum. By constant pressure, this position enlarges and deepens the socket and stretches the supporting muscles.

Treatment is achieved by placing both legs in abduction. Treatment varies with the age of the child and with the severity of the defect. When the defect is diagnosed soon after birth, simple abduction by means of double diapering is enough to produce a stable joint. Older infants may need an abduction device made of plastic or a soft pillow (Frejka splint) that can be removed for bathing.

When abduction contracture is present, the hips are slowly and gently stretched to full abduction using a variety of measures such as a modified Bryant's traction on an A-frame or a Putti board. Traction is followed by application of casts or abduction braces until the joint is stable, usually within the first year.

If the defect is not diagnosed until the child begins to walk, traction abduction with casting is prolonged, and open reduction may be necessary to remove soft tissue obstruction, followed by casting. In children older than 4 years of age, reconstruction becomes increasingly difficult. After age 6, reconstruction is not advised because by then there are severe shortening and contracture of muscles and deformity of the bones.

Nevi (birth marks)

Description. Nevi are abnormal markings of the skin that may be present at birth or may appear later in life. There are two general types: pigmented and vascular. Both types are caused by defects in cell growth, probably associated with heredity.

Pigmented nevi. Pigmented nevi are called *birthmarks* when they are present at birth and *moles* when they appear later in life. They vary in size and color from harmless freckles to dark, hairy patches. Pigmented nevi are composed of specialized epithelial cells containing melanin, called *melanocytes.* They are of medical significance because they can change to malignant melanomas, although seldom before puberty. They also can be quite disfiguring.

Treatment is surgical excision. If a nevus is in a place where it is constantly irritated or appears to be growing at a disproportional rate, it is removed because of the danger of malignancy. Disfiguring nevi are removed early in

life to reduce both physical and emotional scarring.

Vascular nevi. Vascular nevi are called *angiomas.* They are localized lesions of the skin caused by an overgrowth of blood or lymph vessels. Those composed of blood vessels are called *hemangiomas;* those composed of lymph vessels are called *lymphangiomas.* Angiomas occur in about one third of all infants. Although most disappear spontaneously, some persist and cause cosmetic problems. Three common types are nevus flammeus, nevus vasculosus, and cavernous hemangioma.

Nevi flammeus, called port-wine stains, are flat, purplish lesions present at birth. They usually do not fade, and there is no effective treatment except hiding them with cosmetic creams.

Nevi vasculosus, called strawberry marks, are raised red lesions that are present at birth or develop soon thereafter (Fig. 12-12). They consist of dilated venules, capillaries, and arterioles that tend to enlarge for a time and then gradually regress, leaving some scarring and pigmentation. If a nevus ulcerates or is near the eye, anus, or urethra, treatment to reduce the size is attempted, including irradiation, electrocoagulation, and injections of sclerosing solutions. Surgical excision may be performed.

Cavernous hemangiomas are raised red and purple lesions composed of large vascular spaces, sometimes containing lymphangiomas, connective tissue, and fat. They seldom regress by themselves; those that do regress are classified as infantile. When regression does not occur or if a life-threatening hemorrhage appears likely, surgical excision with skin grafting is performed.

Lymphangiomas are elevated lesions composed chiefly of lymphatic vessels. They are usually yellowish tan. Treatment is by electrocoagulation or surgical excision.

Assessment and interventions. Nevi that are present at birth are discovered during the ini-

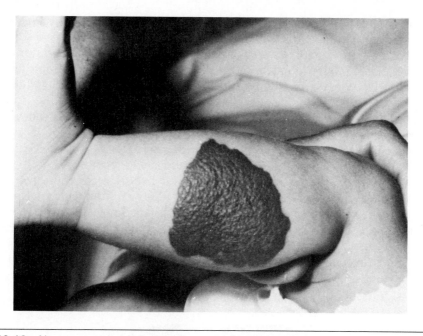

Fig. 12-12 Nevus vascularis, or strawberry mark, on the leg may enlarge after birth but tends to regress with the passage of time.

tial newborn infant examination. If they are large, disfiguring, or life threatening, the infant is referred immediately to a dermatologist. A diagnosis is made and a treatment plan formulated with the parents. A plastic surgeon may be engaged to perform the delicate surgery.

If treatment is deferred in the hope that the lesion will fade with time, nurses may wish to suggest cosmetic preparations to cover the nevi. These preparations are available over the counter in cosmetic stores and drugstores.

Plastic surgery may be done in a brief-stay unit and the child discharged to the home. If skin grafting is required, the child is admitted to the hospital.

Cranial defects

Description. The bones of the fetal skull are separated by fibrous membranes called su-

tures. Normally these sutures gradually fill in with bone and close by the time children are 6 months of age. The soft spot (anterior fontanel) closes by the time they are 16 months of age.

Craniostosis (craniostenosis). In craniostosis one or more of the sutures close too soon. When a suture closes, the bone on both sides stops growing; when sutures remain open, growth continues. Such uneven growth causes various deformed shapes. The condition is serious, not because of the odd-shaped head that results, but because it increases intracranial pressure and interferes with normal brain growth, resulting in mental retardation and blindness.

Microcephaly. This is a condition in which the brain fails to grow. Microcephaly may be caused by a chromosomal defect or result from radiation, toxins, or drugs that damage the developing infant in utero. Brain damage varies from severe to mild. The baby may be completely unresponsive and autistic or may be only mildly motor impaired. Mental retardation is present to some degree in all children with this defect.

Hydrocephaly. Hydrocephalus means "water head." Hydrocephaly is a condition that results in an accumulation of cerebrospinal fluid (CSF) in the ventricles of the brain (Fig. 12-13). It may be present at birth or may occur after birth. Increased CSF can be caused by obstruction of the normal flow, overproduction, or inadequate reabsorption, or it may occur as a result of infection or a space-occupying tumor. The head enlarges from the pres-

sure within because the cranial sutures are not yet closed and the bones are soft.

CSF normally oozes out from the blood vessel tufts in the ventricles within the brain and flows through aqueducts to the subarachnoid space that surrounds the spinal cord and brain. There the fluid is absorbed back into the bloodstream.

Hydrocephalus is classified as noncommunicating and communicating. *Noncommunicating* hydrocephalus results from an obstruction of flow from the ventricles of the brain to the subarachnoid space. The obstruction can occur at any point in the ventricular system. *Communicating* hydrocephalus results when the flow is not obstructed through the ventri-

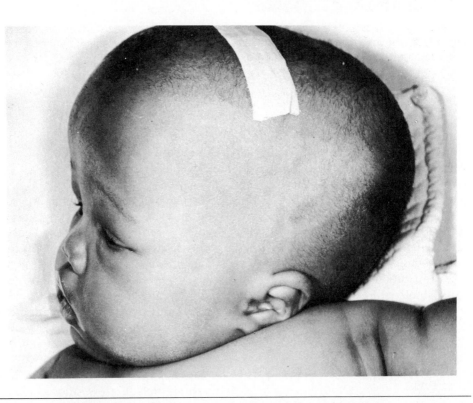

Fig. 12-13 Hydrocephalus. Tape covers site of recent fontanel puncture.

cles but is inadequately circulated or reabsorbed in the subarachnoid space.

In the noncommunicating type, CSF distends the ventricles so that they get larger and larger. Head size increases; cranial bones thin; fontanels bulge; sutures separate; and brain tissue gradually narrows as it is compressed against the skull.

In the communicating type, CSF cannot be absorbed because of congenital malformations or scars from infection or hemorrhage, resulting in an accumulation of fluid outside the brain. The convolutions become flattened; nervous tissue cannot grow; and the fontanels become tense and wide. Pressure of the fluid does not enlarge the head as much as in the noncommunicating type because the brain becomes atrophied, making more space for fluid.

Assessment and interventions. The suture lines of the skull are manually palpated during examination of the neonate. If they are felt to be closed, radiographs are made to confirm a diagnosis of craniostosis. Head circumference is measured at birth and periodically thereafter. Normal measurement at birth is between 13 and 14 inches, or about the same as the crown-to-rump measurement. When head size is greater than normal, diagnostic studies such as transillumination and computed tomographic (CT) scanning may be performed. CSF pressure is measured during aspiration of fluid through a fontanel.

Signs of hydrocephaly depend on the age of onset and amount of increased CSF. When the disorder occurs before birth, the large head may make vaginal delivery impossible. After birth, increase in head size becomes noticeable, and the stretched skin of the scalp appears shiny. The infant is increasingly helpless and unable to lift the head; neck muscles weaken from disuse. The eyes seem to be pushed downward and protrude slightly (setting sun sign). The cry is shrill; the child is irritable, without an appetite. Muscle tone

throughout the body is poor. As the condition worsens, the body becomes emaciated and development is delayed. The child has little resistance to infections. Without medical or surgical intervention, the head becomes enormous and the child dies from malnutrition and infection.

When an infant is born with a defect of such magnitude, the grieving process is complicated and may be prolonged. The family must realistically assess their ability to give home care. If it becomes necessary to place the child in an institution, they may feel guilty. Nurses can help by encouraging family members to express their feelings and by listening with warmth, empathy, and genuine concern. Parents may need approval for such a decision from a health professional or other authority figure.

Neural tube defects

Description. Malformations of the neural tube during embryonic development involve the vertebral column, spinal meninges, and spinal cord. They occur because the midline of the neural plate fails to close as it forms the neural tube during the third and fourth weeks of gestation. These defects range from no symptoms to severe disability. The exact cause is not known, but such defects occur in some families more often than in others.

When the defect is small, marked only by a dimple, port-wine birthmark, or tuft of hair, and if the spinal cord and meninges are normal, the defect is called *spina bifida occulta,* or "hidden."

When the defect is larger, the meninges may protrude through it, forming a sac filled with CSF. This defect is called *spina bifida cystica,* or "saclike." The sac is called a *meningocele.* Because the defect contains no nerve tissue, children are not paralyzed and are able to develop bladder and bowel control. There is potential danger of infection if the sac is torn, and the defect is a cosmetic problem. Therefore, it is surgically corrected as soon as possible.

When a portion of the spinal cord herniates into the meningocele, the condition is called a *myelomeningocele* or a *meningomyelocele* (Fig. 12-14). The sac is covered by a thin membrane that is subject to ulceration and leakage of fluid. Children with this defect suffer partial or complete paralysis and sensory loss below the defect. Hip dislocations and club feet are common. Most children with lumbar or lumbosacral myelomeningocele develop hydrocephalus to some degree, owing to defects of CSF circulation in the brain. They may be incontinent and experience many urinary tract infections as a result of urinary stasis. Lack of bowel tone results in constipation and rectal prolapse. Muscle contractures and osteoporosis from disuse of the limbs make these children more vulnerable to fractures. Convulsions may occur, and mental disabilities are common.

Assessment. The presence of a meningocele is obvious at birth. A complete neurological assessment is made at that time to determine the extent of disability. Head circumference is measured to serve as a baseline for future evaluation, and a CT scan is performed to check for hydrocephaly. A treatment plan is made after consultation with the parents and various specialists.

Medical and surgical treatment. The presence of a spina bifida occulta may not be known at birth. If it is diagnosed, treatment is deferred until a problem arises.

The treatment for meningocele is surgical closure. Treatment of children with myelomeningocele is complex, beginning at birth and continuing throughout their lives. Surgical closure of the myelomeningocele is performed soon after birth to reduce the risk of infection and to prevent further neurological impairment. Skin grafting may be required to close the defect. If hydrocephalus develops, a shunt operation may be performed. The many

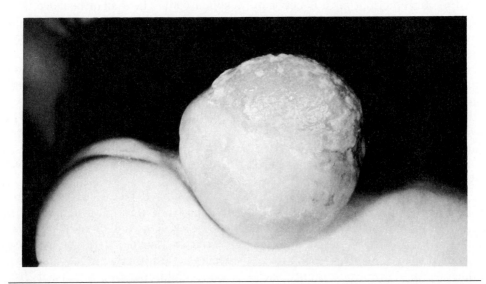

Fig. 12-14 Large myelomeningocele on newborn. *(Courtesy Children's Medical Center, Oakland, Calif.)*

problems created by paralysis, seizures, and mental retardation must be addressed.

Nursing interventions. Nursing interventions involve immediate care after birth and before surgery as well as postoperative and long-term care. The goal of immediate care after birth is to protect the membrane surrounding the meningocele from damage, prevent infection, maintain fluid balance and nutrition, and give the infant human contact.

Careful observations are made of vital signs, degree of incontinence, activity of the legs, signs of increased intracranial pressure, and leakage of CSF. The infant is held for feedings in a sitting position with no pressure on the sac, or the infant may be held with the head over one person's shoulder while another person feeds the infant. When not being held, the infant is positioned on the abdomen or propped on a side with the hips abducted to reduce hip dislocation. The feet are kept in a neutral position to prevent foot deformity, and the ankles are supported by a pad to lift the toes from the bed. Ointment may be applied to the face and knees to prevent chafing.

Diapers are placed beneath, rather than on, the infant. A plastic sheet may be taped to the back below the meningocele to prevent fecal contamination of the sac, and a gauze dressing may be used to cover the meningocele. Parent-infant bonding is encouraged by allowing the parents to participate in the care. Family support and teaching begin with the birth of the infant and continue as the child matures.

Cleft lip and cleft palate

Description, causes, and incidence. Cleft lip and palate are fairly common congenital deformities that appear alone or together in about 1 in 1,000 births. There are many causes, including heredity and teratogens. These defects often are found among children with chromosomal abnormalities.

Cleft lip and palate are defects that result

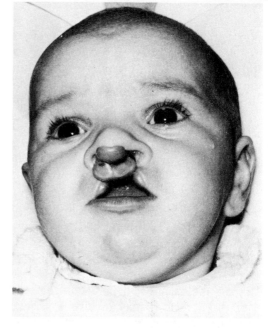

Fig. 12-15 Bilateral cleft lip and palate before repair. *(Courtesy Children's Hospital of the East Bay, Oakland, Calif.)*

from a failure of the embryonic structures of the face to unite. These defects may occur separately or may combine to produce a single unilateral or bilateral cleft from the lip through the soft palate (Fig. 12-15). They interfere with the child's capacity to meet oxygenation and nutritional needs, and they seriously hamper normal parent-child bonding.

Assessment. To determine the extent of abnormality to the soft tissue and hard palate, one must make both visual and manual assessment. In addition, the child is examined carefully to determine if there are defects in other body systems.

Medical and surgical treatment. Initial interventions focus on preventing aspiration of secretions and providing adequate nutrition until surgical intervention is possible. The unnatural openings of the defects make the normal process of sucking and swallowing impossible. These infants cannot create a vacuum in the mouth and therefore cannot suck milk through a nipple. Those with cleft palate cannot control the direction of flow when milk is placed in the mouth because it escapes through the nose or goes down into the trachea. Because of these difficulties, nursing observations and interventions are especially important.

For maximum cosmetic results, surgical intervention to repair the lip defect is performed within the first 2 months of life. A procedure called Z-plasty reduces retraction of the lip and allows for a natural-looking closure of the defect.

Repair of cleft palate depends on the severity of the defect. It may involve a series of procedures that begin when the child is 6 months of age and continue for a number of years.

Nursing interventions. Immediate nursing care after birth involves maintaining an open airway, providing adequate nutrition, and giving emotional support to the parents.

The primary means for maintaining an open airway are positioning, suctioning, and careful feeding. A variety of feeding devices are used to overcome feeding difficulties, including use of a rubber-tipped medicine dropper, Asepto syringe, Brecht feeder, very soft nipple such as a Lamb's nipple, spoon, or cup. Gavage is avoided if possible. Infants must be held in an upright position during feeding to prevent aspiration. They must be burped often because of their increased tendency to swallow air. Suction should be readily available to remove secretions or milk that may block the airway. Some children with cleft palate are fitted with a prosthesis to cover the open palate and guard against regurgitation until corrective surgery can be done. This device also aids children as they learn to speak.

Parents need a great deal of support and information when a child is born with a cleft lip. The face-to-face interaction of the bonding process is disrupted by the deformity. Parents need to talk about their feelings, to see nurses cuddle and talk to the infant as lovable, and to discuss the plan of treatment with the plastic surgeon. Before taking the baby home to await surgery, parents need detailed instructions and opportunities to feed and care for the infant with supervision. Such practice gives parents a sense of control and confidence.

Esophageal atresia and tracheoesophageal fistula

Description and incidence. Esophageal atresia is a congenital defect in which the upper segment of the esophagus ends in a blind pouch. Tracheoesophageal fistula is a defect in which embryonic structures fail to divide into a separate esophagus and trachea, causing an opening (fistula) between the two structures. Although esophageal atresia and tracheoesophageal fistula may occur separately, they often occur together, with the upper portion of the esophagus ending in a blind pouch and the portion just above the stomach connecting to the trachea. Sometimes the esophagus is connected to the trachea so that feedings go directly into the lungs.

Esophageal atresia occurs in about 1 of 3,500 live births. Many of these infants are premature or of low birth weight. About one fourth are born with other anomalies.

Assessment. Depending on the defect, various symptoms appear. Copious oral and nasal secretions may be the first sign of a defect. The infant may cough or choke and become cyanotic. When suctioning or gavage is attempted, the catheter cannot pass into the stomach. Infants with tracheoesophageal fistula may have distended abdomens because of trapped air in the stomach, and they may develop aspiration pneumonia.

The extent and location of the defect are

determined by means of fluoroscopic studies and bronchoscopy.

Medical and surgical treatment. Medical care focuses on prevention of aspiration. A drainage tube may be placed in the blind pouch to suction pooled secretions.

Esophageal atresia is considered a surgical emergency. Surgical repair may be done in a one-stage or two-stage procedure, depending on the defect. Where there is sufficient tissue, the two segments of the esophagus are sewn together in what is called an *end-to-end anastomosis*. If there is insufficient tissue, a section of colon may be transplanted to connect the esophageal stump to the stomach. A feeding tube may be inserted into the stomach through a gastrostomy until the repair heals. A tracheostomy also may be necessary.

A common complication of these surgeries is the formation of esophageal *strictures* (narrowed sections). When strictures occur, the child may need repeated dilations to prevent complete closure of the esophagus.

Nursing interventions. Detection of the defect, prevention of aspiration when diagnosed, and attainment of normal function after surgery are the nursing goals. Nurses in the delivery room and nursery observe infants for symptoms, but even so, defects may not be diagnosed until infants aspirate a feeding. For this reason, many hospitals require the first feeding to be sterile water.

Once diagnosed, infants are placed in a head-up position with continuous suctioning. This is done to guard against aspiration and reflux of acid into the trachea. Intravenous fluids are administered until surgery. When surgery is postponed for more than 48 hours, hyperalimentation may be prescribed.

Postoperative care is given in intensive care nurseries. Gastrostomy feedings are begun, during which infants are given pacifiers to help them retain the sucking reflex and to provide comfort. When possible, infants are held quietly for a time after feedings. As soon as possible oral feedings are begun to reduce the degree of stricture of the esophagus.

Parents of these infants need much support and information. They are encouraged to participate in the care and feeding of the infant to facilitate the normal bonding process and to increase their confidence and skill.

Hernias

A hernia is the protrusion of an organ or part of an organ through the wall of the cavity in which it is normally contained. Hernias are caused by failure of certain normal openings to close during fetal development or from an increase in intraabdominal pressure, such as that occurring during a cough or when lifting a heavy object. The most common types of hernias in children are umbilical hernia, omphalocele, gastroschisis, inguinal hernia, femoral hernia, and diaphragmatic hernia.

Umbilical hernia

Description. During fetal life, the umbilical vessels pass out through an opening in the abdominal wall. Soon after birth these vessels normally shrivel, the peritoneum and connective tissues close, and the skin heals. If the connective tissue fails to close completely and a circular defect remains beneath the umbilicus, a hernia sac may form that is covered by skin and lined by peritoneum. Such defects are relatively common in infants, especially in black children.

Small umbilical defects usually close spontaneously before the second year of life. Larger ones that persist beyond age 5 may need surgical closure. Surgery is required if strangulation occurs.

Assessment and interventions. The infant's abdomen is inspected for a protruding umbilicus. If present, the sac is palpated for abdominal contents and approximate size.

No intervention is needed for most unbilical hernias. If they are large and persist beyond

5 years of age or if strangulation occurs, surgical repair is necessary. For uncomplicated surgical repair, the child may be admitted to the short stay unit and return home immediately afterward.

Nursing interventions are directed toward teaching parents safe, effective care and how to assess the hernia for strangulation. Belly binders are not recommended. They do not reduce hernias and may hold moisture against the skin, causing excoriation. Taping of coins into the hernia may damage the skin and will prevent natural closure. If a portion of bowel enters the sac and cannot be pushed back into the abdominal cavity, the child should be taken to the emergency room immediately.

Inguinal and femoral hernias.

Description. An *inguinal hernia* is a protrusion of peritoneum through the abdominal wall in the inguinal canal. It most often occurs in males, is frequently bilateral, and may be visible as a mass in the scrotum.

As the testes descend during embryonic life, a sac of peritoneum precedes them into the scrotum, forming a canal. After descent of the testes, the canal normally closes and atrophies. If it does not close completely, peritoneal fluid or intestine or both may descend into the canal and produce an inguinal hernia. A collection of fluid in the sac is called a *hydrocele* (Fig. 12-16). Inguinal hernias vary in size, depending on how far they extend into the sac. In girls the anatomy is different, but parallel, in that the inguinal canals are occupied by the round ligaments. An ovary or a loop of intestine may descend into the space, creating an inguinal hernia.

A *femoral hernia* is a protrusion of peritoneum through the wall of the femoral canal, a potential space next to the femoral artery. It occurs more frequently in girls and is felt or seen as a small mass on the anterior surface of the thigh just below the inguinal ligament in the femoral canal.

Assessment and interventions. When a hernia sac is empty, there are no symptoms. If a portion of the bowel descends into the sac, an incomplete bowel obstruction may occur, causing infants to be fretful, lose their appetites, and become constipated. If a loop of intestine becomes incarcerated in the sac, all the symptoms of intestinal obstruction appear. The infant vomits, develops a fever, and has a firm, irreducible swelling in the groin. If the hernia cannot be reduced within 12 hours after it occurs, emergency surgery is required. In severe cases when the blood supply has been cut off, resection of that portion of the bowel may be necessary. Incarceration occurs most frequently in the first 6 weeks of life in infants with inguinal hernia.

Omphalocele and gastroschisis

Description. The word *omphalocele* literally means "umbilical swelling." It is a herniation of abdominal viscera at the point where the umbilical cord connects to the abdomen. It occurs because the abdominal wall fails to develop during embryonic life. More than half of infants born with omphalocele have other congenital defects and 35% die, even with treatment.

Gastroschisis literally means "gastric cleft." It is a relatively uncomplicated failure of the abdominal wall to close, allowing evisceration of abdominal contents. The mortality rate is 15%.

In both omphalocele and gastroschisis the infant is born with all or part of the abdominal viscera exposed, covered only by a transparent membrane. Rupture of that membrane may lead to infection or complete intestinal obstruction as a result of disruption of the intestines.

Assessment, planning, and interventions. The abdomen is examined carefully to determine the extent of the defect, the presence of other defects, and to formulate a plan of action. The general condition is assessed to determine if the infant will be able to undergo immediate surgery.

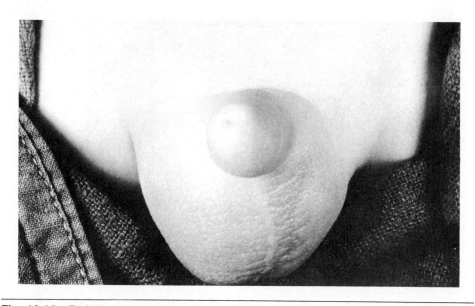

Fig. 12-16 Right inguinal hernia with a collection of fluid in the hernia sac called a *hydrocele. (Courtesy Children's Medical Center, Oakland, Calif.)*

At delivery the omphalocele sac is covered immediately with sterile, moist gauze to reduce drying and contamination by air-borne bacteria. Surgery may then be performed. If a large amount of the bowel has remained outside the abdominal cavity during fetal development, the cavity may be too small to contain the mass. In these cases, a prosthetic sac of synthetic material may be constructed to contain the viscera. The sac is then gently compressed over a period of 5 to 10 days as bowel wall edema lessens and abdominal space expands.

A nonsurgical method of treatment has been found that is less hazardous, especially in cases of large omphaloceles. This treatment consists of repeated applications of 2% Mercurochrome to the sac. A tough layer of scar tissue forms, covers the omphalocele, and converts it into a large ventral hernia, which is repaired later.

Nursing interventions involve protecting the fragile omphalocele sac from rupture and infection and providing the other survival needs of the infant. Until surgery is scheduled the infant is cared for in an intensive care nursery, where the general condition can be evaluated on a continuing basis. Parents are encouraged to visit and cuddle these babies, to talk to them, and to provide them with environmental stimuli such as mobiles, toys, and music until they have recovered enough to go home.

Imperforate anus

Description. During embryonic life the membrane that separates the rectum and anus is normally absorbed, leaving an open, continuous canal. If absorption fails to occur, imperforate anus results (Fig. 12-17). In newborn infants, this defect is the most common one that is incompatible with life.

The anus may appear as a dimple or may look quite normal but end in a blind pouch.

291

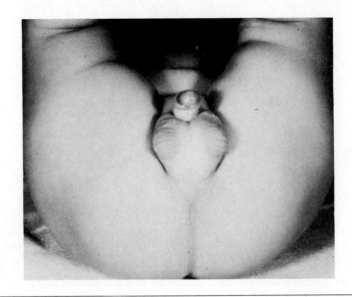

Fig. 12-17 Imperforate anus showing a small dimple where anus should be. *(Courtesy Children's Medical Center, Oakland, Calif.)*

Sometimes an abnormal tube called a *rectoperineal fistula* forms between the rectum and the perineum. A *rectovaginal fistula* may form in girls and a *rectourethral fistula* in boys. When these defects are present at birth, meconium may appear on the perineum, in the vagina, or in the urine. If there is a blind pouch without an outlet, the infant develops abdominal distention and vomits.

Assessment and interventions. Assessment of the newborn infant includes inspecting the anus and checking the rectum for patency. The alert nursery nurse may be the first to note meconium in the vagina or urine, indicating a fistula. The absence of stools during the first 24 hours of life or the development of a distended abdomen may indicate an imperforate anus.

Surgical intervention is necessary for all of these defects. When possible, an anoplasty is performed immediately. If the infant is weak or sick, the anoplasty may be delayed and a temporary colostomy made. In cases of abdominal distention and vomiting, nasogastric suction is begun before surgery.

Exstrophy of the bladder

Description and complications. Exstrophy of the bladder is an extensive defect in the midline closure of the lower abdomen that leaves the pubic bone separated and the bladder completely exposed. It is three times more common in boys than in girls. In boys the defect may extend from the umbilicus to the tip of the penis. In girls the clitoris may be cleft, the labia separated, and the vagina absent. Indirect inguinal hernia and undescended testicles also may occur.

Exstrophy of the bladder is compatible with life, but the complications are serious, and treatment involves complicated plastic surgery. The infant is constantly soaked with urine that drains directly from the ureters, causing excoriation of the skin and considerable discomfort. Infections and ulcerations of the exposed mucosa may occur. Bacteria may invade the kidney, causing pyelonephritis.

Assessment and interventions. Diagnosis is made at birth when the infant's abdomen and genitalia are examined.

The goals of intervention are to preserve kidney function, attain urinary control, and provide reconstructive repair. Initially, sterile petroleum gauze is placed over the exposed bladder and additional diapers are wrapped about the abdomen for more absorbency. A plastic surgeon may be called on to evaluate the infant and to plan a course of repair, which usually involves several procedures. Surgery may be delayed until the infant is several months old.

Diapers are changed frequently, and ointment is applied to the skin to protect it. Because surgical repair will not occur for many months, parents must learn how to care for the child before he or she is discharged. With patience and encouragement, the nurse supervises the parents as they learn to care for their infant. A birth defect as large and deforming as exstrophy of the bladder is difficult to accept. Parents need to feel safe in expressing feelings of guilt, anger, and sadness to the nurse. They may appreciate referral to a community health nurse for home supervision of the infant.

Hypospadias

Description and assessment. Hypospadias is a common deformity in which the urethra of the male opens somewhere along the lower surface of the penis (Fig. 12-18). Because the sphincter is not affected, children can learn urine control. In more extensive defects, a cordlike anomaly called a *chordee* may bow the penis downward so that the tip of the glans lies near the abnormal opening. Diagnosis is made at birth on examination.

Interventions. Soon after birth a plastic surgeon may be called on to plan the repair for

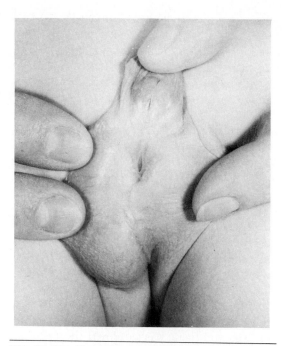

Fig. 12-18 Hypospadias with an undescended left testicle. *(Courtesy Children's Medical Center, Oakland, Calif.)*

hypospadias. If the meatus is near the glans, a high circumcision may be all that is required. For more extensive defects, circumcision is not performed because the foreskin may be needed in a urethroplasty that may involve several successive procedures. Repair is usually planned before school age to avoid the psychological damage of ridicule to the boy.

Epispadias

Epispadias is less common than hypospadias except in conjunction with exstrophy of the bladder. In this defect the urethra opens on the upper surface of the penis. Various degrees may occur: the urethral meatus may lie just behind the glans, or the urethra may lie open along the full length of the penis. As with hypospadias, treatment is surgical repair tailored to the defect. It may be accomplished in one procedure or may take many. The psychological problems of being "different" are similar to those of hypospadias.

Cryptorchidism (undescended testes)

Description and complications. Cryptorchidism, or "hidden testes," is the absence of one testis or both testes from the scrotal sac. It occurs in about 2% of the male population. Because testes normally descend from the abdomen during the seventh to ninth months of gestation, premature infants are more likely to have the defect. There are two types of cryptorchidism: true and ectopic. In *true cryptorchidism* the testis has never been in the scrotal sac but may be found anywhere along the way above the inguinal ring. In *ectopic cryptorchidism*, the testis passed down the inguinal canal through the external ring but moved partly back.

A misplaced testis is more subject to developmental failure, trauma, and tumor formation. Inguinal hernia, hydrocele, and torsion of the vas deferens commonly occur with cryptorchidism. In addition, the developing boy may be the object of ridicule, resulting in a distorted sense of self-worth.

Assessment. Diagnosis of undescended testes is complicated by the normal retraction reflex of the cremaster muscles of the scrotum when they are touched. The reflex is overcome by applying firm pressure on the external ring in the groin before touching the scrotum. Ectopic testes may be felt along the inguinal canal; those in the abdomen cannot.

Interventions. Spontaneous descent sometimes occurs during the first year of life. If it does not, the hormone human chorionic gonadotropin may be prescribed to help enlarge the testes and facilitate descent. If hormone therapy is unsuccessful by the age of 5 years, surgical intervention (orchiopexy) is recommended. If left in the abdomen, spermatogenesis is impaired by the higher body temperature, which results in sterility.

Intersexual defects

Description and incidence. In Greek mythology Hermaphroditus had both male and female reproductive organs. When a child is born with ambiguous genitalia, it is usually one of four conditions: (1) female pseudohermaphroditism (masculinized female), (2) mixed gonadal dysgenesis (chromosomal mosaics), (3) male pseudohermaphroditism, and (4) true hermaphroditism.

The most common, *female pseudohermaphroditism*, is the result of excessive amounts of adrenal androgens. It is most often caused by congenital adrenal hyperplasia, which is an inherited deficiency in the enzymes of adrenal corticoid synthesis. Female pseudohermaphroditism is the only life-threatening intersex problem.

The second most common defect, *mixed gonadal dysgenesis*, is caused by a variety of chromosomal errors, such as the Klinefelter's syndrome.

Male pseudohermaphrodites are true males, but they have not received enough androgen or have responded poorly to what was received. As a result, the male external genitalia do not develop fully and the infant appears to be a girl.

True hermaphrodites are born with both male and female genitalia. The chromosomal sex may be male or female. Although the condition is rare, in all intersexual cases the possibility of true hermaphroditism must be considered.

Assessment. When a child is born whose sex is not immediately obvious, an extensive diagnostic evaluation is performed that includes the following items:

1. The mother's family and prenatal history (includes relatives with ambiguous genitalia, steroid drug ingestion, and profound emotional shock during first 6 weeks of gestation)
2. Physical examination (does not provide enough data)
3. Buccal smears (determine chromosomal sex)
4. Chromosomal studies (determine chromosomal defects and genetic sex)
5. Magnetic resonance imaging (MRI), radiography, or endoscopy (reveals presence and nature of internal genitalia)
6. Gonad biopsy and laparotomy (may be only means for a definitive diagnosis)

Interventions. The assignment of gender sex to an infant whose sex is doubtful is called a "social emergency." Long-term implications are great. The determination of sex should be done before parents announce the child's sex to their family and before a birth certificate is filed. Although this anomaly has little effect on physical health, it has a great impact on emotional health. The social role of a boy is much different from that of a girl. It is harmful for a child to be reared as one sex and find out later that the other is correct.

The decision of which sex to rear a child is made after genetic sex is determined. *The infant's anatomy rather than genetic sex is the primary criterion for assigning gender*. If the genetic sex is male and the infant has an adequate penis, he may be reared as a boy. In this case, testosterone will be administered at puberty, and female organs will be surgically removed.

A functional vagina can be constructed surgically but a functional penis cannot. A female without a uterus or ovaries can lead a relatively normal life, but a male without a penis cannot. For this reason, in most cases it is recommended that infants with ambiguous sex and an inadequate penis be reared as females. Inappropriate internal and external structures are removed, and female hormones are administered at puberty to produce female secondary sex characteristics.

When diagnostic studies are complete, the parents and surgeon decide on a course of action. Meanwhile, parents need a great deal of support and encouragement. They may be confused, anxious, and ashamed. They may appreciate the suggestion that they give the child a unisex name, such as Sidney. Nursing interventions are directed toward providing parents empathetic support and information as the long-term plan is implemented.

Heart malformations

Heart malformations are classified according to whether they produce cyanosis (cyanotic) or not (acyanotic).

Acyanotic diseases are those in which pulmonary circulation and systemic circulation are not connected or, if there is a connection, the pressure is higher in the left side than in the right side of the heart. Some of the most common include patent ductus arteriosus, atrial and ventricular septal defects, coarctation of the aorta, and pulmonic and aortic stenosis (Fig. 12-19). These conditions produce murmurs, retarded growth, heart enlargement, and congestive heart failure.

Cyanotic diseases are those in which there is incomplete oxygen saturation of arterial blood, whether or not the skin and mucous membranes appear blue. Some of these diseases are tetralogy of Fallot (Fig. 12-19), transposition of the great vessels, tricuspid atresia, total anomalous pulmonary venous return, and truncus arteriosus.

Without surgical intervention, prognosis for any of these conditions is extremely poor.

When diagnosis is made at birth, the infant immediately is transferred to a neonatal intensive care unit. Parents need information and empathetic support.

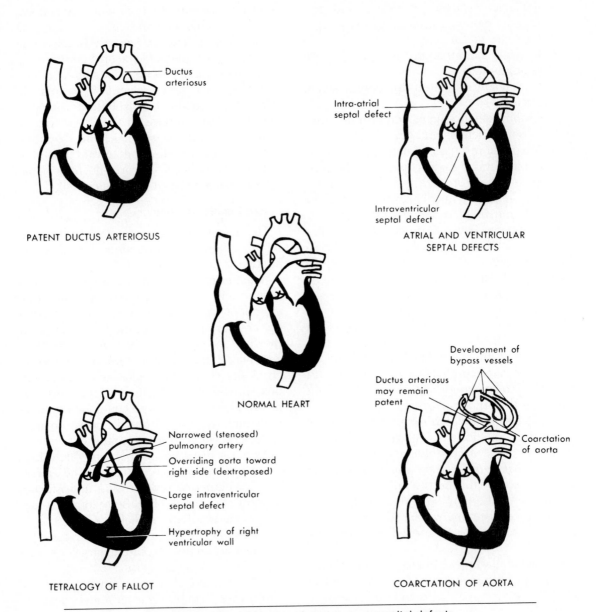

Fig. 12-19 Normal heart and common congenital defects.

Diseases

Because sick babies are seen only briefly in the maternity unit before they are transferred to a neonatal or pediatric unit, only the most common diseases are discussed here.

Diarrhea

Description and causes. Newborn infants usually have four to five stools a day. When stools occur more frequently, the condition is called *diarrhea*. For underdeveloped or sick infants, diarrhea is serious because a loss of water and chemicals can produce fatal electrolyte imbalance.

In infants, two common causes of diarrhea that are not related to illness are overfeeding and a high-fat formula. These problems can be corrected easily by adjusting the ingredients and amount of feedings.

Diarrhea also may be caused by infections anywhere in the infant's body. The most dangerous form is diarrhea caused by pathogenic organisms that invade the intestinal tract. These organisms may be highly contagious, infecting all of the infants in a nursery.

Prevention and interventions. To prevent such epidemics, strict handwashing technique is observed between infants. Linens are sterilized, and overhead antiseptic lights are installed in nurseries.

When symptoms of diarrhea occur in any infant in a nursery, the infant immediately is isolated and the physician notified. Stool cultures and clinical signs are used to diagnose the cause. General treatment includes replacement of body fluids and electrolytes and special skin care to prevent excoriation.

Jaundice

Description and causes. Jaundice is caused by excessive amounts of bilirubin in the tissue. Bilirubin is the pigment found in hemoglobin and bile. It breaks down more quickly in the presence of light and is eliminated largely in the urine. If bilirubin levels become elevated, the excess is deposited in various body tissues. In the skin these deposits cause a yellow color called *jaundice*. In the brain they cause damage to the nervous tissue that may result in mental retardation or even death.

Jaundice may be physiological or pathological. *Physiological jaundice* occurs because there is a normal reduction in the number of red blood cells after birth. As a consequence, free bilirubin levels rise as extra red cells are broken down. *Pathological jaundice* occurs because of abnormal conditions such as erythroblastosis fetalis, bile duct defect, or septicemia. The liver plays an important role in breaking down bilirubin so it can be eliminated from the body. Because their livers are immature, preterm infants are less able to eliminate excess bilirubin than are full-term infants. Preterm infants are therefore more likely to become jaundiced and to suffer the more serious effects of hyperbilirubinemia.

Assessment and interventions. Jaundice is assessed by observing the skin and the whites of the eyes under white light. A more accurate measure of bilirubin levels is obtained from laboratory study of blood samples.

All jaundice is reported at once so that blood levels of bilirubin can be assessed. Depending on these levels, treatment is planned. It includes use of a blue-spectrum lamp to hasten bilirubin breakdown, intravenous fluids, and exchange transfusions when the problem is due to a blood dyscrasia such as erythroblastosis fetalis. When infants are placed under blue-spectrum lamps, it is important to cover their eyes to prevent retinal damage.

Vomiting

Causes and assessment. The most common cause of vomiting in both preterm and full-term infants is too-rapid feeding or overfeeding. Vomiting also may be caused by congenital deformities of the gastrointestinal tract or by increased intracranial pressure.

To determine the cause of vomiting, one should obtain the following information: (1) time in relation to the last feeding, (2) amount of the last feeding, (3) amount of vomitus, (4) color and consistency of the vomitus, (5) odor, (6) force of ejection, and (7) infant's general appearance and response at the time of vomiting, such as cyanosis or pain. Repeated vomiting of feedings can disrupt an infant's fluid balance, quickly causing serious dehydration and electrolyte imbalance. A record of these data must be kept so that a correct diagnosis can be made.

Planning and interventions. Whenever an infant vomits, regardless of cause, there is danger that vomitus will block the airway. Nursery personnel therefore must be prepared to give emergency care.

Emergency interventions are as follows: wipe vomitus out of the infant's mouth, lower the head, milk the trachea toward the mouth, and suction with a bulb syringe. More extensive suctioning can be instituted if necessary.

As a precaution against aspiration, infants never should be left lying with the face straight up. The head is turned to the side, regardless of body position.

The most obvious way to prevent vomiting from too-rapid feeding is to give the baby smaller amounts more slowly. It also is important to hold infants with the head slightly elevated, to burp them frequently, and to return them to bed without excessive juggling. It is helpful to place the infant on his or her right side to enhance the flow of stomach contents toward the small intestine.

If vomiting persists in spite of feeding technique, if it is projectile, or if it is accompanied by other symptoms such as fever, convulsions, or cyanosis, various diagnostic procedures may be prescribed.

Convulsions

Description and causes. Convulsions are paroxysms of involuntary muscular contractions and relaxations that result from central nervous irritation. They are never normal and are a serious sign in any newborn infant. Convulsions are caused by intracranial hemorrhage, congenital cerebral defects, prolonged anoxia, hypoglycemia, hyperglycemia, fever, and overwhelming infection. In a sick or underdeveloped infant, convulsions are especially serious because of the anoxia and stress they produce.

Assessment and interventions. An accurate description of a convulsion helps form the diagnosis. This description includes any preliminary sign, the duration of the convulsion, whether the convulsion is generalized or localized, and what parts of the body are involved.

If a convulsion occurs, the infant is placed under constant observation and a description is reported to the physician at once. Oxygen may be given if there was any prolonged anoxia. Diagnostic studies of the blood and brain are done to determine the cause. Specific medical treatment depends on the findings of these studies.

Retrolental fibroplasia

Description and cause. Retrolental fibroplasia was first recognized in 1942 in children who were premature or small for gestational age and who had received high oxygen concentration during the first 7 to 10 days of life.

In the presence of high oxygen concentrations, immature blood vessels begin a period of accelerated growth that continues for several days or weeks. The extent of growth cannot be detected for 4 to 6 weeks, but by the age of 3 months it is well defined. These overgrown vessels eventually regress but leave scar tissue. Sometimes the swollen veins rupture and the hemorrhaged blood causes the retina to detach from the inner surface of the eye. Glaucoma and corneal opacity may follow, with partial or complete blindness.

Prevention and treatment. Prevention is the only way to reduce the incidence of retrolental fibroplasia. In the past, oxygen concentrations of 40% were considered safe, but recent studies have shown that any concentration of oxygen above the normal 21% atmospheric level is *unsafe* (toxic) for noncyanotic premature infants.

Risk for cyanotic premature infants is high. Laser surgery is being used in some medical centers to reduce vessel growth, thereby limiting vision loss in some infants.

Respiratory distress syndrome (hyaline membrane disease)

Description and cause. Respiratory distress syndrome (RDS) is responsible for more infant deaths than any other disease. It occurs almost exclusively in preterm infants, infants of diabetic mothers, and infants born by cesarean birth. These infants are born before their lungs are ready to function efficiently as gas-exchanging organs. Full-term infants, on the other hand, can usually establish respiratory function without difficulty. The primary reason for this adaptation is maturity of the *surfactant system*.

Surfactant acts as a detergent to reduce the surface tension of the fluids that coat the alveoli and respiratory passages. It permits uniform lung expansion and prevents complete collapse of the lungs after each breath. Surfactant consists of surface-active phospholipids secreted by the epithelium, among which are *lecithin* and *sphingomyelin*. Lecithin is the more active. It is not manufactured in significant amounts, however, until gestational age is 34 to 35 weeks. When the lecithin/sphingomyelin (L/S) ratio is 2 to 1 (stated as 2.0), the likelihood of developing RDS is greatly reduced.

Without surfactant the infant must exert great effort to reexpand the air sacs with each breath. Atelectasis (collapsed lungs), hypox-

emia (inadequate oxygen in the blood), and hypercapnia (excessive carbon dioxide) result. Metabolic acidosis and respiratory acidosis develop. Eventually, damaged lung cells, serum, and white blood cells combine to form a fibrous material called a *hyaline membrane*. This membrane fills the air sacs and further reduces the elasticity of the lungs.

Assessment. The typical infant with RDS is born without obvious respiratory distress. Within minutes or hours, however, a membrane forms within the lungs. The respiratory rate zooms to 60 times a minute or more, and the infant makes a desperate effort to obtain oxygen. The ribs retract, and there is an expiratory grunt, a weak cry, oral bubbling, and deepening cyanosis. If untreated, more than half of the infants with RDS die within 18 hours after birth. With treatment, more than 85% of these babies can be saved, including many who weigh less than 2 pounds (about 900 gm).

Interventions. Prenatal preventive measures help reduce infant mortality. This includes prenatal monitoring of lecithin levels in the amniotic fluid of susceptible infants, such as infants of diabetic mothers. This information indicates the maturity of the fetal lungs. Some physicians administer steroids such as betamethasone to the mother 1 to 2 days before the expected delivery. Steroids enter the fetal bloodstream by way of the placenta and stimulate the lungs to produce surfactant. As a result, the infant is less likely to develop RDS.

When RDS is suspected, the newborn infant is transferred to a neonatal intensive care unit for continuous observation and specialized care. Ordinary respirators usually do not work because the lungs of RDS babies collapse with each breath. The problem is treated with continuous positive airway pressure (CPAP) or positive end-expiratory pressure (PEEP) in which oxygen is given under pressure through an intubation airway or plastic hood. The pressure keeps the lungs from collapsing until the infant begins producing enough surfactant to prevent the membrane from forming.

Phenylketonuria

Description and incidence. Phenylketonuria (PKU) is an inborn error of metabolism that causes severe mental retardation. It occurs in about 1 in 9,000 births and is caused by a deficiency of a liver enzyme that changes phenylalanine to tyrosine. Phenylalanine is an amino acid present in all natural protein foods. In the absence of tyrosine, phenylalanine changes to abnormal by-products that accumulate in the blood; the excess is excreted in the urine and through the skin. High levels of these by-products prevent normal brain development as a result of degeneration of the cells and defective myelination of the nerves. These children are characteristically blonde and blue-eyed with fair skin because their bodies do not convert phenylalanine to tyrosine, which is necessary for the production of the pigment melanin.

The defect is transmitted by inheritance of a recessive gene that is carried by about 1 in 40 members of the population. If two such persons marry, the chances are one in four that one child will be normal, two in four that the child will be a carrier as were the parents, and one in four that the child will have the disease. In some families the proportion of affected children is higher.

Assessment. Diagnosis is made by finding phenylalanine in the blood or its abnormal by-products in the urine. In most states phenylketonuria screening is mandatory for all newborn infants. The most frequently used test is of blood. At birth the serum level of phenylalanine may be normal (1 to 4 mg per 100 ml), but as soon as the baby with PKU begins to take milk the serum level rises rapidly to 15 to 100 mg per 100 ml. The infant *must* have had protein 24 to 48 hours before the test for it to be valid.

Other tests are based on the presence of the abnormal by-products in the urine. Because it takes 2 to 4 weeks for these by-products to be present in sufficient amounts for test accuracy, brain damage already may have occurred. For this reason, early blood tests are preferred.

The prognosis of children with PKU is directly related to how soon they are placed on a low-phenylalanine diet.

Interventions. Medical management focuses on minimizing the intake of phenylalanine. Because children need a certain amount of phenylalanine for normal growth, some must be allowed. Because tyrosine is not being formed, this amino acid must be added to the diet. Infants are begun on a synthetic formula such as Lofenalac that lowers blood levels of phenylalanine. As the child grows older, foods low in phenylalanine are added to the diet. Serum levels are monitored to keep them between 2 and 7 mg per 100 ml to provide adequate nutrition without mental damage.

A low-phenylalanine diet is maintained until the child is 7 to 9 years of age. By then, 90% of brain growth has occurred. Adult women with PKU should be counseled to return to a low-phenylalanine diet during pregnancy because a high level can cause mental retardation in affected fetuses.

Nursing management is directed toward providing dietary education and emotional support. When parents first learn that their infant has this condition, they may be extremely distressed and need to express their feelings. Information about the condition and the special diet required to reduce mental retardation may need to be repeated. When possible, parents may be referred to a nutritionist for additional information.

Umbilical cord infection (omphalitis)

Description. At birth the umbilical cord is clamped or tied, and within a few days it normally shrinks, dried up, and falls off. The small remaining area heals over and forms the umbilicus, or navel. Occasionally bacteria invade the cord stump and an infection, called *omphalitis,* occurs. The first signs are moistness of the cord, a foul odor, and a thin discharge. The area around the cord then becomes inflamed. The discharge increases, is foul in odor, and is more profuse. The baby develops a fever as the infection becomes increasingly toxic. Without treatment, death may occur in a few days.

Assessment and interventions. To prevent such infections, the cord is painted with applications of 70% alcohol until the navel is fully healed. If the cord begins to show evidence of infection and the skin becomes red and swollen, the physician is notified at once. A culture and sensitivity test is done to identify the organism and antibiotics to which it is sensitive. Treatment depends on how far the infection has advanced and includes both systemic and local antibiotic applications.

The danger of omphalitis is greater when babies are dismissed from the hospital soon after they are born. Mothers should be instructed to keep the navel dry and to paint the area daily with 70% alcohol until it is fully healed. If the skin around the navel becomes red, the mother is instructed to report it at once.

Sexually transmitted diseases

Newborn infants may be infected by sexually transmitted diseases (STD) from their mothers before or during passage through the birth canal. These diseases are caused by a variety of pathogens that produce especially serious disorders in newborns. These include gonorrhea, chlamydia, herpesvirus, syphilis, thrush (candidal or monilial infection), and acquired immunodeficiency syndrome (AIDS).

Gonorrhea. Gonorrhea is caused by gram-negative diplococci called *Neisseria gonorrhoeae.* It is contracted by the fetus during vaginal delivery and usually is manifested as an eye infection called ophthalmia neonatorum. The baby's eyes become inflamed with purulent discharge. Corneal ulcers develop that produce permanent scars and eventual blindness. Because of the serious results of such an infection, prophylactic (preventive) silver nitrate 1% or antibiotic ophthalmic ointment is instilled in the conjunctiva of the eyes of newborns.

Chlamydial infections. *Chlamydia trachomatis,* a bacteria-like organism, is transmitted by direct contact as the baby passes through the birth canal. The mucous membranes are most susceptible to infection, especially the urethra and the conjunctiva of the eyes. The infection causes mucopurulent discharge from infected areas. The treatment of choice is tetracycline; penicillin is not effective.

Herpesvirus infections.

Description and incidence. Herpesvirus types I and II cause lesions of the skin, throat, conjunctiva, liver, central nervous system, and other body organs of newborn infants. The infant may be infected before or during birth. About one third of infected infants exhibit vesicular skin lesions in small clusters all over their bodies at or soon after birth. The disease may affect only the central nervous system, or it may appear as an isolated eye or skin infection.

If the mother has recurrent genital lesions at the time of delivery, and if her membranes are either intact or have been ruptured less than 4 hours before, the physician may recommend cesarean birth to prevent infection of the baby.

Assessment and interventions. When it is believed that the neonate is infected, diagnosis is confirmed by cultures from the throat, urine, blood, CSF, skin lesions, or conjunctiva. If diagnosed, the infant is treated with intravenous vidarabine or acyclovir. Even when treated, the virus may cause microcephaly, seizures, paralysis, blindness, deafness, or death.

Isolation measures are instituted for all infants born to mothers with genital herpes lesions. Suspected herpetic infants require gown and glove isolation with linen precautions. Rooming-in may be a helpful solution. The mother is taught proper handwashing technique, which is to be used both in the hospital and at home.

Syphilis

Description. All pregnant women are screened to determine if they are infected with *Treponema pallidum,* the spirochete that causes syphilis. Fortunately the spirochete does not infect babies before the fifth month of gestation, affording time to test and treat syphilitic mothers before their infants can be harmed. If a mother goes untreated, organisms enter the fetal bloodstream and gain immediate access to all body tissues, particularly attacking the nervous system, liver, lungs, skin, bones, kidneys, and pancreas. The fetus may die in utero or be born with obvious disease. More often, symptoms appear at a later time. For this reason congenital syphilis is classified as early and late. In early syphilis symptoms appear during the first 2 years of life; in late syphilis symptoms appear after the child is 2 years old.

Assessment and interventions. In early congenital syphilis, even in infants who appear normal at birth, 75% show signs of the disease within 3 months. Typical signs are positive serology, anemia, skin rash, failure to thrive, persistent rhinitis (called *snuffles*), vesicular lesions on palms and soles, joint inflammation, enlarged liver and spleen, jaundice, and generalized edema.

At birth, cord blood is obtained from all infants whose mothers had positive prenatal serology test results. A repeat test at 6 months is more definitive than one made from cord blood. Repeated tests are recommended at intervals throughout childhood for all children who had abnormal serology at birth.

Treatment of congenital syphilis is both spe-cific and supportive. Penicillin is given in large doses as soon as the disease is diagnosed. Supportive treatment includes blood transfusions for anemia, regulated feedings for malnutrition, prevention and treatment of secondary infections, immobilization of inflamed joints, and fever control.

Thrush (candidal or monilial infection)

Description and assessment. Thrush is caused by *Candida albicans,* a one-celled fungus. It is contracted from a yeast-infected vagina during delivery or when a mother does not thoroughly wash her hands after touching her perineum.

Thrush appears as white patches on the buccal mucosa inside the cheeks and on the tongue, gums, and lips. It resembles milk curds, but when a cotton-tipped applicator is used to wipe away the patches, a raw bleeding area is exposed. The infection may be seen in the diaper area, and it sometimes becomes generalized.

Interventions. Cleanliness of hands, bedding, clothing, diapers, and feeding equipment is essential, because *Candida albicans* is present in oral secretions and stool. Breast-feeding mothers are taught to treat their nipples with topical nystatin; otherwise a cycle of reinfection will occur, as well as sore nipples and breakdown of nipple tissue.

Gentian violet 1%, a purple dye that irritates normal mucosa, or nystatin is swabbed on oral lesions once daily, usually an hour after feeding. Topical nystatin is also used for skin lesions. Parents are taught how to apply these medications.

Acquired immunodeficiency syndrome (AIDS)

Description and incidence. AIDS is caused by a retrovirus, Human T-lymphotropic Virus (HTLV-III) or human immunodeficiency virus (HIV). It enters the fetus through blood and blood products and affects specific T cells, decreasing the body's immune responses. This makes the infected baby susceptible to opportunistic organisms such as *thrush,* herpes, and other pathogens. The incubation period for AIDS can be as long as 5 to 7 years, so infants born to women with AIDS are not necessarily free of the disease, even if they show no symptoms at birth. Current statistics indicate that of the infants born to women with a positive HTLV-III, less than half have the disease at birth.

Assessment and interventions. Signs of AIDS in infants are failure to thrive, enlarged liver and spleen, interstitial pneumonia, recurrent infections, neurological defects, and SGA weights. Babies infected at birth may have severe neurological defects. Within 2 years, 80% to 90% of all infants born with AIDS will die.

At delivery the newborn is suctioned with a disposable bulb syringe. DeLee mucous traps are not used because of the infant may ingest secretions. Blood and secretion precautions are necessary. If their conditions permit, rooming-in is recommended for the mother and her baby because it promotes bonding and facilitates precautions and teaching.

Infants of diabetic mothers

Description. Diabetes in pregnancy is discussed in Chapter 6. It may be remembered that 25% of these pregnancies end unfavorably. Mothers with severe diabetes of long duration may give birth to SGA infants. More often, their babies are LGA, macrosomic (big bodied), and fat. The large size of these infants is *not* caused by edema; in fact, infants of diabetic mothers (IDMs) have decreased extracellular body fluid. The large appearance results from fat and the increased size of all body organs except the brain.

Excessive fetal growth is caused by high levels of maternal glucose, which readily crosses the placenta. The fetus responds and increases its insulin production by hyperplasia (growth) of pancreatic beta cells. Since the main action of insulin is to facilitate entry of glucose into muscle and fat cells, in infants insulin functions similar to a growth hormone.

Once in the cells, glucose is converted to glycogen and stored. Insulin inhibits the breakdown of fat and increases the uptake of amino acids, thus promoting protein synthesis (formation) and tissue growth.

Complications. IDMs are usually large, but their physiological functions are immature. They have many of the problems of preterm infants, including the following.

Hypoglycemia. After birth the most common problem of IDMs is hypoglycemia. Even though the supply of maternal glucose has stopped, the baby continues to produce high levels of insulin for some time, depleting his or her blood glucose within hours after birth. Of all IDMs, 2% to 75% are hypoglycemic, depending on the length of labor, on maternal blood sugar at delivery, and on the class of maternal diabetes.

Hypocalcemia. Low calcium levels cause tremors, a common symptom of IDMs and result from prematurity and the stress of a difficult pregnancy, labor, and delivery. Because diabetic women tend to have higher calcium levels at term, their infants may have a secondary lack of parathyroid endocrine, the hormone that regulates calcium metabolism and muscle control.

Polycythemia. IDMs usually have a greater number of red blood cells than other neonates, probably because during fetal life there is less available oxygen for their tissues. In response, their bodies produce more red blood cells to carry more oxygen.

Hyperbilirubinemia. Seen 48 to 72 hours after birth, hyperbilirubinemia may be caused by the number of red blood cells or traumatic delivery. At birth the extra cells begin to break down, freeing bilirubin in the bloodstream.

Birth trauma. Because these babies are large for gestational age, they are more likely to suffer traumatic deliveries caused by long labors, forceps use, and other procedures.

Respiratory distress. This condition is common among IDMs whose mothers have diabetes classified by White as A to C (see Table 6-2). It is thought that infants whose mothers have more severe diabetes (White D to F) may have been stressed enough to produce steroids, which caused their lungs to mature.

Congenital birth defects. IDMs are more likely to have a variety of defects of the heart, blood vessels, colon, and spinal cord.

Medical treatment and nursing interventions. Prenatal care of the mother is directed toward control of hyperglycemia, thus reducing complications in the infant.

At birth, hypoglycemia in IDMs occurs within 2 hours. For this reason blood glucose is determined at 1, 2, 4, 6, 12, and 24 hours. Babies who have symptoms are given 10% to 15% glucose intravenously, beginning immediately after birth. Once blood glucose has been stable for 24 hours, intravenous glucose gradually is reduced.

Because IDMs are at risk for so many complications, they are transferred to intensive care nurseries immediately after birth. As a result, the survival rate of these babies has been increased greatly.

Infants of substance-abusing mothers

When an addictive substance such as alcohol or heroin is taken by a pregnant woman, it enters the fetus through the placenta. With continual absorption, the baby becomes physically addicted to the substance. When the infant is born the source of the substance is gone, and signs of withdrawal begin to appear. Also of great concern are the *teratogenic* (defect-producing) effects of these substances.

Infants of alcohol-dependent mothers

Alcohol withdrawal. Infants who are addicted to alcohol at birth are wakeful and irritable. They may suffer tremors and seizures. If the mother is known to be an alcoholic, the baby is monitored closely, including vital signs, signs of tremors or seizure activity, level of activity and rest, intake and output, and ability to suck. Intravenous glucose and sedatives

may be necessary to reduce symptoms. Acute withdrawal response usually subsides by the third day.

Fetal alcohol syndrome

DESCRIPTION AND COMPLICATIONS. Fetal alcohol syndrome (FAS) is a group of malformations frequently found in infants born to women who have been chronic and severe alcoholics. Partial or complete FAS occurs in about 5 live births per 1,000. It is believed that acetaldehyde, a break-down product of alcohol, causes much of the damage. Abstinence from alcohol is advised for all pregnant women, because some of them unknowingly have an inherited metabolic defect that causes dangerously high acetaldehyde levels after even modest alcohol intake.

Complications of FAS include growth deficiency, failure to thrive, poor sucking, and persistent vomiting until 7 months of age. Since the brain is most sensitive to damage during fetal life, the FAS infant may suffer from mild to severe mental retardation, hyperactivity, and speech and language dysfunction.

ASSESSMENT AND INTERVENTIONS. Characteristics of FAS newborns are growth deficiency, central nervous system dysfunction, and distinctive facial defects (receding chin, small cheekbones, small upper lip that lacks a median groove, tiny fissures on the eyelids). Various anomalies of the heart, eyes, kidneys, and joints are also common.

The goal of nursing care is to promote the infant's physical well-being by avoiding the loss of body heat by protecting the infant from injury during seizures, by monitoring intravenous fluid therapy, and by reducing environmental stimuli. A quiet, dimly lit environment is most comfortable for these babies. Because FAS infants have feeding problems, nurses need extra patience and time for feeding these babies. Nurses monitor vital signs, evidence of seizure activity, and respiratory distress. They also provide support for the parents by teaching feeding techniques, by referring families to social services, and by encouraging positive parenting activity.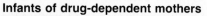

Infants of drug-dependent mothers

Drug withdrawal. Withdrawal symptoms develop in infants after birth at different times for different drugs. Withdrawal symptoms for heroin, for example, develop in 1 to 2 days; for cocaine, 4 to 5 days, and for barbiturates, 3 to 5 days. Methadone withdrawal symptoms may not appear until 14 to 21 days after birth, but they can occur earlier. Narcotic withdrawal from heroin or methadone produces the most serious problems. For most infants, withdrawal peaks about the third day after it begins and subsides by the seventh day. About half of the newborns of addicted mothers experience withdrawal symptoms severe enough to require treatment.

The most serious problem for the fetus of a drug-dependent mother during pregnancy is intrauterine asphyxia, which occurs as a direct result of the mother's withdrawal. For this reason, heroin-addicted mothers are not encouraged to withdraw completely but are placed on methadone maintenance during pregnancy. These mothers have a high incidence of pregnancy-induced hypertension (PIH), abruptio placentae, and placenta previa, all of which lead to placental insufficiency and fetal asphyxia. Heroin-addicted mothers are also at risk as carriers of the AIDS virus.

Assessment. Nursing assessment of infants includes discovering the mother's last intake and dose (history and laboratory tests); noting signs of SGA, intrauterine withdrawal (asphyxia), and prematurity; and assessing the infant for signs of withdrawal. Signs of withdrawal are as follows:

1. Central nervous system—hyperactivity, high-pitched cry, increased muscle tone, exaggerated reflexes, tremors, seizures, fitful sleep, fever
2. Respiratory system—rapid breathing, excessive secretions
3. Gastrointestinal system—entire system disorganized; strong sucking, vomiting, drooling, sensitive gag reflex, diarrhea, cramps
4. Vasomotor system—stuffy nose, yawning, sneezing, flushing, sweating, sudden circumoral (around the mouth) pallor
5. Skin—excoriated buttocks, facial scratches, pressure point abrasions

Interventions. The goals of nursing care are to promote the physical well-being of the infant and to facilitate family adaptation.

Special precautions are required because infants of drug-dependent mothers may be infected with the AIDS virus. Discharge planning is of prime importance. Because these infants are born with a parent-induced disorder, nurses may need help coping with their own feelings of anger and sadness.

Parents of infants at risk
Needs assessment

Parents of a preterm or sick baby may have difficulty adjusting to their unnatural roles. The baby is placed in an incubator at birth and often transferred to a neonatal intensive care unit many miles away. The parents may have difficulty identifying with the tiny stranger who bears their name but whom they have never held or seen very closely. They may develop feelings of inadequacy or show evidence of mourning (as if the child were dead) or reluctance to "become attached" because they fear the baby will not survive.

Interventions and evaluation

Nurses can do much to help parents overcome their fears. They can encourage parents to phone the nursery regularly for progress reports. They can speak of the infant by his or her given name. This helps parents think of the infant as a real child, their own child. When the mother's milk comes in, she may be encouraged to express it for her baby. As soon as possible, parents are invited to come to the nursery to hold and feed the baby. Nurses use every opportunity to instruct the parents in infant care so that when their baby is ready to go home, they will feel competent to take over the care.

The decision of the pediatrician to dismiss the baby from the intensive care unit is based on two factors: the condition of the baby and the home environment. When the baby is feeding well, is gaining weight, and has no life-threatening defect, the infant is usually ready to leave the nursery. To evaluate the home situation, the discharge planning nurse or home health nurse may be asked to make a home visit. The nurse assesses not only the physical facilities but also the attitudes of the parents toward health teaching, cleanliness, and continued medical supervision. It would be folly to send a fragile newborn baby to a home if he or she would be neglected and exposed to disease. The baby is dismissed when a favorable report has been received.

CIRCUMCISION
Purposes

Circumcision is a surgical procedure by which the foreskin or prepuce is separated from the glans penis and then excised. It is done to facilitate cleaning and to prevent future complications. Circumcision is also performed as a religious rite. It was once performed on most male newborns in the United States. In 1975, however, the American Academy of Pediatrics stated that there are no valid medical reasons for routine circumcision. It is *not* performed if a newborn is premature or sick, has a bleeding problem, or has a birth defect, such as hypospadias, where the prepuce may be needed for later plastic repair.

In the interest of cleanliness, the foreskin of the uncircumcised male newborn is regularly retracted and the glans gently washed with soap and water. If retraction is not possible, circumcision may be required to correct the unusual narrowing, called *phimosis*.

Procedure and nursing interventions

Parents are informed of the risks and outcome of circumcision. There is potential for pain, hemorrhage, infection, difficulty in voiding, and damage to the urethra. An operative permit must be signed. The procedure usually is performed during the infant's first week of life. It may be done before or after he is discharged from the hospital.

The nurse is responsible for restraining the infant on a circumcision board (Fig. 12-20) or frame, preparing equipment for the surgeon, and comforting the baby. Pain relief can be achieved by using lidocaine to block the penile dorsal nerve. Various devices, such as the Gomco clamp (Fig. 12-21) and Plastibell, are used. Vaseline gauze may then be applied to control bleeding.

Postoperatively, voiding is monitored for amount and stream. If bleeding occurs, the nurse should apply light pressure and notify the physician. The diaper is applied loosely to prevent undue pressure, and the baby is turned on his side. He may be fretful and may feed poorly for a few hours.

Before the baby is discharged, parents are told to observe his penis for bleeding or signs of infection. If the Plastibell is used, parents are informed that it usually remains in place for 3 to 4 days before it falls off.

RELIGIOUS RITES

In the United States, religious freedom is the birthright of every person. In our effort to protect this right, we often ignore the religious needs of patients. Maternity nurses should remember these needs and conscientiously seek to fill them.

If a baby becomes ill yet no emergency exists, parents are asked their wishes regarding religious rites. If, however, a baby suddenly becomes critically ill, nurses should be familiar with the rites of the major religious groups in their community and seek to follow the wishes of the family.

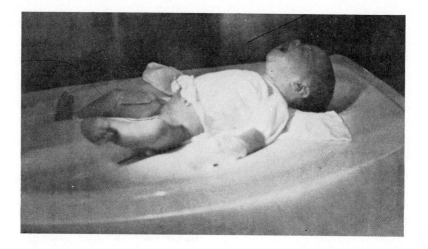

Fig. 12-20 Molded circumcision board on which the infant is restrained before being covered with sterile drapes.

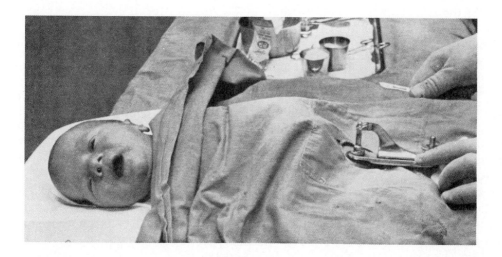

Fig. 12-21 Circumcision, using a Gomco clamp. Sterile equipment and supplies are on nearby tray.

Jewish

Historically, circumcision is a Jewish religious rite performed on the eighth day after birth unless it is postponed until the baby is stronger. All branches of Judaism practice the rite, which is presided over by a rabbi, to which all male members of the family are invited, and at which the boy receives his name.

The procedure is performed by a *mohel,* one trained in ritual circumcision, although some liberal groups permit any male physician to perform the circumcision. It may be performed in the hospital, physician's office, clinic, or synagogue.

If a baby of a Jewish family becomes critically ill or dies, the rabbi may be called to comfort the bereaved parents. No particular ritual is necessary for the baby. Orthodox Jews do not permit autopsy except in unusual circumstances.

Roman Catholic

The rite of baptism is especially significant to Roman Catholics, some Episcopalians, and members of the Greek Orthodox Church. They believe that baptism makes the infant a member of the Christian household of faith. If an infant becomes critically ill, every effort should be made to baptize the infant. In the case of abortion or fetal death, the expelled products of conception are also baptized unless there is obvious evidence of decay. Although the family prefers that a priest administer the rite, in an emergency a Catholic nurse or any other person can baptize an infant. Water should be poured over the head or some skin area and the following words spoken, "I baptize thee, Baby _____ , in the name of the Father, of the Son, and of the Holy Spirit."

After baptizing an infant, the nurse reports the fact to the family and to the priest if he arrives later. The rite is recorded on the infant's chart together with the time and name of the nurse who did the baptizing.

The Catholic church does not officially disapprove of autopsy after death. However, individuals may object for personal reasons.

Protestant

In general Protestants do not require special religious rites for infants. If a baby becomes critically ill or dies, parents may be comforted by a visit from the minister or pastor. Some Protestant groups strongly disapprove of autopsy, whereas others have no official position. The individual family will make known its wish if the question arises.

ADOPTION

Adoption is a procedure by which a person becomes a legal member and heir of a new family. Each state has its own laws that follow federal guidelines. In general terms, there are five types of adoption: independent, relinquishment, intercountry, stepparent, and adult.

Independent

Independent adoption is adoption in which a parent selects a new family for the child and places the child directly with that family.

In California the process occurs in two steps. (1) In the presence of a representative of the State Department of Social Services (SDSS) or a licensed private agency, the natural parents sign a consent to adopt and place the child in the custody of the adoptive parents, who file a petition to adopt with the court. (2) Within 180 days the SDSS makes a study of the adoptive home to determine if the new parents are able to provide an environment that will enable the child to develop to his or her best potential. The SDSS also determines if the child is legally free to be adopted. The court examines the study and response to the petition by granting or denying a decree of adoption.

Natural parents must petition the court to rescind the consent after it is signed. Adoptive parents may change their minds and return the child to the natural parent at any time before the decree is granted.

In recent years the issue of surrogate mothering has been debated hotly. As a result, new laws are being written. As of this time, where it is legal, these adoptions fall under independent adoption laws. A woman agrees to be impregnated with a man's sperm, to carry the baby to term, and to relinquish the infant to the father after the birth through the independent adoption process.

Relinquishment

Relinquishment means that the natural parent signs a legal document relinquishing the child to a licensed agency that has agreed to accept the child for placement. Relinquishment ends parental responsibility for the child and transfers it to the agency.

A natural parent interested in the possibility of placing a child for adoption or one who has made that decision may go to an adoption agency for help. There, experienced social workers discuss the issues in confidence. Referrals are made for medical care and other needs. The natural mother is under no obligation to give up her child. In fact, she is not permitted to sign a relinquishment until after she has left the hospital and recovered from the birth experience. When a parent signs a relinquishment, the adoption agency becomes the child's legal guardian and is responsible for the child's care and support. Only in rare circumstances, by mutual agreement, can relinquishment be nullified.

Agency services to adoptive parents and children include the following:

1. Assessing the needs and capabilities of children
2. Compiling social and medical history of children
3. Establishing that children are free for adoption
4. Studying and approving adoptive appli-

cants before placing children in their homes
5. Providing continuing services to adoptive parents

Persons wishing to adopt contact an adoption agency. They are interviewed, and they make application for a child. The agency investigates the home and through a state registry seeks to match children to parents. When a potential match is made, the foster parent who has been caring for the child brings the child to meet the prospective parents. If it is agreeable, the child is placed in the adoptive parents' home. The family is given time to feel satisfied that it is a good match before they petition the court to adopt. At a subsequent time the court responds to the petition by granting or denying a decree of adoption.

Original birth records are sealed away. A new birth certificate is issued with the adoptive parents' names. In recent years this practice has been challenged on the grounds that it violates civil rights of citizens to know their natural heritage.

The demand for perfectly formed white babies far exceeds that supply. However, there are thousands of racially mixed and physically or emotionally disabled older children who need loving homes. More and more people are adopting these "special kids" or are seeking children from other countries.

Intercountry

Eligible orphans and half-orphans may be adopted by families in the United States through intercountry adoption. These adoptions take place through the services of the Intercountry Adoption Program, various licensed adoption agencies, and the federal Department of Immigration and Naturalization.

Stepparent

A stepparent may petition the court for custody of a child. Both of the natural parents and the stepparent must sign the consent. A study is made on behalf of the child by a state agency for social services, and the court responds to the petition by granting or denying a decree of adoption.

Adult

An adult may adopt another adult by an agreement of adoption in a superior court. If the court is satisfied that the adoption will serve the best interests of all parties concerned the agreement is approved, and a decree of adoption is granted.

▶ **KEY CONCEPTS**

1. Signs of physiological distress in infants include cyanosis, jaundice, dyspnea, tachycardia, bradycardia, absent or watery stools, vomiting, excessive salivation, poor sucking, abdominal distention, discharge from umbilicus or eyes, shrill or weak cry, bulging or sunken fontanels, convulsions, twitching, facial grimacing, and lack of voiding.

2. Handicaps of preterm infants involve respiration, body temperature regulation, gastrointestinal development, elimination of wastes, resistance to disease, nutrient storage, blood cell production, bleeding tendency, and the surfactant system.

3. Postterm infants suffer degrees of hypoxia and malnutrition because of placental aging.

4. Interventions to overcome handicaps of preterm and postterm infants are directed toward maintaining an open airway, providing adequate oxygen, conserving energy, maintaining body temperature, ensuring safety, preventing infection, and meeting nutritional needs.

5. Birth injuries seen in newborn infants include forceps marks, caput succedaneum, cephalohematoma, intracranial hemorrhage, subdural hematoma, brachial plexus palsy, and facial nerve paralysis.

6. Congenital defects of all body systems may occur. Nurses need to assess infants to identify these defects.

7. Symptoms of disease that typically affect infants are diarrhea, jaundice, vomiting, and convulsions. Early nursing assessment and interventions are vital.

8. Retrolental fibroplasia occurs because blood vessels in the eyes of premature infants respond to oxygen with excessive growth. The resulting scar tissue or other complications may cause blindness.

9. Respiratory distress syndrome is caused by an immature surfactant system. Prevention, assessment, and interventions can help to reduce the death rate.

10. Phenylketonuria is an inherited defect of metabolism that causes mental retardation if phenylalanine is not eliminated from the diet. Blood and urine tests are done after the first feedings; parent education is essential to successful treatment.

11. Sexually transmitted diseases are passed from mothers to their infants before, during, or after birth and cause damage to various body systems of infants. These diseases include gonorrhea, chlamydial infections, herpes virus infections, syphilis, thrush, and AIDS. Nurses assess, intervene, and take precautions to prevent or control these infections.

12. Infants of diabetic mothers are fat and large, yet they are at risk for hypoglycemia and immature physiological development.

13. Infants of substance-abusing mothers are at risk for immediate withdrawal and for long-term effects, such as fetal alcohol syndrome, mental retardation, and AIDS.

14. Parents of infants at risk need empathy, information, and education. Also, they need the opportunity to bond with their infant.

15. Circumcision is surgical removal of the prepuce. It is done for cleanliness, as a religious rite, and to correct phimosis. Circumcision is not a routine necessity. Nurses should assess the infant for bleeding and infection.

16. Religious rites, such as circumcision and baptism at death, need to be respected by nurses.

17. Adoption is a procedure for becoming a legal member of a new family. There are five types of adoption: independent (includes surrogate mothers), relinquishment, intercountry, stepparent, and adult.

■ *ANNOTATED SUMMARY*

I. High-risk infants
   A. Terminology—based on gestational age and growth: LGA, SGA, etc.
   B. Assessment of neonates
      1. Scoring systems—Apgar and characteristic growth and neuromuscular signs
      2. Physical examination—using inspection, palpation, auscultation, percussion
      3. Signs of physiological distress—measures of function, symptoms, and laboratory tests
   C. Description
      1. Preterm infants—underdevelopment; handicaps—all body systems immature
      2. Postterm infants—suffer malnutrition and hypoxia
      3. Asssessment of needs and interventions
         a. Airway and oxygen—monitored with various devices
         b. Conservation of energy—handle as little as possible
         c. Maintenance of body temperature—equipment varies
         d. Safety and prevention of infection—asepsis essential
         e. Provision of nutritional needs—feedings begin a few hours after birth
            (1) Intravenous feeding—hyperalimentation may be needed
            (2) Oral feedings—by soft nipple, gavage tube, or dropper
            (3) Feeding techniques—small amounts are given slowly and recorded
   D. Perinatal injuries
      1. Forceps marks—disappear soon after birth
      2. Caput succedaneum
         a. Description—swelling between scalp and skull
         b. Assessment and interventions—swelling gradually subsides
      3. Cephalohematoma
         a. Description—blood between skull bones and periosteum
         b. Assessment and interventions—not aspirated; blood is gradually absorbed
      4. Intracranial hemorrhage
         a. Description and assessment—bleeding into brain
         b. Interventions—monitor vital and neurological signs
      5. Subdural hematoma—bleeding below dura mater of brain
      6. Fractures—humerus, clavicle, femur
      7. Brachial plexus palsy (Erb-Duchenne paralysis)
         a. Description—upper arm paralysis caused by damage of fifth and sixth cervical spinal nerves
         b. Assessment and interventions—weakness and loss of reflex; corrective positioning
      8. Facial nerve paralysis (Bell's palsy)
         a. Description—caused by damaged seventh cranial nerve
         b. Assessment and interventions—cover affected eye
   E. Congenital defects
      1. Developmental anomalies of the extremities
         a. Description and causes—result from teratogens
         b. Assessment and interventions—varying disabilities
      2. Clubfoot (talipes)
         a. Description and causes—equinus and calcaneus
         b. Assessment and interventions—repositioning feet
      3. Hip dysplasia—most common defect
         a. Description—various degrees of underdevelopment
         b. Assessment—restricted abduction and other tests
         c. Interventions—repositioning until bone forms
      4. Nevi (birthmarks)
         a. Description

(1) Pigmented nevi—melanin in skin

(2) Vascular nevi—overgrowth of blood and lymph vessels

b. Assessment and interventions—depends on type and size

5. Cranial defects

a. Description

(1) Craniostosis (craniostenosis)—sutures close too soon

(2) Microcephaly—brain fails to grow

(3) Hydrocephaly—cerebrospinal fluid accumulates

b. Assessment and interventions

6. Neural tube defects

a. Description—vary in severity and size

b. Assessment—spina bifida occulta to myelomeningocele

c. Medical and surgical treatment—depends on severity

d. Nursing interventions—immediate care to long-term care

7. Cleft lip and cleft palate—failure of embryonic facial structures to close

a. Description, causes, and incidence—multiple problems

b. Assessment—varying degrees of abnormal opening

c. Medical and surgical treatment—repair of palate and lip

d. Nursing interventions—keep airway open; provide food

8. Esophageal atresia and tracheoesophageal fistula

a. Description and incidence—trachea and esophagus connected

b. Assessment—mucus, cyanosis

c. Medical and surgical treatment—surgical repair

d. Nursing interventions—head-up position with continuous suctioning

9. Hernias

a. Umbilical hernia

(1) Description—protrusion through abdominal opening

(2) Assessment and interventions—surgery after 5 years

b. Inguinal and femoral hernias

(1) Description—protrusion through abdominal wall

(2) Assessment and interventions—incarcerated bowel

c. Omphalocele and gastroschisis

(1) Description—herniation through umbilical opening

(2) Assessment, planning, and interventions

10. Imperforate anus

a. Description—various degrees; no visible anus

b. Assessment and interventions—surgery required

11. Exstrophy of the bladder

a. Description and complications—bladder exposed

b. Assessment and interventions—degrees of defect

12. Hypospadias

a. Description and assessment—urethra opens on lower side of penis

b. Interventions—surgical repair may be needed

13. Epispadias—urethra opens on upper side of penis; less common

14. Cryptorchidism (undescended testes)

a. Description and complications—hidden testes; may cause sterility

b. Assessment—firm pressure overcomes reflex

c. Interventions—surgical repositioning before puberty

15. Intersexual defects—true hermaphroditism and pseudohermaphroditism

a. Description and incidence—hormonal, genetic, true

b. Assessment—history, examination, cytology, chromosomal studies

c. Interventions—depends on nature of defect

16. Heart malformations—various defects at birth

F. Diseases

1. Diarrhea

a. Description and causes—overfeed-

ing, high-fat formula, infection
 b. Preventions and interventions—
  barriers; no overfeeding
2. Jaundice
 a. Description and causes—physiological, pathological
 b. Assessment and interventions—
  laboratory tests
3. Vomiting
 a. Causes and assessment—common
  cause is too-rapid feeding
 b. Planning and interventions—danger of aspiration
4. Convulsions
 a. Description and causes—never
  normal; many causes
 b. Assessment and interventions—
  describe accurately
5. Retrolental fibroplasia
 a. Description and cause—blindness
  resulting from growth of blood vessels
 b. Prevention and treatment—oxygen less than 21%
6. Respiratory distress syndrome (hyaline membrane disease)
 a. Description and cause—immature
  surfactant system
 b. Assessment—lecithin/
  sphingomyelin ratios: 2:1
 c. Interventions—CPAP or PEEP
7. Phenylketonuria (PKU)
 a. Description and incidence—inherited metabolic error
 b. Assessment—blood and urine
  tested for phenylalanine
 c. Interventions—low-phenylalanine
  diet until puberty
8. Umbilical cord infections (omphalitis)
 a. Description—pathogenic invasion
 b. Assessment and interventions—
  culture and sensitivity test antibiotics
9. Sexually transmitted diseases (STD)
 a. Gonorrhea—causes corneal ulcers
  and blindness
 b. Chlamydial infections—conjunctivitis, urethritis
 c. Herpesvirus infections—from

mother's vagina at birth
 (1) Description and incidence—
  minor to major effects
 (2) Assessment and interventions—lesions; IV acyclovir
 d. Syphilis—infects fetus after fifth
  month of gestation
 (1) Description—dangerous; goes
  to all body organs
 (2) Assessment and interventions—serology; penicillin
 e. Thrush (candidal or monilial infection)
 (1) Description and assessment—
  white patches in mouth
 (2) Interventions—gentian violet
  1% on lesions
 f. Acquired immunodeficiency syndrome (AIDS)
 (1) Description and incidence—
  infected from mother
 (2) Assessment and interventions—blood tests; signs
10. Infants of diabetic mothers (IDMs)
 a. Description—fat, LGA; not edematous
 b. Complications—hypoglycemic after birth; others
 c. Medical treatment and nursing interventions—cord blood tested often; IV glucose given
11. Infants of substance-abusing mothers
 a. Infants of alcohol-dependent mothers
 (1) Alcohol withdrawal—irritable,
  tremors
 (2) Fetal alcohol syndrome (FAS)
  (a) Description and complications—pinched face,
   poor sucking, organ defects, mental retardation
  (b) Assessment and interventions—history, physical
   examination
 b. Infants of drug-dependent mothers
 (1) Drug withdrawal—symptoms
  develop at various times
 (2) Assessment—CNS, respiratory, GI tract, vasomotor, skin

      (3) Interventions—IV fluids; supportive measures
   G. Parents of infants at risk
      1. Needs assessment—degree of parents' attachment to sick infant
      2. Interventions and evaluations—closeness, time together
II. Circumcision
   A. Purposes—cleanliness, religious rite, phimosis
   B. Procedure and nursing interventions—restrain and comfort
III. Religious rites
   A. Jewish—circumcision
   B. Roman Catholic—baptism last rites
   C. Protestant and other religions—various preferences
IV. Adoption
   A. Independent—mother directly to adoptive parents
   B. Relinquishment—mother to agency to adoptive parents
   C. Intercountry—wards of court placed in adoptive homes
   D. Stepparent—both natural parents and stepparents sign agreement
   E. Adult—adult adopts another adult

● *STUDY QUESTIONS AND LEARNING ACTIVITIES*

1. Define preterm, SGA, LGA, IUGA, and LBW.
2. Describe 10 signs of physiological distress in an infant.
3. What special handicaps must preterm infants overcome? What nursing interventions can be used to help them?
4. Compare the tissues involved in, seriousness of, and nursing interventions for forceps marks, caput succedaneum, cephalohematoma, intracranial hemorrhage, and subdural hematoma.
5. Describe the nursing interventions for infants with brachial plexus palsy and facial nerve paralysis.
6. How would you explain clubfoot and hip dysplasia and their treatments to an anxious parent?
7. Through role playing, tell a parent about the

two major types of birthmarks and their possible treatments.
8. Compare the defects in craniosynostosis, microcephaly, and hydrocephaly.
9. Compare spina bifida occulta and spina bifida cystica, and describe the immediate nursing interventions.
10. Describe the immediate nursing interventions for infants with cleft palate and lip, esophageal atresia, omphalocele, imperforate anus, and exstrophy of the bladder.
11. If a child's sex is ambiguous, what assessment measures are performed?
12. Which of the heart malformations might be obvious at birth?
13. What causes respiratory distress syndrome, and why is it most often seen in premature infants?
14. Through role playing, explain PKU and its treatment to the parent of a baby whose tests show a serum level of 50 mg per 100 ml.
15. Compare the causative agent, potential danger, and treatment for each of the sexually transmitted diseases.
16. Even though IDMs are large and fat, they have many problems. Describe those problems and explain why they occur.
17. What are the nursing goals for care of infants with FAS?
18. What are the reasons circumcision is performed? What are the dangers?
19. Describe four types of adoption. Which one is used by surrogate mothers?

REFERENCES

Babson SG, and others: Management of high-risk pregnancy and intensive care of the neonate, ed 4, St Louis, 1979, The CV Mosby Co.

Centers for Disease Control: Report on caution about AIDS Virus, NAACOG Newsletter, 13(6):5, Atlanta, 1986, CDC.

Fanaroff AA, and Martin RJ, eds: Neonatal-perinatal medicine: diseases of the fetus and infant, ed 4, St Louis, 1987, The CV Mosby Co.

Hamilton PM: Basic pediatric nursing, ed 5, St Louis, 1987, The CV Mosby Co.

Jensen MD, and Bobak IM: Maternal and gynecologic

care: the nurse and the family, ed 3, St Louis, 1985, The CV Mosby Co.

Korones SB: High-risk newborn infants: the basis for intensive nursing care, ed 4, St Louis, 1986, The CV Mosby Co.

Olds SB, London ML, and Ladewig PA: Maternal-newborn nursing, ed 3, Menlo Park, Calif, 1988, Addison-Wesley Publishing.

Pierog SH, and Ferrara A: Medical care of the sick newborn, ed 2, St Louis, 1976, The CV Mosby Co.

Tranmer J: Fetal alcohol syndrome, J Obstet Gynecol Neonat Nurs 14(6):484, 1985.

Whaley LL, and Wong DL: Nursing care of infants and children, ed 3, St Louis, 1987, The CV Mosby Co.

Who Keeps Baby M? Newsweek, Jan 19, 1987, p. 44.

UNIT FIVE
POSTPARTUM CARE

Nursing Care of the Mother

LEARNING OBJECTIVES

- Discuss the fourth stage of labor, including dangers, goals, diagnoses, assessment, and interventions.

- Describe continuing needs of the postpartum woman, including goals, diagnoses, assessment, and interventions.

- Discuss involution of the uterus, lactation, ambulation, elimination, nutrition, abdominal and pelvic muscles, prevention of Rh sensitivity, sexual intercourse, menstruation, ovulation, and emotions of the postpartum woman.

- Describe stages of the development of the parental role.

- Describe the discharge instructions given to new mothers and give rationales for them.

The postpartum period is a time of healing and change, a time of return to the nonpregnant state and adjustment to a new family constellation. Although the body undergoes continual change as it recovers from childbirth, nursing care is divided into three periods of time: (1) the critical 2 to 4 hours immediately after delivery, (2) the following 3 days, and (3) the next 4 to 6 weeks. Today healthy mothers and babies usually leave acute care facilities sometime during the 3 days following delivery.

FOURTH STAGE OF LABOR

Even though childbirth is the climax of pregnancy, the first 2 to 4 hours afterward are considered more dangerous. For this reason the period is called the *fourth stage of labor.*

Danger

During the fourth stage of labor the primary danger for mothers is hemorrhage. The safety of mothers depends on frequent assessments and timely interventions of alert nurses.

Goals of nursing care

The goals of nursing care during this fourth stage are to:
1. Prevent hemorrhage.
2. Provide physical comfort, nutrition, hydration, safety, and elimination.
3. Encourage the mother and family to begin to integrate the birth process into their life experience.
4. Foster attachment process to the newborn.

In some hospitals the mother is moved directly from the delivery room to an obstetrical recovery room equipped and staffed to give intensive care. In other hospitals the mother is moved to her postpartum room where an experienced nurse cares for her during the critical fourth stage. The baby may be brought to the mother's room or may be kept in the nursery for observation during all or part of this period. In alternate birthing centers mother and baby usually remain in the same room for all stages of labor.

Immediately after delivery and perineal repair, the mother's perineum is gently washed and dried, and sterile perineal pads are put in place with a T binder. The gown is replaced with a warm clean one, and the mother is covered with a warm bath blanket. These measures are taken to refresh her and counteract the chill that often follows a strenuous labor and delivery. The mother's uterus should be firm and hard as a result of oxytocic drugs administered after the placenta was expressed.

Assessment

In the intensive care unit or in her own room, the mother is made comfortable. The following observations begin at once:

1. Blood pressure: *check every 15 minutes for 1 hour or until stable, then every 30 minutes for another hour.* The mother's blood pressure may be slightly elevated from delivery effort and excitement; it returns to normal within 1 hour.

2. Pulse: *check every 15 minutes for 1 hour or until stable, then every 30 minutes for another hour.* Pulse returns to normal rate within 1 hour; slight bradycardia may occur (50 to 70 beats per minute).

3. Temperature: *check once, at 1 hour, then as per hospital protocol.* Temperature may be elevated if dehydrated or fatigued.

4. Fundus: *check every 15 minutes for 1 hour or until stable, then every 30 minutes for another hour.* The fundus should be in the midline, firm and 2 cm below or at the umbilicus. If the uterus is soft, massage until firm and express clots until contracted to midlevel. If fundus is to the right of the midline, check bladder for distention (Fig. 13-1).

5. Bladder: *check every time fundus is assessed.* Mother's bladder fills quickly because of postdelivery diuresis and intravenous fluids.

6. Lochia: *check every 15 minutes in conjunction with fundus.* There should be moderate flow. If blood comes in spurts, suspect cervical tear.

7. Perineum: *check in conjunction with assessment of lochia.* The episiotomy and perineum should be clean, discolored, and edematous, and the sutures should be intact.

8. Discomfort: *pay attention to complaints of pain.* Any severe pain in the perineum should be investigated; a hematoma may be forming under the episiotomy. Headache may warn that eclampsia is near. Afterpains are expected in multiparas.

9. Parent-child interaction: *if the infant is in the room, note parents' facial expression as they look at their baby, what they say, and what they do.* Strongly negative responses signal problems.

10. Emotional status: *note the mother's emotional status.* Exaggerated negative or

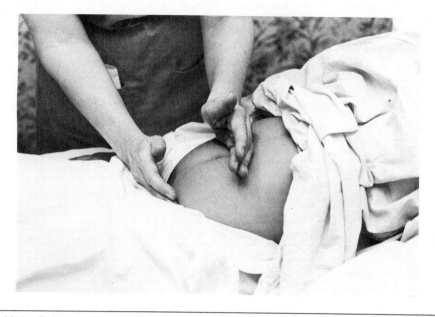

Fig. 13-1 Palpating the uterus during the first hour after delivery. Note that the upper hand is placed over the fundus. Lower hand presses in above the symphysis pubis, supporting the uterus as it is massaged. *(From Phillips, CR: Family-centered maternity/newborn care, ed 2, St Louis, 1988, The CV Mosby Co.)*

positive emotions or lack of emotional expression may be cultural or personality traits. Such emotions also may indicate maladaptive symptoms.

Nurses may wish to use a worksheet to collect assessment data, such as the one in Table 13-1.

Nursing diagnosis

Typical nursing diagnoses for women during the fourth stage of labor are:
1. Potential for hemorrhage related to uterine atony and trauma.
2. Potential for urinary retention related to childbirth trauma.
3. Alteration in comfort related to afterpains and childbrith trauma.
4. Self-care deficit: bathing/hygiene; re-

lated to fatigue and medications given during childbirth.
5. Potential for injury related to ambulating without assistance and/or impaired mobility related to postanesthesia paralysis.
6. Potential fluid volume deficit related to restrictions during delivery.
7. Potential altered parenting related to fatigue and postpartum discomfort.
8. Potential distress of the human spirit related to lack of a support system.

Interventions

During the fourth stage of labor mothers need rest in order for the natural resources of the body to begin the healing process. Bed rest during this period is recommended. In fact,

Table 13-1 Sample worksheet for the fourth stage of labor

Name _____ T _____ P _____ A _____ L _____ Room # _____

Time of delivery _____ Type of delivery _____ Anes/anal _____

Epis/lac _____ Baby: Sex _____ Apgar _____ Mother's MD _____

	Admit	15 m	30 m	45 m	1 h	1 h 15 m	1 h 30 m	1 h 45 m	2 h
Time									
Temperature, pulse, respirations									
Fundus									
Bladder									
Intake/output									
Lochia									
Perineum									
Discomfort: type and location									
Parent-child inter- action									
Emotions, rest, activity									

many mothers fall into a deep sleep, bothered little by frequent nursing assessments. Nursing interventions appropriate for the identified nursing diagnoses follow.

Potential for hemorrhage related to uterine atony and trauma. Normally the fundus remains or becomes firm with intermittent gentle massage. Such massage helps express the accumulated blood and clots so that the uterus can contract again. If the uterus does not respond and bleeding continues, oxytocic drugs such as intravenous pitocin are administered.

Lochia is described by amount and character. During the fourth stage it is bright red in color and is described as *scant, light moderate,* or *heavy (profuse).* Later lochia becomes *serosanguinous* (serum and blood) and then *serous* (serum).

Nurses assess the amount of flow on the perineal pad. They also check under the mother's buttocks because blood may miss the pad and flow between the buttocks onto the linens below. A perineal pad that is soaked through from tail to tail contains about 100 ml of blood. Loss of 100 ml of blood in 15 minutes is considered a heavy flow. Such loss signals a need for continuous monitoring of vital signs, maternal color, and behavior.

If large clots are passed, they are saved together with saturated pads so that the amount can be estimated. If tissue is passed, it also is saved for inspection by the physician. Discharge of tissue may indicate retained placenta. If bleeding comes in spurts or in a steady trickle, laceration of the cervix or vagina is suspected. The physician is notified, and the woman is taken to the delivery area for inspection and possible surgical repair.

Potential for urinary retention related to childbirth trauma. A full bladder forces the uterus upward and to the side. Such a position interferes with sustained uterine contraction and leads to hemorrhage. This adds to the discomfort and can result in atony of the bladder wall, urinary retention, and eventual infection.

Because of recent trauma and swelling of the urinary meatus, a mother may find it difficult to void. Warm water poured over the vulva and water allowed to trickle into a basin may help her relax the sphincter. If these measures fail, catheterization may be prescribed.

Alterations in comfort related to afterpains and childbirth trauma. During the first few hours after delivery, uterine contractions may be quite strong and painful, especially in multiparas. Nursing interventions are:

1. Explain normal physiology of afterpains to the mother.
2. Encourage the mother to empty her bladder frequently.
3. Cover her abdomen with a warmed blanket.
4. Administer analgesics as prescribed.
5. Encourage self-relaxation techniques learned prenatally.

The episiotomy and hemorrhoids may cause considerable discomfort. Nursing interventions include:

1. Encourage side-lying position.

2. Apply ice packs for the first 2 hours.
3. Apply sprays or ointments as prescribed.
4. Administer analgesics as prescribed.
5. Encourage self-relaxation.

Self-care deficit: bathing/hygiene; related to fatigue and medications given during childbirth. Because of fatigue or the effects of analgesics during delivery, a woman cannot cleanse or warm herself. When a nurse washes the mother's face and hands and places a warm blanket over her, the mother feels cared for and safe and is able to rest more comfortably.

Potential for injury related to ambulating without assistance and/or impaired mobility related to postanesthesia paralysis. During the fourth stage of labor bed rest is recommended to allow the body to recover from the effects of labor and delivery.

If a woman has had a saddle block or caudal anesthesia, her legs will be numb and paralyzed for some time afterward. Until the effects of the anesthesia have worn off, the mother needs help to place them in a position of comfort. For several hours the head of the bed is kept flat or in a low Fowler's position, and the woman is encouraged to roll from side to side to avoid postspinal headache. Remember to place the call bell within reach because the mother cannot get out of bed.

Potential fluid volume deficit related to restriction during delivery. Because oral fluids are often restricted during labor, many women are thirsty and request fluids soon after delivery. Usually clear fluids in moderate amounts are permitted; however, drinking too much and too quickly may cause vomiting. After the first hour most woman tolerate a light diet without difficulty. As a precautionary measure, a "keep open" intravenous infusion may be prescribed during the fourth stage of labor. Accurate records of intake and output are maintained.

Potential altered parenting related to fatigue and postpartum discomfort. No matter how pleased a woman is with her baby, if a labor is long and difficult and she is exhausted, the woman may not be able to sustain enthusiasm for the baby. At birth, if the mother smiled, talked directly to the baby, made positive statements, or reached out for and established eye contact with the baby, her responses are considered strongly positive and signs that successful bonding has begun. Such reactions probably will return with her strength. If, however, the mother's initial response was strongly negative, as indicated by the bonding assessment score, she may need time and encouragement to form an attachment and bond with her baby.

Potential distress of the human spirit related to lack of a support system. When a woman goes through pregnancy, labor, and delivery without a support system, the birth of the baby may not be a joyful event. It may be a nightmare of physical and psychic pain. The woman may feel fearful, sad, and angry. She may say little, interact minimally with the baby, and seem preoccupied, distant, and depressed. Nurses need to be alert for the mother who has no visitors or is relinquishing a baby for adoption. Nurses can offer special attention, encourage the mother to share her painful emotions, inquire if she wants a visit from the chaplain, and refer her to social services.

Nurses need to remember that reactions of mothers vary widely depending on personal characteristics and culture. Some women express emotions freely. Others express emotions in more restrained ways or not at all. By offering accurate empathy, genuineness, and nonpossessive warmth, nurses provide the acceptance all woman need regardless of circumstances or personal characteristics.

MATERNAL-CHILD CARE UNIT

The maternal-child care unit of the hospital includes labor, delivery, and recovery rooms, nurseries for the babies, rooms for mothers, and the alternate birthing center (ABC). The entire unit is considered "clean" in contrast to other parts of the hospital. To prevent infec-tious organisms from crossing to mothers and infants, movement between the maternal-child care unit and the rest of the hospital is discouraged.

If the mother and infant do not go home soon after delivery, there are two arrangements for postpartum and infant care. In the traditional arrangement, mothers and infants are housed in separate rooms and nurseries except for brief feeding and viewing times. In the *rooming-in* arrangement, babies and mothers share the same room except for brief periods during which babies are cared for in the nurseries. In the *modified rooming-in* plan, infants are housed in the nursery during times when the mother is sleeping.

The advantages of rooming-in are that mothers and infants are not separated for long periods. As a result, parent-child bonding is hastened. Rooming-in is especially desirable for new parents, since it gives them an opportunity to learn child care skills such as how to diaper and bathe with the support and guidance of an experienced nurse.

CONTINUING POSTPARTUM CARE
Nursing care goals

By the end of the fourth stage of labor, the mother's condition usually has stabilized. Nursing care goals are broaden to match the mother's changing needs. They are to:

1. Prevent infection.
2. Promote tissue healing.
3. Promote uterine involution and comfort.
4. Promote rest, activity, and safety, and prevent complications of immobility.
5. Promote adequate food and fluid intake.
6. Promote establishment of lactation or its suppression.
7. Promote normal patterns of elimination.
8. Prevent Rh isoimmunization in Rh-negative mothers.
9. Meet learning needs of mothers: per-

sonal hygiene, perineal care, breast care, infant care, parenting, muscle-strengthening exercises, sexual intercourse, and contraception.

10. Promote self-esteem and a positive body image, and stress reduction.

11. Encourage continued health maintenance through use of community health resources.

Assessment

If a mother has been cared for in a postpartum recovery room area during the fourth stage of labor, she will be transferred to the postpartum nursing care unit when her condition has stabilized.

Initial assessment includes a report to the receiving nurse. The woman's record is reviewed for information from the prenatal and labor records that will affect her continuing care. The prenatal record alerts the health care team to a possible need by the woman for rubella vaccination or protection against Rh isoimmunization. A fetal cord blood test confirms a need for Rh_o (D) immune globulin.

The nurse interviews the woman informally to determine her emotional status, energy level, location and degree of discomfort, hunger, thirst, her knowledge about self-care and infant care, and whether she will breast-feed or bottle-feed her baby. Ethnic and cultural factors such as language or dietary variations are assessed as they affect care and recovery.

Assessment of vital signs, fundus, lochia, bladder, intake/output, perineum and episiotomy, breasts, bowels, and emotional status is made at this time. Unless problems develop, laboratory tests are rarely prescribed. Assessment continues every 4 to 8 hours until discharge.

Nursing diagnoses

Typical nursing diagnoses for women during this stage of postpartum recovery are:

1. Potential for infection related to unhealed tissue and uterine involution.
2. Potential self-care deficit.
3. Alteration in comfort related to afterpains, unhealed episiotomy, and breast engorgement.
4. Alterations in bowel or urinary elimination related to postpartum discomfort.
5. Sleep distrubance related to discomfort and infant feeding schedule.
6. Potential cracked nipples and mastitis related to breast-feeding practices.
7. Alterations in activity related to episiotomy and afterpains.
8. Potential thrombosis related to hemostasis.
9. Potential knowledge deficit regarding breast-feeding, sexual intercourse, contraception, and use of community resources.
10. Depression related to hormone levels, discomfort, and posttraumatic shock.

Interventions
Asepsis

After the initial danger of hemorrhage has passed, the second danger is infection. Puerperal sepsis, called "child bed fever," was once the curse of hospital obstetrics. It still is a potential menace for all postpartum women. The most effective ways to prevent infections are for hospitals to maintain clean facilities and supplies, for nurses to practice aseptic technique, and for mothers to learn good personal hygiene, especially handwashing.

The battle against infection is an ongoing effort that requires participation of all hospital personnel. Fixtures, floors, instruments, and linens must be free of pathogens. Food, fluids, and drugs must be pure. Wastes must be discarded properly.

The greatest source of infection for postpartum mothers is the staff, especially their hands, noses, and mouths. At delivery sterile gowns and gloves are worn. Face masks help prevent airborne organisms from infecting the mother's birth canal. Thereafter, nurses must conscientiously wash their hands between patients. Because of current concerns for spread of secretion-borne pathogens, nurses must protect themselves from body secretion as well as prevent cross contamination between patients.

Personal hygiene

Personal hygiene of mothers helps remove sources of infection and promotes their feeling of well-being. As soon as they are strong enough to walk, mothers are assisted to the shower. They are instructed to wash their nipples first, then the body, and finally the perineum. Clean perineal pads and gown are provided.

Perineal care

Special perineal care for women after childbirth relieves discomfort, cleanses, prevents infection, and promotes healing. Although procedures vary from hospital to hospital, the basic principles are universal, as follows: (1) prevent contamination from the rectum, (2) deal gently with traumatized tissue, and (3) thoroughly remove bacteria-laden discharge and odor. Applying these principles, a suggested procedure follows.

Nurses teach mothers to:
1. Wash their hands.
2. Fill individual plastic bottles with warm water.
3. Remove soiled perineal pads with a downward movement toward the rectum and place pads in a plastic bag.
4. Void or defecate into the toilet.
5. Spray perineum generously with water.
6. Pat perineum dry with tissue from front to back.
7. Apply perineal pads from front to back.
8. Wash hands again.

Nurses wear gloves when they give perineal care to mothers.

Sitz baths

Sitz baths are useful because the moist heat not only increases circulation to promote healing, but also relaxes tissues to promote comfort and decrease edema. Sitz baths may be given in a tub, a specially constructed sitz chair, or a disposable unit that fits inside the toilet. The nurse makes certain the water temperature is comfortable at about 105° F (40.5° C) and that the woman has a call bell at hand should she feel faint. Some research suggests that cold sitz baths may be even more effective than warm ones. Women are encouraged to use a sitz bath three or four times a day for about 20 minutes.

Dry heat

Dry heat from a heat lamp is sometimes used to promote perineal healing. The perineum first should be cleaned to remove secretions. The patient lies on her back with her knees flexed and apart, and the lamp is positioned 20 inches from the perineum. Heat lamps generally are used three times a day for about 20 minutes.

Topical anesthetics

Topical anesthetics such as Dermoplast Aerosol Spray or Nupercainal Ointment may be used to relieve perineal discomfort. The woman is advised to apply the medication after sitz baths or perineal care. To avoid tissue burns, she should not apply medications before using a heat lamp.

Hemorrhoid care

Some mothers experience hemorrhoidal pain after delivery. Measures that provide relief include sitz baths, anesthetic ointments, rectal suppositories, and witch hazel pads. Women may be taught to replace external hemorrhoids into the rectum with a gloved finger. They may find it helpful to maintain a side-lying or prone position and to avoid prolonged sitting. Women are encouraged to maintain adequate fluid intake and to take stool softeners to ensure greater comfort with bowel movements. Hemorrhoids usually disappear a few weeks after delivery if the woman did not have them before the pregnancy.

Elimination

Most women void spontaneously within 8 hours after delivery. During pregnancy there is a 50% increase in extracellular fluid. After delivery this fluid is eliminated as urine. Acetone may appear in the urine of women who have had long labors or who are dehydrated. When lactation begins, lactose may appear in the urine.

Defecation usually is suspended for 2 to 3 days after delivery because of a predelivery enema, a liquid diet, analgesic drugs during labor, and a painful perineum. The resumption of regular meals and ambulation is usually enough to reestablish regularity. Adequate fluid intake and a high-roughage diet are recommended. For breast-feeding mothers, stool softeners such as docusate or bulk laxatives that act locally on the bowel are preferred to laxative food.

Uterine involution

Immediately after delivery the uterus is about the size and consistency of a small melon and the fundus is located just below the umbilicus (Fig. 13-2). Thereafter the fundus subsides 1 to 2 cm per day until the end of the first week, when it is at the level of the pubic bone. By the sixth week the uterus normally returns to its nonpregnant form as a small, pear-shaped organ deep in the pelvis. Uterine muscle tone is maintained by nervous control and can be stimulated by massage or by nipple stimulation. The cervix regains its shape within a week after delivery and by the sixth week has healed and appears as a crosswise slit typical of multiparas. Uterine in-

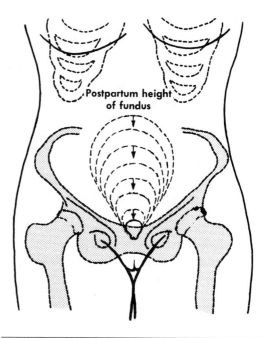

Fig. 13-2 Uterine involution showing descent of the fundus into the pelvis during the first week following delivery.

volution is slowed if the uterus becomes infected.

Lochia

Lochia is the uterine discharge that follows delivery. It is composed of blood, old cells, and bacteria. At first lochia is bloody and may include clots. The amount and character change from day to day. At first the amount of lochia is profuse, then moderate, then scant, and usually stops within 2 weeks. Its color is described by the Latin words *rubra* for bright red, *serosa* for brownish serum, and *alba* for whitish yellow. Total discharge following delivery is 400 to 1,200 ml. Normal lochia has a musty odor. A foul or putrid odor indicates infection. Menstrual periods usually begin again about 6 to 8 weeks after delivery for nonnursing mothers and 3 or more months after delivery for nursing mothers. The first menses may be heavier than those that follow.

Episiotomy

Nurses inspect the episiotomy for signs of infection and evidence of healing at least every 8 hours. Healing rate depends on the location and depth of the incision. Most episiotomies heal before the sixth week postpartum. As already described under perineal care, sitz baths, heat lamps, and topical medications promote healing and relieve discomfort of the episiotomy.

Afterpains

Afterpains are painful contractions experienced by multiparas during the first 3 to 4 days postpartum. They are unusual after the first pregnancy, but with each succeeding pregnancy they become more severe. Since breast-feeding stimulates uterine contractions, afterpains are common at nursing times. Analgesic drugs give some relief.

Breasts

During the 9 months of pregnancy, breast tissue grows and prepares for its function of providing food for the newborn infant. After delivery, when placenta-producing hormones are no longer present to inhibit it, the pituitary gland sends out *prolactin (lactogenic hormone)*. By the third day after delivery, prolactin's effect on breast tissue is evident. Vessels in the breast become engorged with blood, causing heat, swelling, and pain. Milk-producing cells begin to function, and milk begins to reach the nipples through milk ducts, replacing the colostrum that preceded it. Thus lactation begins.

When the baby sucks the nipple, a nervous reflex stimulates the posterior lobe of the pituitary gland to secrete *oxytocin hormone*. Oxytocin stimulates the "let-down" reflex, causing ejection of milk from the lactiferous sinuses in the breast to the ducts of the nipple.

(Oxytocin also stimulates uterine contractions, hastening uterine involution and producing afterpains.) When milk is drawn off by the baby's sucking or by pumping, lactating cells in the breasts are stimulated to produce more milk. This process can go on for months and even years. If milk remains in the ducts, increased back pressure develops; less and less milk is produced, and eventually none at all. This is how "drying up" occurs naturally.

If, for various reasons, a mother decides not to breast-feed her infant, various drugs may be given to inhibit prolactin production. These are given during the first hours after delivery before lactation begins. Among these drugs are bromocriptine (Parlodel), a dopamine agonist, and testosterone enanthate (Deladumone), a hormone. These drugs are of little value once lactation begins.

Nonnursing mothers. Even when lactation-inhibiting medications are prescribed, some degree of engorgement may occur. A well-fitted brassiere or a tight binder that lifts upward and inward is recommended. Ice may be applied but should be removed periodically to permit normal nerve reflex function and blood flow within the skin. Analgesic medications also may be prescribed to reduce discomfort.

Nursing mothers. For mothers who are breast-feeding, nipple care is especially important. Breasts should be washed carefully every day during the shower and again just before each feeding. This removes dried colostrum or milk crusts and helps prevent bacteria from accumulating and entering either the nipples or the baby's mouth. Special ointments and creams may be used to help prevent nipple cracking.

If nipples become cracked, nursing is temporarily suspended until they can heal. Milk then is manually or electrically expressed but saved and given to the baby. Continued nursing on cracked and bleeding nipples may lead to mastitis, a serious complication discussed in Chapter 14. Mothers of premature infants may need to express their milk until the baby is strong enough to nurse.

Breast-feeding technique. Nurses have great influence on breast-feeding experiences of new mothers. The following suggestions for nurses working with new mothers and babies are adapted from Ocasio and Strokamer (1982) and Velasquez (1984).

1. Establish rapport with the mother, support her in a nonjudgmental way; and answer her questions.

2. Assess the breasts, areola, and nipples. Treat hard areas with warm soaks and massage. Expose tender nipples to the air, apply creams, and reduce nursing time.

3. Encourage mothers to wear well-fitting nursing brassieres.

4. Teach mothers to massage breasts from chest wall to areola, thus facilitating movement of milk and/or colostrum from milk-producing glands to collection sinuses under the areola.

5. Explain the value of a relaxed atmosphere for breast-feeding. Assist mothers to assume a comfortable, well-supported position, without distractions, in a warm, quiet, private area.

6. Assist mothers to position their babies comfortably with skin contact. Express a little colostrum or milk to interest the baby in nursing and guide the nipple into the baby's mouth. To be positioned correctly, most of the areola must be in the baby's mouth (Fig. 13-3). Encourage mothers.

7. Educate mothers to respond to the cues of their infants and switch breasts when babies become agitated. End feedings when babies fall asleep or detach from the breast.

8. Explain how to remove a baby from the breast without damaging the nipple. The mother inserts her little finger in the corner of the baby's mouth to break the suction and gently pulls away.

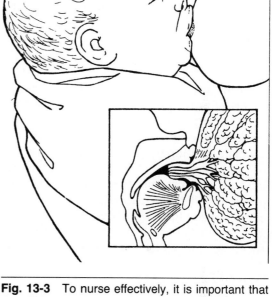

Fig. 13-3 To nurse effectively, it is important that the infant's mouth cover most of the areola to compress the ducts below. *(Reprinted with permission of Ross Laboratories, Columbus, Ohio, 43216.)*

9. Remind mothers to facilitate burping by holding babies in an upright position after each feeding, stroking the back.

10. Because breasts need to be stimulated frequently, both breasts are used at each feeding until the milk is well established. Nursing should be on demand, every 2 to 3 hours, for as long as the baby wishes to nurse.

Support and encouragement. It is not unusual for a mother who is breast-feeding for the first time to become discouraged. Her breasts are painfully swollen, and the baby does not know how to suck. At first there is no milk, only colostrum. Then there is far too much milk. In addition, painful uterine cramps occur every time the baby goes to breast.

Nurses can do much to help such a mother. They can assist her to hold her infant properly. They can explain that engorgement will gradually decrease and milk supply will adjust to the baby's appetite. Nurses can help the mother relax and just enjoy holding her infant.

Activity and rest

Most women can ambulate as soon as the effects of drugs given at birth have worn off. Such activity is beneficial to all body systems, especially the function of bowels, bladder, circulation, and lungs. It helps prevent clot formation (thrombosis) of leg vessels and assists the mother to progress from a dependent sick role to an independent healthy one. Likewise, mothers need to recover from their labor and to allow the body to heal. Therefore, they are encouraged to assume activities gradually, to space their activities, and to rest before they become overly tired.

Muscle-strengthening exercises

When their strength returns, after the initial period of adjustment following childbirth, women can begin muscle exercises to strengthen pelvic floor and abdominal muscles. Kegel's exercises, described in Chapter 5, are taught to mothers during prenatal care. As soon as it feels comfortable, mothers are encouraged to resume these exercises. Likewise, they can begin abdominal muscle exercises (Fig. 13-4) as their strength returns. Women should remember that for 5 to 6 months their muscles have been relaxed and that it will take as many months to restore their former tonus.

Food and fluids

New mothers need a well-balanced diet. A good general guide for an adequate diet includes two to four servings each day from the basic food groups: dairy foods, meat and protein foods, vegetables and fruits, and breads and cereals. Nursing mothers need extra proteins, minerals, and fluids. They can obtain these by adding 4 to 6 cups of low-fat milk to their diet each day. Mineral and multivitamin supplements also may be recommended.

Skin

The striae that result from stretching of abdominal skin may remain long after delivery, but they fade to lighter shades. If a linea nigra or a mask of pregnancy (chloasma) is present, it usually blanches and disappears with time.

Prevention of Rh-factor sensitivity

As part of antepartum care, blood typing for ABO and Rh factor is performed. If a woman is $Rh_o(D)$ negative, antibody levels are monitored throughout her pregnancy. (See Chapter 6.) When $Rh_o(D)$ immune globulin (such as RhoGAM) is given at 28 weeks prenatally and again within 72 hours after delivery, the incidence of isoimmunization is significantly reduced.

If a woman has had no antepartum care, blood type determination is done on admission to the hospital. She is considered a candidate for RhoGam if (1) she is Rh negative, (2) her baby is Rh positive as determined from cord blood, and (3) the baby has a negative reaction to the Coombs' test, indicating that the mother probably is not yet sensitized to Rh factor.

If it is decided that a mother is a candidate for RhoGam, (1) she signs an informed consent, (2) the Rho Gam is ordered from the laboratory, (3) a compatibility test is performed, and (4) the Rho Gam is delivered to the postpartum unit for administration. In giving Rho Gam, nurses follow the same precaution as for whole blood. Two nurses double-check

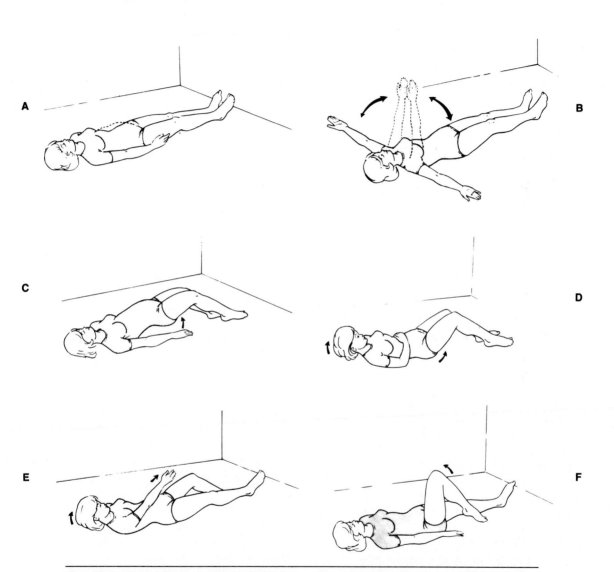

Fig. 13-4 Postpartum exercises. **A,** First day; **B,** second day; **C,** third day; **D,** fourth day; **E,** fifth day; **F,** sixth day; **G,** seventh day; **H,** eighth day; **I,** ninth day; and **J,** tenth day. *(From Bobak, IM, and Jensen, MD: Essentials of maternity nursing: the nurse and the childbearing family, ed 2, St Louis, 1987, The CV Mosby Co.)* *Continued.*

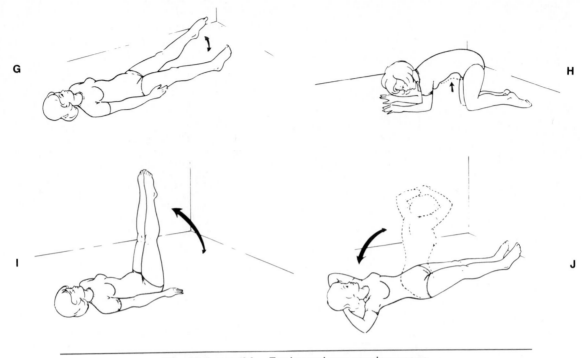

Fig. 13-4, cont'd. For legend see previous page.

the woman's name and identifying numbers on the vial of RhoGam against the laboratory slip. RhoGam is injected intramuscularly, usually into the buttocks. Reactions are rare, but the injection site is checked for signs of local inflammation; vital signs are measured at least twice during the next 4-hour period.

Sexual intercourse

Sexual intercourse can be resumed safely when the perineum heals and lochial discharge stops. Because of lower estrogen levels in the weeks immediately after delivery, secreting cells in the vagina may produce less natural lubrication. Therefore, lubricating cream may be helpful. Some women experience a milk "let-down" response with sexual orgasm. They also may experience sexual arousal with breast-feeding. These physiological responses may distress women unless they understand that they are normal.

Menstruation and ovulation

In non-breast-feeding women, menstruation begins 6 to 8 weeks after delivery. Ovulation may occur at this time. Thus conception is possible. In breast-feeding mothers menses may not commence for 3 or more months after delivery. Continued production of prolactin *may* inhibit release of follicle-stimulating hormone (FSH) from the pituitary gland and delay ovulation. However, FSH *may not* be inhibited and ovulation may occur. For this reason breast-feeding is not a reliable contraceptive. If abstinence is not possible and another pregnancy is unwanted, some form of contraception should be used.

Emotions

Emotional responses of women to pregnancy, delivery, and the puerperium are discussed in Chapter 4. As described, when the time for delivery approaches, women experience increasing elation, climaxed by birth of the baby. Often the emotional high undergoes rapid decline after delivery. Progesterone and estrogen levels within the body fall. Women are exhausted from labor, and they have a sore perineum, engorged breasts, and afterpains. They feel strangely depressed and may be found in tears they do not understand. This depression is termed *postpartum blues*.

Nurses comfort mothers by explaining the physical causes for postpartum depression. They assure mothers that such depression is common and soon it will disappear, just as do the other discomforts of childbirth. Their feeling of joy and hope will return as it was before the birth.

Parenting

Initial assessment of the interaction between parents and their baby is made in the delivery room. (See Chapter 9.) This "claiming process," called *bonding*, occurs as the mother and father accept and identify with the infant. Strongly positive reactions include talking to the baby, smiling at, cuddling, examining, and making positive remarks about the infant. Strongly negative reactions include declining to hold or look at the baby, being apathetic, and making disparaging remarks about the infant. When parents feel positively about their infant, they are more likely to gain skills in child care and are less likely to abuse or neglect the infant in the future.

According to some researchers, assuming the parenting role is a process that occurs in three stages: (1) dependence, (2) dependence-independence, and (3) interdependence.

Stage 1: dependence. For new mothers this stage occurs on days 1 and 2 after childbirth. Rubin (1961) described these days as the "taking in" phase, a time during which the mother needs nurturing and protecting. She focuses her energy on the new baby. She may need to verbalize the birth experience over and over, "taking in" the facts of her new role. This preoccupation narrows her perceptions and reduces her ability to concentrate on new information. Nurses may need to repeat instructions during this stage.

Stage 2: dependence-independence. The second stage begins about 3 days after the birth and lasts for 4 to 5 weeks. Rubin called this the "taking-hold" stage. By the third day the mother is ready to assume her new role and learn all about her new challenge. However, her body is undergoing significant change. As a result of powerful hormonal action, breast milk appears. The uterus and perineum still are healing. The woman becomes fatigued by her energetic efforts. Her independent energies dissolve into dependent exhaustion. When she returns home, she may feel overwhelmed.

During this time a support system is especially valuable to the first-time mother who needs a source of information and physical relief so she can rest. The woman's coping mechanisms are important resources during this stage when postpartum blues are common. Visiting nurse services are recommended, especially for first-time mothers.

Stage 3: interdependence. Beginning about 5 or 6 weeks after the birth, the family system has adjusted to its new member. The woman's body has healed, feeding routines have developed, and sexual activity between parents has been reestablished. Extended family and friends, although useful as a support system at first, no longer alter normal family interactions, and daily routines have been established. The mother is physically able to resume normal responsibilities and no longer assumes a "sick" role. This interdependence stage continues on until it is interrupted by other periods of dependence.

HEALTH TEACHING

During the days that follow a birth, nurses seize opportunities for health teaching, which should be part of every care-giving function. In addition, many maternal-child units offer group instruction, including classes on infant bathing, feeding, safety, cardiopulmonary resuscitation (CPR) for infants, and parenting skills.

Discharge examination and follow-up care

Most healthy mothers and babies go home 2 to 5 days after delivery. A nurse, midwife, or physician performs a physical examination and interviews the mother before discharging her. Physical examination includes assessment of major body organs, breasts, pelvic organs, and perineum. The interview gives mothers an opportunity to discuss problems and ask questions.

Some physicians and midwives provide a printed list of discharge instructions for mothers, including the following:

1. *Activity.* Reasonable activities are recommended. Frequent naps should be taken to conserve strength for the really important things. Moderation is the key.

2. *Bathing.* A daily shower or tub bath is recommended.

3. *Sexual intercourse.* Intercourse should be avoided until the episiotomy is healed. With resumption of intercourse, gentleness is vital. Since it is possible to become pregnant again in less than 6 weeks, contraceptive precautions may be desired.

4. *Diet.* A well-balanced diet is encouraged, including meat or meat substitutes, fruit and vegetables, bread and cereals, and dairy foods every day. Weight reduction diets are accept-able if they are balanced and there is adequate fluid intake. The nursing mother needs an added quart of low-fat or whole milk each day.

5. *Exercise.* Any abdominal muscle-strengthening exercises may be undertaken, but moderation is the key. Kegel's exercises to tighten muscles of the pelvic floor are recommended.

6. *Danger signs.* Any fresh bleeding or foul discharge from the vagina should be reported to the physician at once. Menstruation may begin again as early as 6 weeks after delivery. Fever or prolonged abdominal or pelvic pain should be reported. A telephone number to call in case of danger signs is provided.

7. *Six-week checkup appointment.* The date, time, and place of the checkup are indicated on the appointment slip.

▶ *KEY CONCEPTS*

1. The first 2- to 4-hour period after delivery is called the fourth stage of labor, during which the greatest danger is hemorrhage.

2. Nursing assessments include vital signs for evidence of hypovolemic shock, fundus for contraction, bladder for distention, lochia for amount and nature, perineum for hemostasis, discomfort, parent-child interaction for bonding, and emotional status.

3. Interventions focus on preventing hemorrhage, urinary retention, discomfort, providing rest, safety, adequate fluid intake, and emotional support.

4. The maternal-child care unit is maintained as a "clean" unit with areas for labor, delivery, recovery, infant nurseries, and rooms for mothers and their infants. Rooming-in means that the mother and infant share the same room.

5. Goals of continuing care following the fourth stage of labor include prevention of infection; promotion of healing; uterine involution; comfort; safety; rest and activity; adequate food and fluid intake; elimination; establishment of lactation or suppression, as desired; prevention of Rh isoimmunization; meeting learning need of mothers; promoting self-esteem; and encouraging health maintenance.

6. Interventions focus on preventing infection and

supporting the healing process of mothers by asepsis, personal hygiene, perineal care, and hemorrhoid care; promoting elimination; assessing uterine involution, lochia, episiotomy healing, and afterpains; and teaching breast care for both nonnursing and nursing mothers and breast-feeding techniques. Nurses also provide information on activities, rest, exercises, food, fluids, skin care, prevention of Rh sensitivity, sexual intercourse, menses, postpartum emotions, parenting, and health teaching.

7. Discharge instructions to mothers include information about activity, bathing, sexual intercourse, diet, exercises, danger signs, and appointment for 6-week checkup.

■ ANNOTATED SUMMARY

I. Fourth stage of labor—first 2 to 4 hours after birth
   A. Danger—hemorrhage
   B. Goals of nursing care—prevent hemorrhage; provide physical comfort, nutrition, hydration, safety, and elimination; encourage integration of birth into life experience; foster infant bonding
   C. Assessment—vital signs, fundus, bladder, lochia, perineum, discomfort, parent-child interaction, emotional status of mother
   D. Nursing diagnoses—potential for hemorrhage, urinary retention, injury related to ambulation, fluid volume deficits, altered parenting, distress of human spirit, alterations in comfort, and self-care deficit
   E. Interventions—address specific diagnoses

II. Maternal-child care unit—considered more clean, separate from other hospital areas. Rooming-in allows infant to be in same room as mother; may be modified to give mother rest

III. Continuing postpartum care
   A. Nursing care goals—broadened to meet mother's changing needs; include prevention of infection, Rh isoimmunization, promotion of tissue healing, uterine involution, comfort, rest, activity, safety, adequate food and fluid intake, establishment of lactation or its suppression, normal elimination, self-esteem, meeting learning needs of mother, and encouraging continued health maintenance

   B. Assessment—continues until mother and infant are discharged
   C. Nursing diagnoses—potential for infection, self-care deficit, cracked nipples, thrombosis, knowledge deficit; alterations in comfort, bowel or urinary elimination, sleep, activity, and depression
   D. Interventions—address specific problems
      1. Asepsis—helps decrease infections
      2. Personal hygiene—taught to mothers
      3. Perineal care—principles: prevent rectal contamination, be gentle, be thorough to remove discharge
      4. Sitz baths—both cleansing and comfort producing
      5. Dry heat—promotes healing
         Topical anesthetics—sprays and ointments
      7. Hemorrhoid care—moist heat, side lying, stool softeners, topical anesthetics
      8. Elimination—adequate fluid intake, stool softeners, roughage in diet
      9. Uterine involution—continuous process, speeded by nipple stimulation, slowed by infection
      10. Lochia—rubra, serosa, alba
      11. Episiotomy—moist and dry heat promote healing
      12. Afterpains—common in multiparas
      13. Breasts—lactogenic hormone stimulates milk-producing cells to begin to function, oxytocin stimulates let-down reflex, causing milk to go to ducts of nipple
         a. Nonnursing mothers—lactation inhibiting medications, brassiere or breast binders, ice, analgesics
         b. Nursing mothers—wash nipples, apply creams, wear supporting brassiere
            (1) Breast-feeding technique—proper technique prevents cracked nipples and facilitates lactation
            (2) Support and encouragement—important
      14. Activity and rest—assume activities

gradually; ambulation helps prevent thrombosis

15. Muscle-strengthening exercises—Kegel's and abdominal muscle exercises help mothers regain strength

16. Food and fluids—balanced diet with added milk for lactating mothers

17. Skin—striae, linea nigra, and chloasma gradually fade

18. Prevention of Rh-factor sensitivity—RhoGam administered at 28 weeks and within 72 hours of delivery to Rh-negative mothers who have Rh-positive infants; helps prevent Rh-factor sensitization.

19. Sexual intercourse—resumed gently after perineum heals

20. Menstruation and ovulation—non-breast-feeding women: begins in 6 to 8 weeks; breast-feeding women: begins in 3 or more months; ovulation may not be inhibited, need some form of contraceptive to prevent pregnancy.

21. Emotions—postpartum depression is common because of hormone drop and trauma of childbirth

22. Parenting—three-stage process: dependence (taking in), dependence-independence (taking hold), interdependence

IV. Discharge and follow-up care—discharge interview and instruction

● *STUDY QUESTIONS AND LEARNING ACTIVITIES*

1. What is the fourth stage of labor? Why is it considered a dangerous period? Describe nursing assessment that should be made during this period.

2. State goals of nursing care during the fourth stage.

3. What are the principles of perineal care? How are they carried out in the hospitals where you are working?

4. Of what is lochia composed? What words are used to describe its color and quantity?

5. Where does the fundus of the uterus lie immediately after delivery? What effect does breast-feeding have on the involution of the uterus? What effect does uterine infection have on involution?

6. What are the benefits of early ambulation after delivery?

7. What daily assessments should be made of each mother during continuing care following the fourth stage of labor?

8. List and describe the three stages of the development of the parental role.

REFERENCES

Bobak, IM, and Jensen, MD: Essentials of maternity nursing: the nurse and the childbearing family, ed 2, St Louis, 1987, The CV Mosby Co.

Ocasio, IT, and Stokamer, CL: Supporting the breast-feeding mother, Newborn Nursery 1(2), 1987; Pampers Disposable Diapers.

Olds, SB, London, ML, and Ladewig, PA: Maternal-newborn nursing: a family-centered approach, ed 3, Menlo Park, Calif, 1988, Addison-Wesley Publishing.

Rubin, R: Maternal behavior, Nurs Outlook 9:682, 1961.

Tsikouris, C: Increasing your milk; information sheet #85, 1982, Franklin Park, Ill. LaLeche League International.

Velasquez, S: Lactation update (unpublished newsletter), 1984.

Complications and Surgery

LEARNING OBJECTIVES

- Discuss postpartum hemorrhage, its causes, nursing assessment, and interventions.

- Describe disseminated intravascular coagulation (DIC), its causes, and nursing interventions.

- Discuss thrombophlebitis, its incidence, assessment, and interventions.

- Describe puerperal infection, sites, causative agents, and nursing interventions.

- Discuss mastitis, its causes, assessment, interventions, prevention, and implications for breast-feeding mothers.

- Describe urinary tract infections, their assessment, medical treatment, and nursing interventions.

- Discuss postpartum mental illness, stressors that trigger its development, its assessment, and interventions.

- Describe surgical procedures that produce sterility and appropriate nursing interventions.

- Describe the various surgical procedures and nursing interventions for early, interim, and late abortions.

COMPLICATIONS

Complications of pregnancy, labor and delivery have been discussed in Chapters 6 and 10. Although some of those conditions continue beyond delivery, others are unique to the postpartum period. These include bleeding and clotting disorders, infections, and mental illness.

Bleeding and clotting disorders
Hemorrhage

Description and causes. Postpartum hemorrhage is one of the three most common causes of maternal death; preeclampsia/eclampsia and thrombophlebitis are the other two. Although some blood loss is normal at every delivery, loss of 1% or more of body weight is considered life threatening. Thus a 110-pound (49.90 kg) woman should not lose more than 499 ml (1 pint) of blood. Such loss is especially serious if the general condition of the mother is poor from a long labor or a preexisting disease. Often these women are the ones most likely to bleed excessively. Postpartum hemorrhage may be *early,* within the first 24 hours, or *late,* from 24 hours until the twenty-eighth day.

Common causes of postpartum hemorrhage are:

1. Uterine atony
2. Retained placenta
3. Lacerations of the birth canal
4. Disseminated intravascular coagulation (DIC)
5. Tumors of the uterus or cervix
6. Uterine inversion (turning inside out)
7. Medical complications such as vitamin K deficiency
8. Infections
9. Subinvolution of the uterus (late bleeding).

Uterine atony often follows long or precipitate labor, polyhydramnios, and multiple pregnancy. When any one of these predispos-

ing conditions is present, physicians may prescribe an oxytocin intravenous drip for several hours after delivery.

During pregnancy large blood sinuses develop under the placenta. After delivery the uterine muscle contracts, squeezes closed the blood vessels, and prevents major blood loss. When tissue remains within the uterus or if the muscle has been stretched excessively, it cannot contract fully and hemorrhage results. Thus retained placenta, uterine inversion, and tumors can cause serious postpartum bleeding.

When there are lacerations (tears) of the cervix or vagina from which blood is flowing, no amount of uterine contraction will stop the hemorrhage. After delivery physicians inspect the birth canal closely for lacerations. If one is found, it is repaired immediately. Sometimes an exposed vessel may be overlooked, and hemorrhage results.

Assessment. Nurses assess all postpartum women for signs of hemorrhage. This includes checking the (1) uterine fundus for sustained firmness, (2) lochia for quantity, (3) and vital signs for symptoms of hypovolemic shock. A tremendous amount of blood can be lost in a short time. Signs of hemorrhage are rapid and weak pulse, pallor, excessive amount of bright-red lochia with or without clots, maternal thirst, dizziness, restlessness, weakness, and unconsciousness. Even with treatment, hypovolemic shock is more difficult to reverse in postpartum women, and death may result.

Interventions. Medical treatment of hemorrhage includes treatment of hypovolemic shock by prescribing intravenous fluids, plasma, and whole blood, finding the cause of the bleeding, and stopping the blood loss.

When uterine atony is the cause, a continuous intravenous oxytocin drip usually is prescribed. If the hemorrhage is still not controlled, the mother may be returned to the delivery room or surgical suite. There the physician inspects the cervix and vagina for lacerations and bleeding vessels. If found, they are sutured. If the bleeding is caused by a retained placenta, it is removed.

Nursing interventions involve continuous assessemnt of vital signs, level of consciousness, and lochia; administration of intravenous fluids; and obtaining laboratory tests as prescribed. Through all the activity that such an emergency creates, the mother and her family cannot help but realize the unusual nature of the situation and be frightened. They need support and assurance that the welfare of the mother is of prime importance. Uncomplicated explanations by nurses and a calm reassuring presence can allay their fears.

Disseminated intravascular coagulation

Description and causes. Disseminated intravascular coagulation (DIC) is a condition characterized by abnormal clotting. DIC is triggered by bacteremia (bacterial infection in the bloodstream), amniotic fluid embolism, immune reactions, intrauterine fetal death, preeclampsia/eclampsia, hydatidiform mole, and saline abortions. As a result, numerous clots form in the bloodstream throughout the body. These clots block the flow of blood to the tissue, causing damage wherever the blockage occurs. Because of the abnormal coagulation, factors responsible for clotting, such as platelets and fibrinogen, are used up so that normal clotting cannot take place and widespread bleeding results.

Assessment and interventions. Initial symptoms of DIC develop as a result of blocked blood flow to such tissues as the brain, lung, kidneys, and heart. Symptoms of bleeding into the tissue follow. The patient is critically ill, may be unconscious and anoxic, and have reduced urinary output. Hemorrhages may appear in the skin. She is transferred to an intensive care unit.

Medical treatment consists of:
1. Removing the causative factor, such as treatment of a bacterial infection

2. Initiating supportive care such as administration of oxygen
3. Administering whole blood or blood components such as factor VIII, fibrogen, and platelets
4. Giving heparin to stop abnormal clotting (Fig. 14-1).

Nursing interventions include:
1. Provision of skin care, personal hygiene, elimination, range of motion, body alignment, and emotional support
2. Monitoring of vital signs, level of consciousness, and intake and output
3. Administration of intravenous oxygen and heparin therapy
4. Continuous assessment for signs of bleeding; ecchymosis, pallor or cyanosis of body parts, oliguria, or changes in mental status

If the woman survives the initial crisis, permanent kidney, liver, and brain damage may limit the quality and length of her life. Discharge planning is essential and may include home health nursing services, homemaker services, counseling, and vocational rehabilitation.

Thrombophlebitis

Terminology and description. The following terms are useful in the understanding of thrombophlebitis:

thrombus Blood clot.
embolus Moving mass such as a clot in the bloodstream.
occlusion Blockage of a vein.
phlebo- Blood vessel.
-itis Inflammation.
stasis Standing still.
Homan's sign Pain produced by compression of tibial vein.
Homan's test Dorsiflexion of foot at ankle as if standing on toes; if action of muscles compressing tibial veins produces pain, Homan's sign is present.

Thrombophlebitis is an inflammation of a vein with clot formation. It occurs most often in the femoral (leg) veins and pelvic (uterine,

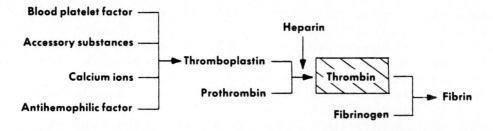

Fig. 14-1 Mechanism of heparin in preventing blood coagulation. It inhibits the conversion of prothrombin to thrombin, which in turn prevents the conversion of fibrinogen to fibrin. Heparin does not alter the blood's normal components significantly. It only prolongs normal clotting time, not bleeding time. *(Adapted from Nyman, JES: Thrombophlebitis in pregnancy, Am J Nurs 80:1, 1980.)*

ovarian, hypogastric) veins. Major concerns are that the clot will (1) cause local inflammation and occlude the vein and (2) break loose, become an embolus, and move up into vessels of the heart and lung, blocking those vessels. Often the condition has an abrupt onset, with fever, chills, severe pain, and swelling of the affected leg. Arterial spasm may give a bluish white appearance, called "milk leg." Homan's sign may or may not be present. Its presence indicates the likelihood of a thrombus.

Incidence. The incidence of thrombophlebitis during pregnancy is low, occurring in only 1.8 to 20.9 cases per 10,000 women. When it develops, usually it is after week 26 of gestation, with 40% of the women having a history of thrombophlebitis. On the other hand, the incidence of thrombophlebitis following pregnancy is relatively high, occurring more often after cesarean birth and postpartum infection. It is the third leading cause of maternal death. Because occurrence of thrombophlebitis is associated with venous stasis, early ambulation is an important factor in its prevention.

Assessment and interventions. Interventions are aimed at resolving the acute episode and preventing complications, namely, pulmonary embolism and chronic venous insufficiency. Medical treatment includes:

1. Anticoagulation therapy using heparin (Fig. 14-1)
2. Bed rest with the affected leg elevated
3. Moist heat to increase peripheral circulation and relieve discomfort
4. Avoidance of massage of affected legs to prevent dislodging clots
5. Elastic stockings, worn for at least 6 months after the acute attack

Clotting time is prolonged in patients who receive heparin. Therefore signs of hemorrhage must be noted and reported. Repeated subcutaneous injections of heparin result in tender, bruised skin areas. A heparin lock may be prescribed instead. Vital signs may be elevated; if so, they are checked for accuracy and reported. Lochia may be heavy for 3 to 4 days; pads are counted and heavy flows reported. Cracked nipples may bleed and cause pain in women who are nursing. A nipple shield may help reduce the discomfort until they heal. Hematomas may form in the pelvis or perineal region from severed blood vessels, causing pressure on the urethra and bowel. The size of the swelling is measured at intervals and reported. Surgical evacuation of accumulated blood may be necessary.

Fear, discouragement, and impatience to return home are normal responses of the mother. She is kept informed of her progress, given support, and taught the importance of wearing support hose and not massaging her legs. Her family is encouraged to visit. Ambulation is attempted cautiously as soon as pain and swelling subside. Because ambulation must be resumed gradually, the mother needs assistance to care for the new baby and assume her role as mother and wife when she is discharged.

Infections
Puerperal infection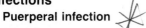

Description. Puerperal infection is a general term for infections of the birth canal and pelvis following delivery. These infections are caused by bacteria common to the vagina and by pathogens introduced from the outside, such as streptococci, staphylococci, *Escherichia coli*, and various sexually transmitted diseases. Occasionally tetanus, diphtheria, typhus, and gas gangrene bacteria gain access to the birth canal, with disastrous consequences.

Puerperal infections may occur anywhere in the pelvis or birth canal. They are named for the involved area, as follows:

endometritis Infection of endometrium (most common site).
parametritis Infection of connective tissue around uterus.
peritonitis Pelvic cavity infection.
vaginitis Vaginal infection.
vulvitis Vulval infection.

Normally the uterine cavity remains free of bacteria for 2 to 3 days after delivery. This period allows time for the raw inner surface to seal over with a layer of new cells before natural bacteria of the vagina move up into the uterus. The outward flow of lochia helps wash bacteria away during these crucial days of healing. This normal protection is breeched and the likelihood of infection is increased when:

1. Membranes rupture long before delivery.
2. Labor is prolonged and many examinations are performed.
3. Unsterile gloves or instruments are used.
4. The birth canal is exposed to droplet infection from noses or mouths of birth attendants.

Assessment. The first and most obvious symptom of infection is fever. Any elevation of temperature over 100.4° F (38° C) for 2 successive days during the first 10 days postpartum is considered a puerperal infection. If the episiotomy becomes infected, cardinal signs of an infection appear: pain, heat, swelling, and purulent discharge, especially along the incision line or around the sutures. If the endometrium becomes infected, the uterus may become tender and not show its normal involution. Lochia is green or yellow and has an unusual foul odor.

Interventions. Treatment consists of prescribing one or more antibiotics. Before selecting one of these drugs, the physician may order a culture of the discharge to determine what organisms have invaded the birth canal and which drugs will be most effective in destroying them. *Culture and sensitivity (C and S) tests* have become increasingly necessary because many pathogens have grown resistant to the common antibiotics. If treatment is urgent, a *broad-spectrum antibiotic* (one that is effective against many organisms) may be prescribed before the 48 to 72 hours needed for C and S test results.

Additional interventions include bed rest with the head of the bed elevated, forced fluids, frequent monitoring of vital signs, and local treatment of the infection by such measures as warm sitz baths.

Universal precautions are carried out to protect newborn infants, other patients, and staff from infection. Most mothers continue to breast-feed their infants unless the infection is overwhelming or their milk is contaminated.

Fortunately the woman's body begins to work against organisms soon after they invade. White cells rush to the area to combat the pathogens. Often the infection is walled off by tissue layers and kept from spreading into other areas. Local lymph nodes enlarge as cells within them fulfill their function of engulfing and destroying pathogens. With the aid of antibiotics, women today have a much better chance of surviving puerperal infection than they did in the past. However, availability of antibiotics is no reason for lax technique. The best defense against puerperal infection is prevention. Conscientious use of aseptic technique is essential.

Mastitis

Description. Mastitis is an inflammation of the breast. It is usually seen in first-time breast-feeding mothers. The infection primarily is caused by *Staphylococcus aureus*, which enters through cracked nipples. The most common bacterial source is the infant's nose and throat; other sources are the mother's hands or bloodstream. The infection usually occurs unilaterally, several days or weeks postpartum.

Assessment and interventions. The mother may have a high fever, chills, tachycardia, and headache. The affected breast becomes extremely tender, with one or more red, warm, and firm areas. If treatment is not begun at once, abscesses may develop. A culture is taken and antibiotics prescribed. If abscesses develop, they usually must be incised, drained, and packed open until they heal from below.

Opinion varies about whether mothers should continue to breast-feed. Some suggest that they stop breast-feeding temporarily, pump the breasts to relieve engorgement until they are afebrile, and then resume feeding. Others suggest that breast-feeding should be discontinued and that the breast be pumped just enough to relieve engorgement.

Often cracked and fissured nipples are caused by ignorance of correct breast-feeding and aseptic practices. (See Chapter 12 for breast-feeding technique.) Important learning needs of new mothers include proper breast-feeding technique and handwashing. If abscesses develop and mothers must stop breast-feeding, they are encouraged to express their disappointment and take pleasure in holding and nurturing the baby.

Urinary tract infections

Description. After delivery the woman is at increased risk of developing urinary tract problems because of normal postpartum diuresis, decreased bladder sensitivity, and possible inhibited nervous control following anesthesia. She may have difficulty initiating voiding because of tissue trauma, swelling, and perineal pain. Even when she is able to urinate, it may be in small amounts at frequent intervals, indicating retention with overflow. When urine is retained, it provides an ideal setting for bacterial growth. Cystitis and pyelonephritis may result.

Cystitis is an inflammation of the bladder. In 73% to 90% of the cases *Escherichia coli* is the causative bacteria. *Pyelonephritis* is an inflammation of the renal pelvis that is usually caused by infection. In most cases the infection has ascended from the lower urinary tract. Either kidney may be affected. If untreated, the renal cortex may be damaged and kidney function impaired.

Assessment and interventions. Frequent assessment of the bladder for distention following delivery is essential. If an infection is suspected, a clean-catch specimen is obtained for microscopic examination and culture and sensitivity. Catheterization is avoided to reduce the increased risk of infection. If it is necessary, strict sterile technique must be maintained.

Symptoms of cystitis often appear 2 to 3 days after delivery. These include frequency, urgency, cloudy urine, pelvic pain, and a bacterial concentration of 10,000 or more microorganisms per milliliter. When the infection progresses to pyelonephritis, systemic symptoms often occur. The woman becomes acutely ill with chills, high fever, flank pain on one or both sides, and nausea and vomiting, in addition to all the signs of cystitis.

Medical treatment for cystitis includes antibiotic therapy based on the C and S findings, antispasmodic drugs, and forced fluids. Pyelonephritis is treated vigorously with antibiotics. Bed rest, careful monitoring of intake and output, forced fluid or intravenous fluids if nausea and vomiting is severe, antispasmodics, and analgesics are prescribed. Antibiotics are continued for 2 to 4 weeks after signs and symptoms disappear. A clean-catch urine culture is done 2 weeks after treatment and periodically for 2 years.

Nurses play a significant role in preventing urinary tract infection (UTI) by avoiding overdistention of the woman's bladder, teaching proper perineal care and wiping techniques to avoid fecal contamination, and using scrupulous aseptic technique if catheterization becomes necessary. Women with pyelonephritis need to understand the importance of follow-up care after discharge to prevent recurrence or complications.

Mental illness
Incidence and description

Postpartum mental illnesses range from transitory depression to severe psychosis. Some depression, called *postpartum blues,* is experienced by up to 80% of all women. (See Chapters 4 and 13). It lasts for various periods, from a few hours to a year after childbirth.

Psychosis severe enough to require hospitalization occurs in about 0.1% of postpartum women. Of women with histories of mental illness, one fourth develop mental illness with subsequent pregnancies. Most postpartum mental illness appears as an affective, schizophrenic, or paranoid disorder.

The cause of postpartum mental illness is *not* pregnancy. However, it is believed that pregnancy-induced physiological and psychosocial stressors trigger mental illness in women who are predisposed to developing it. Physiological stressors include hormone changes, traumatic labor and delivery, preeclampsia, and similar factors. Psychosocial stressors include self-concept, interdependence, and role changes brought about by pregnancy.

Affective disorders may be unipolar depression or bipolar mania and depression. Symptoms include depression, mania, confusion, delusions (false ideas), hallucinations (false perceptions), anxiety, suicidal thinking, and sexual dysfunction. Symptoms may appear immediately after delivery, or they may appear gradually. Hospitalization becomes necessary if the woman is seriously disabled or a danger to herself or her infant.

Schizophrenic and *paranoid reactions* to pregnancy meet criteria for various schizophrenic, paranoid, and psychotic disorders found in the Diagnostic and Statistical Manual III-R. Usually symptoms appear within 10 days of delivery and include delusional thinking, flight of ideas, distortion of reality, and agitation. In some women symptoms appear more gradually, with increasing hostility, fear, suspiciousness, anxiety, and aversion to sexual activity. Some women exhaust themselves or become violent, physically harming their infants and others.

Assessment and interventions

A history of previous psychiatric problems should alert nurses to the possibility of another episode. Nurses observe mothers for signs of depression, including tearfulness, lack of facial expression or energy, and statements of hopelessness, worthlessness, or helplessness. Behavior or statements that are bizarre or indicate a potential for violence are noted and reported. Nurses need to establish a trusting relationship with mothers during the antepartum period, labor, delivery, and puerperium. Mothers are encouraged to share their understandings, feelings, and concerns. If caregivers doubt a mother's emotional stability, they may refer the mother and her family to community health resources for follow-up care.

When a specific mental illness is identified, psychotropic medications and hospitalization may be prescribed. Patient teaching about drug therapy is imperative. Family planning issues need to be addressed, especially when psychotic reactions to pregnancy recur. Adult family members are encouraged to participate in parenting classes and assume responsibility for infant care as soon as the mother's symptoms subside.

SURGERY

Sterilization surgery and induced abortions are two types of surgical procedures frequently encountered by nurses in the course of providing care to maternity patients.

Sterilization surgery

Sterilization is a procedure by which a person is made incapable of reproduction. In women this is accomplished by removing the ovaries or uterus or by interrupting the fallopian (uterine) tubes through which ova travel to the uterine cavity. In men sterilization is accomplished by severing the vas deferens or removing the testes. Because surgery to reopen uterine tubes and vas deferens is only rarely successful, the decision to undergo sterilization should be made with informed consent after due consideration. A signed consent

for such surgery from both spouses usually is required by hospitals and physicians.

Common indications for sterilization of women are multiple cesarean births, multiparity (many pregnancies), repeated serious complications of pregnancy, acute or chronic diseases, and economic or emotional stressors.

Tubal ligation

Description. The most common type of sterilization surgery for women is tubal ligation. This is done by ligation (cutting and tying) or by cautery (burning) of the tubes. The tubes are reached through a small abdominal or vaginal incision. A puncture is made through the umbilicus, and a periscope-like instrument called a *laparoscope* is inserted. Through it the tubes are located and severed or cauterized. Often tubal ligation is performed within a few hours after an uncomplicated delivery while the uterus is high in the abdomen and the tubes are easily located.

Interventions. Preoperative nursing care of the person who is to undergo tubal ligation is the same as for any abdominal surgery. An informed consent is signed, food and fluid withheld, and preoperative medication given. If general anesthesia is used, the woman recovers in the recovery room. Often the procedure is done under local anesthesia; postoperative recovery is rapid and usually uneventful.

Hysterectomy

Description. Removal of the uterus obviously causes sterility, but indications for hysterectomy usually are not strictly contraceptive. Indications for this procedure following pregnancy include:

1. Ruptured or inverted uterus
2. Fibroid and malignant tumors
3. Placenta accreta
4. Severe intrauterine infection
5. Uncontrolled postpartum hemorrhage
6. Abdominal pregnancy when the abdom-

inal organs and supporting tissues are the site of placental implantation
Cesarean birth of the fetus followed by hysterectomy may be performed at the same time, such as in the last of a series of cesarean births.

Interventions. When hysterectomy is planned, there is time to prepare both the mother and her family. Preoperative and postoperative nursing care are similar to that of cesarean birth, described in Chapter 10.

When hysterectomy is performed because of an obstetrical emergency such as a ruptured uterus, however, there is little time for preparation of the mother and her family. An informed consent is obtained, and surgery is begun at once. Postoperative care is intense because of conditions surrounding the decision to perform surgery, such as hemorrhage or infection. Assessment is made of vital signs, intake and output, pain, and the incision. Intravenous therapy, antibiotics, and analgesics usually are prescribed. Interventions include comfort measures, attention to elimination, relief of pain, and meeting the mother's emotional needs.

Postoperatively the mother may undergo an acute grief reaction from the loss of so significant a body part. If the baby did not survive, her grief is even more profound because she can will not be able to have another baby. Interventions for loss and grief are described in Chapter 10.

Induced abortion
Description

Induced abortions are categorized according to when they are performed: *early* (until week 12 of gestation), *interim* (13 to 16 weeks), and *late* (16 or more weeks). The risk of complications increases with weeks of gestation. Procedures used for abortions are vacuum aspiration, dilation and curettage (D and C), saline instillation, prostaglandin injection, and hysterotomy.

Uterine vacuum aspiration is the procedure most often used for early abortions. The cervix is dilated with a laminaria tent or dilating sounds, and a small tube is inserted into the uterus. Suction is applied to the tube, and contents of the uterus are emptied. The procedure usually is performed in an outpatient clinic or office using local anesthesia.

Dilation and curettage (D and C) is a procedure used for both early and interim abortions. The cervix is dilated with a laminaria tent or dilating sounds, and the uterine lining is scraped with a curet. Contents of the uterus is aspirated with suction. The procedure is done in a clinic, office, or hospital surgical suite using local or general anesthesia.

Saline instillation (salting out) is a procedure used for late abortions. After cleansing the abdomen and injecting local anesthetic, a needle with a stylet is inserted midline through the lower abdomen into the uterus. As much as 250 ml of amniotic fluid is withdrawn and up to 240 ml of 23.4% salt solution is injected and the needle removed. Fetal death occurs within 1 hour of the injection, probably because of dehydration. Six hours after the salt injection an intravenous infusion containing oxytocin is started at 10 drops per minute and increased to produce active labor. The cervix usually must dilate to 4 cm before abortion occurs. If no oxytocic drugs are given, spontaneous labor usually begins within 8 to 48 hours. In about 10% of cases reinjection of salt is necessary to initiate labor.

Prostaglandin injection is the preferred technique for late abortions, except for asthmatic women, who may suffer from the bronchoconstricting action of the drug. Prostaglandins are fatty acids that occur naturally in the body tissues of animals and humans. When injected into the pregnant woman, they produce strong uterine contractions with rapid dilation of the cervix. Dinoprost tromethamine (Prostin F2 Alpha) is the drug of choice. A dose of 40 to 60 mg is instilled in the uterine cavity or amniotic sac. Labor begins soon thereafter, and abortion occurs in 18 to 24 hours. If it does not, the procedure is repeated using half the dose.

Hysterotomy is the removal of the fetus through an abdominal incision resembling a mini–cesarean birth with the mother under regional or general anesthesia. This procedure is done only when no other option is available, such as when the fetus is large and grossly deformed.

Nursing interventions

Before any procedure is scheduled, counseling is provided to discuss the risks and alternatives to abortion. A description of the procedure is given, and an informed consent is signed. Preoperative instructions are provided, and the woman is encouraged to bring a support person who will stay with her during and after the abortion. Because the decision to have an abortion may be especially painful, nurses need to understand the grieving process discussed in Chapter 10 and to provide ongoing emotional support in every possible way.

Early abortions usually are performed in an outpatient surgical suite. After the procedure a single dose of oxytocin is administered to control bleeding. Antibiotics may be prescribed to prevent infection and oral analgesics administered to reduce discomfort. The woman is observed for hemorrhage for 3 to 4 hours. Discharge instructions include information about complications, an emergency number to call, community counseling services, alternative contraceptive methods, and a return appointment in 4 to 6 weeks.

Interim abortions may be performed in an outpatient or hospital surgical suite using either local or general anesthesia. Postoperatively, oxytocin, antibiotics, and analgesics are prescribed, and the woman is observed closely for hemorrhage for 6 to 18 hours. Discharge instructions include information about com-

plications, an emergency number to call, alternative contraceptive methods, community counseling services, and a return appointment in 4 to 6 weeks.

Late abortions are performed in a hospital where emergency care is available. When saline or prostaglandin instillation is used, labor may not begin for several hours. Because labor for an abortion is joyless work, discomfort is increased. Nurses may be the sole source of emotional support. They also provide basic hygiene, adequate fluids, and pain relief; keep output records; help conserve the woman's energy; and observe vital signs and the progress of labor.

Delivery often is signaled by rectal pressure. If the cervix has dilated to 4 cm, the woman is instructed to push. Expulsion of the placenta usually follows the fetus within 2 hours. Drugs may be administered to promote uterine contraction, prevent infection, suppress lactation, and control discomfort. The woman is observed closely for hemorrhage for several hours. Discharge instructions are similar to those for postpartum women, including information about complications, an emergency number to call, community counseling services, and a return appointment in 4 to 6 weeks.

▶ KEY CONCEPTS

1. Postpartum hemorrhage of 1% or more of body weight is life threatening. Nursing assessment includes checking the fundus for firmness, lochia for quantity, and vital signs for hypovolemic shock.

2. Disseminated intravascular coagulation (DIC) is characterized by abnormal clotting and widespread bleeding and is triggered by bacteremia, amniotic fluid embolism, immune reactions, and other disorders. Intensive care is needed.

3. Thrombophlebitis is inflammation of a vein with clot formation, often occurring in femoral and pelvic veins. A major concern is occlusion or embolism. Treatment involves heparin ther-

apy (may cause heavy lochia, bleeding nipples, and pelvic hematoma), bed rest, moist heat, avoidance of leg massage, and elastic stockings worn for 6 months. Nursing interventions are patient teaching, emotional support, and discharge planning.

4. Puerperal infection is caused by invasion of bacteria into the uterine cavity or episiotomy. Symptoms are fever, foul lochia, tender uterus, and inflamed episiotomy. Interventions include antibiotics, fluids, monitoring of vital signs, and sitz baths. Prevention is the best defense against infections.

5. Mastitis (inflammation of the breasts) is usually seen in first-time breast-feeding mothers and often results from improper technique. Symptoms include high fever, local redness, tenderness, and heat. Antibiotic therapy is instituted; if abscesses develop, they are incised and drained.

6. Increased risk of urinary tract infections results from postpartum diuresis, decreased bladder sensitivity, and inhibited nervous control causing retention with overflow. Infection ascends from the bladder to kidneys, resulting in frequency, urgency, cloudy urine, pain, and bacteria in urine. Treatment includes antibiotics and fluids. Prevention measures: avoid bladder distention, give proper perineal care, and use aseptic technique.

7. Mental illnesses range from transitory depression to severe psychosis. Their cause is *not* pregnancy, but physical and psychosocial stressors that trigger affective, schizophrenic, and paranoid disorders. Nurses assess for signs of depression and bizarre statements or behavior. If severe, treatment involves psychotropic medications and hospitalization.

8. Tubal ligation is a common sterilization procedure done immediately after delivery with few complications.

9. Hysterectomy for an obstetrical emergency is especially difficult for parents when infant dies because it may produce an acute grief reaction.

10. Induced abortions are categorized as early (until week 12 of gestation), interim (13 to 16 weeks), and late (16 or more weeks). Vacuum aspiration is used for early abortions; dilation and currettage for early and interim; saline instillations, prostaglandin injections, and hysterotomy are used for late abortions. Pre- and postabortion counseling is important. Postoperative concerns are hemorrhage, infection, and contraceptive information.

■ *ANNOTATED SUMMARY*

I. Complications—unique to postpartum period
   A. Bleeding and clotting disorders
      1. Hemorrhage
         a. Description and causes—one of most common causes of maternal death; 1% of body weight is life threatening
         b. Assessment—check fundus, lochia, signs of hypovolemic shock
         c. Interventions—IV oxytocin, continued assessment, emotional support
      2. Disseminated intravascular coagulation (DIC)
         a. Description and causes—abnormal clotting occurs; clotting factors used up, causing widespread bleeding
         b. Assessment and interventions—transfer patient to ICU; remove causal factor; initiate supportive care; give whole blood, plasma and heparin
      3. Thrombophlebitis
         a. Terminology and description—inflammation of veins with clot formation; dangers are local inflammation and embolism
         b. Incidence—low during pregnancy, high after delivery
         c. Assessment and interventions—heparin therapy, bed rest, moist heat, no leg massage, elastic stockings; ambulation is begun slowly
   B. Infections
      1. Puerperal infection
         a. Description—caused by bacterial invasion of uterine cavity and episiotomy
         b. Assessment—fever, foul discharge, signs of inflamed episiotomy

c. Interventions—administer antibiotics and fluids; monitor vital signs; universal precautions; prevention is best defense

2. Mastitis
   a. Description—infection of breasts; usually seen in first-time breast-feeding mothers, often because of improper breast-feeding techniques
   b. Assessment and interventions—fever, pain, heat, redness; antibiotic therapy; abscesses incised and drained and breast-feeding stopped

3. Urinary tract infections
   a. Description—ascending infection from bladder to kidney; results from diuresis, decreased bladder sensitivity, inhibited nervous control causing retention with overflow
   b. Assessment and interventions—frequency, urgency, cloudy urine, pain, bacteria in urine; antibiotic therapy, fluids; prevention: aseptic technique

C. Mental illness
   1. Incidence and description—postpartum blues are common; severe psychosis in 0.1% of cases: affective, schizophrenic, and paranoid reactions
   2. Assessment and interventions—bizarre action or statements, may injure infant; psychotrophic drugs, psychotherapy, sometimes hospitalization

II. Surgery
A. Sterilization surgery
   1. Tubal ligation
      a. Description—fallopian tubes cut or cauterized; often done soon after delivery
      b. Interventions—few complications
   2. Hysterectomy
      a. Description—removal of uterus; usually done for reasons other than sterilization
      b. Interventions—postoperative care as for any abdominal surgery; if done for obstetrical emergency and baby dies, acute grief reaction

B. Induced abortion
   1. Description—categorized as early (to 12 weeks' gestation), interim (13 to 16 weeks), late (16 or more weeks); vacuum aspiration for early; dilation and curettage for interim; saline instillation, prostaglandin injection, or hysterotomy for late.
   2. Nursing interventions—pre- and postoperative counseling, postoperative concern for hemorrhage, infection, and contraceptive information

● **STUDY QUESTIONS AND LEARNING ACTIVITIES**

1. What are the causes and signs of postpartum hemorrhage? What amount of blood loss is considered life threatening for a woman who weighs 150 pounds (68 kg)?
2. If DIC occurs as a result of clotting, why is there widespread bleeding?
3. Describe two major concerns in thrombophlebitis and symptoms that might be seen at its onset. List the treatment and rationale for each.
4. Where might puerperal infection occur? What increases the likelihood that it will occur?
5. What are the initial signs and symptoms of mastitis? Who is a likely candidate for acquiring this infection, and what can be done to reduce this likelihood?
6. What can nurses do to prevent urinary tract infection? Why is a bladder infection especially dangerous?
7. If pregnancy is not the cause of postpartum psychosis, what is? Describe signs of mental illness in postpartum mothers.
8. What is the optimum time for tubal ligation? Describe the procedure as you would to a mother.
9. How would you describe a vacuum aspiration to a pregnant woman? When might a hysterectomy be performed?

REFERENCES

Affonso D: Postpartum depression. In Fields P, ed: Recent advances in perinatal nursing, New York, 1984, Churchill Livingstone.

American Psychiatric Association: Diagnostic and Statistical Manual of Mental Disorders, ed 3, rev, Washington, DC, 1987, APA.

Bobak IM, and Jensen MD: Essentials of maternity nursing: the nurse and the childbearing family, ed 2, St Louis, 1987, The CV Mosby Co.

Fagnant RJ, and Monif G: Septic pelvic thrombophlebitis, Contemp OB/GYN, 29(2):129, 1987.

Hillard PA: Postpartum hemorrhage, Parents 62(1):104, 1987.

Nyman JE: Thrombophlebitis in pregnancy, Am J Nurs 80:1, 1980.

Olds SB, London ML, and Ladewig PA: Maternal-newborn nursing: a family-centered approach, ed 3, Menlo Park, Calif, 1988, Addison-Wesley Publishing.

Sciarra JJ, ed: Gynecology and obstetrics, vol 2, Philadelphia, 1982, Harper & Row, Publishers.

CHAPTER 15

Care of the New Family

LEARNING OBJECTIVES

- Describe the adjustments necessary to meet the needs of each family member after the newborn is at home.

- Describe the care of the newborn infant at home, including sleep, bathing, feeding, positioning, handling, and medical supervision.

- Describe the various methods of contraception, including abstinence, prevention of the sperm from reaching the ovum, prevention of ovulation and spermatogenesis, and prevention of implantation.

- Discuss the relative effectiveness of each contraceptive method.

- List the professional persons who are prepared to offer social service referrals for families.

FAMILY ADJUSTMENT
Intrafamily relationships

As the mother and baby come home from the hospital or birthing center, they and their family begin a new life together. Each member must make major adjustments.

Children

If there are older children, the new baby's arrival may be particularly disturbing, especially to the youngest child. Such children may seem shy or distant as a result of their feelings of having been abandoned by mother when she was away. When the mother and baby first arrive home, it may be wise for father to carry the new baby into the house so that mother's arms are free to embrace the "older" baby.

As children see how much time their mother spends with the new baby, they may feel resentment and develop open hostility. The mother can provide evidence of her con-

tinuing love by giving them individual attention. Sometimes it helps to give older children
a doll with the same name as the new baby.
The doll can be "their baby." If the mother
notices them spanking or mistreating the doll,
she can repeat their words or verbalize their
actions with such remarks as, "Andy is getting
a spanking. What did he do? Did he hurt you?"
Such questions opens the way for a mother to
reassure older children that she understands
and continues to love and care for them.

A father, too, can help older children accept
the new baby. He can give his "first" attention
to older children when he comes home from
work. When visitors come to see the new baby,
older children may feel ignored and "show
off" in an effort to be noticed. To avoid such
behavior and the reproof it may bring, parents
need to seek ways to recognize older children
in meaningful ways that promote self-esteem.

Father

Father may become the forgotten family
member, especially if this is the first child.
Before the baby arrived, he was the other half
of a family of two. Daytime activities were easily negotiated with his partner and night time
was undisturbed. Now the house is dishev-
eled, meals are unscheduled, sleep is interrupted, and coitus is temporarily forbidden.
Fathers need to be included in child care and
home maintenance activities. By sharing
these responsibilities, they become part of the
parenting experience. As a result, the couple
are drawn closer together.

Mother

The ability of the mother to cope with her
new role depends on her physical health, pre-
formed attitudes, living patterns, and workload. If she had a normal pregnancy and delivery, prepared for her new role, and is a fairly
organized homemaker, care of the new baby
probably will not overwhelm her. If, however,

she is recuperating from a complication of
childbirth, was unprepared for child care, or
is unaccustomed to managing a home, she
may need to call on family or community resources to help her meet these responsibilities.

Maternal postpartum needs

Mothers need adequate rest, even if they
must get it in small naps. They need a balanced diet, including extra milk if they are
breast-feeding. Mothers need to maintain personal hygiene and grooming. Douching and
intercourse are not advised until the uterine
lining and episiotomy are fully healed. This
takes about 4 to 6 weeks after delivery. Mothers may want to begin abdominal muscle-
strengthening exercises after that time, but
they should not overdo and exhaust themselves. (See Chapter 13.)

The postpartum checkup usually is scheduled about 6 weeks after delivery. At this visit
a thorough physical examination is performed,
including vital signs, weight, general appearance, breasts, nipples, lungs, heart, abdomen,
extremities, episiotomy repair, cervix, vagina,
and uterus. Lochia should have ceased by this
time. The physician or nurse discusses breast
care, diet, weight gain or loss, exercise, elimination, rest, return to work outside the home,
bathing, douching, return of menses, intercourse, and contraception. Laboratory tests
are performed if indicated.

Newborn infant care

It may seem to older children that all the
new baby does is eat and sleep. Indeed, this
is true. The newborn infant primarily needs
sleep, nutrition, nurturance, and protection
from harm.

Sleep

Newborn infants sleep about 20 to 22 hours
per day. The baby's bed should have a firm
mattress, be easily cleaned, and have sides

high enough to keep the baby from falling out. If the sides are made of slats, they should be close enough together so that the small head will not become wedged between them. The first crib need not be elaborate; a dresser drawer serves well. Most babies sleep best on their abdomens with the head turned to the side. If babies always lie on their backs, the back of the head will flatten because the bones of the newborn's skull are soft and easily molded.

Nutrition

Breast- or bottle-feeding is begun in the hospital before the baby and mother are discharged. Since milk does not come into the breasts until about the third day, mother and baby often are at home when the milk comes in. At first there is much more milk than the baby needs. Soon the supply adjusts to the baby's appetite. Before discharge mothers should be instructed in proper breast-feeding technique. (See Chapter 13.) An "on demand" feeding schedule is recommended by most authorities.

If a baby is bottle-fed prepackaged formula, only sterile bottles are needed. If the formula is made by the family according to a recipe, special care must be taken to sterilize both the formula and the equipment. Because bacteria multiply rapidly in warm, sweet milk, formula should be refrigerated until it is used. The American Academy of Pediatrics recommends the introduction of solid food when the baby is 4 to 6 months of age.

Bathing

Classes on how to bathe a baby may be taught in the postpartum unit or preparation-for-childbirth classes. Newborn infants should be bathed regularly with warm water; a mild soap may be used. Until the navel heals, sponge baths are recommended with application of alcohol to the umbilical site.

An elaborate bathinette is not necessary. A plastic tub on the kitchen table is perfectly acceptable. The room should be free of drafts and the infant protected from falls. All bathing equipment and clean clothing are assembled before the infant is undressed.

The bath begins with the face and head, then upper torso, arms, abdomen, back, legs, and finally buttocks. When the navel is healed, the baby can be carefully placed into the warm water. Because the infant cannot sit up alone, the bather's arm supports the baby from slipping under the water. To avoid chilling, bath time is brief; the baby is dressed quickly and wrapped in a warm blanket.

There is no "correct" time for bathing a baby; however, it should be done before a feeding rather than after to avoid movement that may cause regurgitation.

Handling and holding

Newborn infants need to be held but not handled. If they are wrestled about excessively, they become fretful and tired and may regurgitate their feedings. On the other hand, the comforting security of being firmly held in someone's arms is vital to emotional development (Fig. 15-1). For this reason, breast-feeding is promoted, and parents of bottle-fed infants are encouraged to hold babies for every feeding.

Medical supervision

As the infant is discharged from a birthing center or hospital, parents are given an appointment for the baby's first medical checkup, usually in about 4 weeks. If the infant is small or sickly, medical followup is scheduled sooner. Parents are given an emergency telephone number to call in case problems arise.

The baby's first office or clinic visit includes an examination by a nurse practitioner or physician. The baby is weighed, measured, and

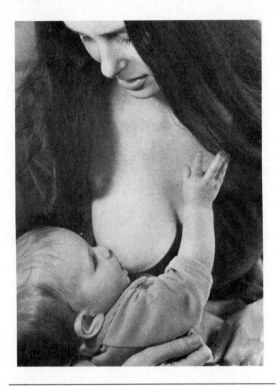

Fig. 15-1 Breast-feeding is one of the best ways to promote emotional development in the newborn infant.

examined. Infant care is discussed, including feeding, elimination, sleep, skin condition, and any problems that may have been identified.

Monthly medical checkups are scheduled for the first year of life. If a family cannot afford a private physician, low-cost well-child conferences are offered by local public health departments. Immunizations usually are begun when the baby is 8 to 10 weeks of age. Sick infants should not be taken to well-child conferences but to physicians' offices or pediatric clinics.

FAMILY PLANNING

Planning the number and spacing of children has been possible since the advent of

effective contraceptive (birth control) methods. In the United States 90% of couples use or intend to use some form of contraception. Religious creeds, cultural values, economic pressure, and career goals play a part in the decision of couples to use birth control. If couples use no contraception, 60% to 80% of the women will become pregnant within the first year, and 10% will not conceive.

Methods of contraception

The ideal contraceptive method is safe, effective (reliable), economical, simple to use, aesthetically acceptable, and promptly reversible. Although no method has been found that achieves all these objectives, progress is being made. At this time there are four basic ways to prevent pregnancy temporarily: (1) abstinence (no coitus), (2) prevention of fertilization, (3) prevention of ovulation or spermatogenesis, and (4) prevention of implantation.

Abstinence

Abstinence means refraining from coitus, either periodically or permanently. It is the only method of birth control fully approved by the Roman Catholic Church. Periodic abstinence, also called *continence,* is employed in a number of systems, including:
1. Coitus interruptus (withdrawal)
2. Mutual masturbation without coitus
3. Rhythm or calender method
4. Basal body temperature (BBT) method
5. Cervical mucus (Billings, ovulation) method
6. Symptothermal method
7. Fertility awareness method
8. Predictor test for ovulation

Coitus interruptus. This method involves the withdrawal of the penis before ejaculation. It is probably the oldest method of birth control. Because sperm are emitted in various amounts in the seminal fluid before ejaculation, this method is not reliable.

Mutual masturbation. This method is sex play to climax without genital contact. Although this method may be temporarily useful for both partners, it is not considered a long-term solution to family planning.

Rhythm (calendar) method. Principles underlying most periodic abstinence methods are that (1) human ovum can be fertilized for about 18 to 24 hours after ovulation, and (2) if a menstrual cycle is 28 days long, ovulation usually occurs at about day 14. If menses are not regular, this method is not effective. In this method the couple abstain from intercourse for 3 days before the expected ovulation day and 3 days afterward.

Basal body temperature method. This method is based on the fact that 1 to 2 days before ovulation the basal body temperature (BBT) may drop 0.2° to 0.3° F (0.1° C). Then, 1 to 2 days after ovulation, BBT may rise 0.7° to 0.8° F (0.3° to 0.4° C). BBT continues on at that level until the temperature drops to the low levels recorded during the previous menses. Abstinence from day 10 to 19 is recommended. Illness, activity, hydration, and emotions can also elevate body temperature, invalidating the data.

Cervical mucus (Billings), ovulation method. This method is based on changes in the consistency of cervical mucus 3 days before ovulation. The woman checks her cervical mucus; if it is sticky, ovulation is about to occur or has occurred. This method depends on the ability of the woman to judge relative stickiness of cervical mucus and abstain from intercourse for at least 6 days after the stickiness first is noticed.

Symptothermal method. This method combines BBT and cervical mucus evaluation with awareness of other secondary symptoms such as mood changes. Detailed records and cooperation of both members of the couple are necessary.

Fertility awareness. This method combines the symptothermal method and barrier contraception. During the fertile period the couple have a choice of abstinence or use of a barrier contraceptive such as condoms.

Predictor test for ovulation. This test detects the sudden surge of luteinizing hormone (LH) that occurs about 12 to 24 hours before ovulation. The test is not affected by illness, activity, or emotions. Available for home use, the test kit contains enough material for several tests during each cycle. An LH surge produces an easily read color change. During the fertile period the couple have a choice of abstinence or use of a barrier contraceptive such as condoms. The test also is useful for couples who desire conception.

Prevention of fertilization

A number of physical and chemical barriers are used to prevent conception, including the condom, diaphragm, cervical cap, vaginal sponge, and spermicidal preparations.

Condom. A condom is a soft rubber sheath that is placed over the erect penis before coitus. A half-inch "pocket" should be maintained at its end. At ejaculation the sperm are contained and prevented from entering the cervix. Recently this method has enjoyed great popularity because the condom also serves as a physical barrier to prevent pathogens from infecting either partner.

Diaphram. A diaphragm is a soft rubber disk that is placed over the cervix. To be effective, the correct size must be fitted to the woman. The diaphragm must be inserted no more than 1 hour before intercourse with a fresh spermicidal agent and left in place for at least 8 hours afterward.

Cervical cap. Recently approved for sale in United States, the cervical cap is a small plastic cap about an inch in diameter. A small one-way valve in the center permits menstrual flow to escape but bars semen from entering. The cap is held in place by cervical mucus and is designed to remain in place for 1 year. Its effectiveness is increased if a spermicidal agent also is used.

Vaginal sponge. The vaginal sponge is a mushroom-shaped device made of soft polyurethane that is positioned over the cervix. It prevents conception in three ways: (1) by a slow but constant release of spermicide, (2) by blocking the cervical opening, and (3) by absorbing semen and destroying sperm. A vaginal sponge does not require special fitting or a prescription.

Spermicidal preparations. A variety of foams, jellies, creams, suppositories, and tablets are available over the counter. They destroy sperm and provide a physical barrier as well. They must be applied immediately before intercourse, (their maximum duration is 15 to 60 minutes) and must be allowed to remain in the vagina for 8 hours after intercourse.

Progestin. Progestin acts to thicken cervical mucus and prevent sperm from entering the uterus. It is administered as a "minipill" every day of the year, an injection that is effective for 3 to 6 months, and as an implant in a Silastic container effective for up to 5 years.

Douches. Douching is not an effective contraceptive method because sperm may enter the cervix 10 to 90 seconds after ejaculation. Douching actually may help force sperm into the uterus.

Prevention of ovulation and spermatogenesis

Estrogen and progesterone tablets ("the pill"). The combination of estrogen and progesterone produces a condition similar to pregnancy. Even in tiny amounts these hormones act to suppress pituitary hormones necessary for ovulation. As a result, ovulation does not occur. When the pill is discontinued, normal monthly ovulation returns, just as it does after pregnancy. To be effective, the pill must be taken daily from day 5 to day 28 of the menstrual cycle. It is stopped to allow a menses and begun again on day 5.

Correctly followed, this method is 99% to 100% effective. However, the pill is expensive; requires intelligent, consistent use; causes undesirable symptoms in some women, such as fluid retention; and is associated with thrombosis. Long-term studies show that women who take the pill have a lower incidence of cervical, endometrial, and breast cancer.

Spermatogenicidal drugs ("male pill"). Not yet on the market, these drugs prevent the development of sperm. They do not affect potency, and their effects stop when the man stops taking them.

Prevention of implantation

Morning-after pill. Several drugs are being tested that make it impossible for a fertilized ovum to undergo nidation. One such preparation is diethylstilbestrol (DES); it must be taken within 72 hours of unprotected coitus during the fertile period. Another drug, designated RU 486, was released by a French firm in 1988. It is not yet available in the United States. RU 486 acts by blocking the action of progesterone, the hormone needed by the uterus to support development of a fertilized ovum. An effective abortient, it safely can end an early pregnancy in 85% of women who take it within 10 days of a missed menses.

Intrauterine devices. Interuterine devices (IUDs) are inert plastic forms placed inside the uterus. A variety of shapes are made, including the loop, spiral, cone, and coil (Fig. 15-2). Medicated IUDs are loaded with various drugs, such as copper or progesterone, which are released continuously into the endometrium. The presence of an IUD interferes with implantation of a fertilized ovum but not with normal menstrual cycles. Unlike contraceptive drugs, an IUD does not need constant or even periodic attention. It does not alter the hormone cycle of the body. Once in place, an

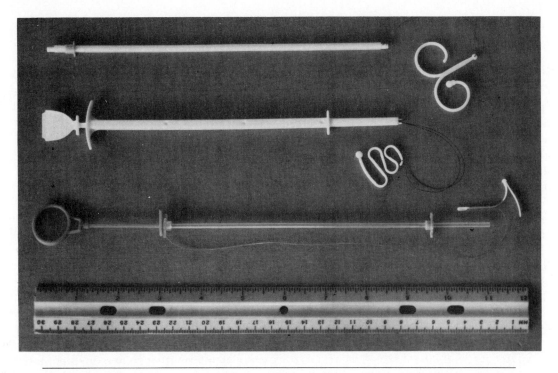

Fig. 15-2 Types of intrauterine devices (IUDs) with their inserters. From top down: Saf-T-Coil, Lippes Loop, and "Cu 7." *(From Ingalls, AJ, and Salerno, MC: Maternal-child health nursing, ed 6, St. Louis, 1987, The CV Mosby Co.)*

IUD can remain until the woman desires pregnancy.

Serious complications can result from an IUD, including a higher incidence of infections, severe cramping, heavy menses, and loss of the device without the woman's knowledge. An IUD may become embedded in the uterine wall or in the products of conception. Even with these drawbacks, IUDs are highly effective (95%), are inexpensive, require no special knowledge, and do not interfere with normal coitus.

Abortion

Abortion has been a means of birth control for centuries, although a risky one. With the legal barriers removed and modern techniques improved, the dangers of abortion have been greatly reduced, but not eliminated. (See Chapter 14 for a description of surgical abortion methods.) Although a variety of contraceptive methods have been developed, abortion continues to be a measure of last resort, used when other methods of birth control fail.

Sterilization

Sterilization might be called "terminal" contraception, since it renders the man or woman permanently infertile. It has become an exceedingly popular method of family planning as men and women grow weary of using devices and drugs that are less than 100% effective and cause so many complications. (See

Chapter 14 for a description of sterilization procedures.)

Effectiveness of contraceptive methods

The reliability of a contraceptive method is of prime importance to the couple as they plan their family. Remembering that a method is only as effective as the consistency and accuracy of its use, the various methods can be ranked as follows:

Most reliable:
   Total abstinence
   Predictor test for ovulation
   Estrogen-progesterone tablets (the "pill")
   Progestin
Highly reliable:
   Intrauterine device
   Cervical cap with spermicidal agent
   Condom with spermicidal agent
   Diaphragm with spermicidal agent
   Vaginal sponge
      Moderately reliable:
   BBT, cervical mucus, symptothermal, and
      fertility awareness methods
   Spermicidal agents only
Least reliable:
   Rhythm (calendar)
   Coitus interruptus
   Douches

COMMUNITY RESOURCES
Recognition of need

Although the family is the basic unit of most human societies, it does not exist alone. It is interdependent with the community and, as such, gives and receives services to and from others. In older societies, neighbors helped each other in every way. They harvested crops, tended children, delivered babies, built barns, cooked meals, and even settled arguments.

In our mobile, impersonal society a variety of specialized agencies have replaced neighbors. These agencies are available to every individual and family, yet many people are not

benefited by them because they are ignorant of their existence or function. Nurses are in a unique position to help, since they can recognize needs and realize that there are certain community agencies that may help. They cannot be expected to know all the community resources, but they can see that patients are directed to informational resources.

Sources of information

The professional specialist in the field of social services who is available to the family and its members is the *social worker*. Many hospitals employ medical social workers for the primary purpose of helping their patients use the tremendous number of community agencies to their best advantage. Together with the social worker, the *discharge planner* helps patients with transition back to their homes.

In addition to services, the hospital agencies serve as information centers to direct families to other appropriate sources for help. Some organizations exist specifically for the purpose of providing information, counseling, and guidance, such as federal, state, and local family service agencies.

EPILOGUE

Members of the maternal-child care team enjoy a privilege not known in any of the other medical specialties. They witness the miracle of birth and participate in one of the most critical of family experiences. This unusual privilege demands unusual responsibility. It requires that health care providers use their knowledge and skill with genuine concern, acceptance, and warmth. Such is the challenge of maternity nursing.

▶ *KEY CONCEPTS*

1. When a new baby enters the family, each member must make major adjustments. Older children learn to share parental attention; father accommodates to a new schedule and respon-

sibilities; mother assumes a new role and may need outside help for awhile.

2. Maternal postpartum needs are for a balanced diet, personal hygiene, grooming, rest, gradual activity, medical care, and family planning information.

3. Newborn infants need sleep (20 to 22 hours per day), nutrition (breast or bottle feedings), nurturance (to be held, not handled), and protection (to be bathed, sleep in a safe firm bed, and receive medical supervision).

4. Family planning of some kind is practiced by 90% of couples in United States. There are four basic types: abstinence, fertilization prevention, ovulation or spermatogenesis prevention, and implantation prevention.

5. Types of abstinence are absolute, coitus interruptus (withdrawal), mutual masturbation without coitus (sex play), rhythm or calendar (based on menstrual cycle), BBT (based on body temperature change before and after ovulation), cervical mucus (based on consistency of mucus), symptothermal (combination of BBT and cervical mucus), fertility awareness (combination of symptothermal and barrier contraception), and predictor test for ovulation period.

6. Types of fertilization prevention are condom (rubber sheath), diaphragm (rubber dome for cervix), cervical cap (plastic cap with one-way valve), vaginal sponge (spermicidal-saturated polyurethane), spermicidal agents (destroying sperm), progestin (minipill; thickens cervical mucus), and douches (ineffective).

7. Types of ovulation and spermatogenesis prevention are estrogen-progesterone tablets (pill; suppresses pituitary hormone for ovulation) and spermatogenicidal drugs (male pill; not yet available).

8. Types of implantation prevention are morning-after pill (DES), RU 486, and intrauterine devices (plastic forms inserted into uterus).

9. Abortion is a contraceptive method of last resort; sterilization is "terminal contraception."

10. Reliability of contraceptive methods: most reliable are total abstinence, predictor test for ovulation, estrogen-progesterone tablets, and

progestin; least reliable are rhythm, coitus interruptus, and douches.

11. Families may need help from community resources. Nurses should recognize needs and make referral to social workers and discharge planners who specialize in knowledge of these resources.

■ ANNOTATED SUMMARY

I. Family adjustment
  A. Intrafamily relationships—major adjustments necessary for all family members
    1. Children—need extra demonstrations of parental concern
    2. Father—needs to be included in child care and home responsibilities
    3. Mother—must adjust to new role; may need outside help
  B. Maternal postpartum needs—rest, personal hygiene, grooming, gradual activity, postpartum checkup, family planning method if desired
  C. Newborn infant care
    1. Sleep—20 to 22 hours per day
    2. Nutrition—on demand, formula should be sterile; solid food at 4 to 6 months
    3. Bathing—before feeding, but any time of day
    4. Handling and holding—gentleness, always for feedings
    5. Medical supervision—at 4 weeks of age
II. Family planning—90% of U.S. couples use some form
  A. Methods of contraception—four types
    1. Abstinence—no coitus, may be periodic
      a. Coitus interruptus (withdrawal)—sperm may be emitted before ejaculation
      b. Mutual masturbation—sex play to climax
      c. Rhythm or calendar method—based on ovulation and menstrual cycle
      d. Basal body temperature (BBT)—based on slight changes in body temperature during menstrual cycle
      e. Cervical mucus (Billings, ovulation) method—based on changes in consistency of mucus
      f. Symptothermal method—combines

BBT and cervical mucus evaluation
g. Fertility awareness method—combines symptothermal and barrier contraception
h. Predictor test for ovulation—tests for LH
2. Prevention of fertilization
   a. Condom—rubber sheath for penis
   b. Diaphragm—rubber dome for cervix
   c. Cervical cap—plastic cap with one-way valve
   d. Vaginal sponge—mushroom-shaped, polyurethane sponge
   e. Spermicidal preparations—destroy sperm
   f. Progestin—thickens cervical mucus, "minipill," injected, implanted
   g. Douches—ineffective
3. Prevention of ovulation and spermatogenesis
   a. Estrogen-progesterone tablets ("the pill")—suppress pituitary hormones for ovulation
   b. Spermatogenicidal drugs ("male pill")—not on market yet
4. Prevention of implantation
   a. Morning-after pill—prevents nidation
   b. Intrauterine devices (IUDs)—plastic forms inserted into uterus
5. Abortion—measure of last resort
6. Sterilization—"terminal contraception"
B. Effectiveness of contraceptive methods—methods ranked according to reliability

III. Community resources
   A. Recognition of need
   B. Sources of information—social workers and discharge planners
IV. Epilogue

● *STUDY QUESTIONS AND LEARNING ACTIVITIES*

1. How can the older child be helped when the new baby arrives home from the hospital?
2. Describe an "ideal" sleeping, bathing, and feeding routine of daily care for the 2-week-old infant at home. Give your rationale.
3. What are four basic ways currently available to families to control human reproduction? Give examples.
4. Discuss the means by which each of the following contraceptive methods works: pill, IUD, diaphragm, foam, condom, and rhythm.
5. What professionals could a staff nurse call on in the hospital for referral information to community agencies?

REFERENCES

Bachrach CA: Contraceptive practices among American women: 1973-1982, Fam Plann Perspect 16:253, 1984.

Bobak IM, and Jensen MD: Essentials of maternity nursing: the nurse and the childbearing family, ed 2, St Louis, 1987, The CV Mosby Co.

Ingalls AJ, and Salerno MC: Maternal-child health nursing, ed 6, St Louis, 1987, The CV Mosby Co.

Kols A, and others: Oral contraceptives in the 1980's, Popul Rep A (6), 1982.

Willson JR, and others: Obstetrics and gynecology, ed 8, St. Louis, 1987, The CV Mosby Co.

Zatuchni G: New devices for intrauterine contraception, Contemp OB/GYN 24:77, 1985.

Glossary

abortion Termination of pregnancy.

abruptio placentae Partial or complete separation of a normally implanted placenta after viability and before delivery.

abstinence Refraining from sexual intercourse periodically or permanently.

AIDS Acquired Immunodeficiency Syndrome

afterbirth Lay term for the placenta and membranes.

afterpains Painful uterine contractions that occur intermittently in multiparas for 3 to 4 days after delivery.

albuminuria Presence of albumin, a protein, in the urine.

alveoli Air sacs of the lung.

amenorrhea Absence of menstruation.

amnesia Loss of memory.

amniocentesis Puncture of the amnion to draw off amniotic fluid.

amnion Inner of the two fetal membranes forming the sac that encloses the fetus within the uterus.

amniotic fluid Fluid secreted by the amnion that surrounds the fetus.

anesthesia Absence of feeling, with or without loss of consciousness.

anomaly Abnormality or defect.

anoxia Absence of oxygen.

antibody Substance of the body fluids that exerts specific restrictive or destructive action on bacteria or toxins.

apnea Cessation of respirations.

areola Pigmented ring around the nipple.

asphyxia Decreased oxygen and/or excessive carbon dioxide.

ataractics Tranquilizing drugs that potentiate analgesic drugs.

atelectasis Imperfect expansion of the lungs.

atony Lack of muscle tone.

attitude Posture of the fetus, especially the degree of extension or flexion of its spine.

auscultation Listening for sounds within the body.

bag of waters Lay term for fetal membranes that enclose the amniotic fluid and fetus.

ballottement Rebound of fetus within amniotic fluid when displaced by examiner's fingers.

Bandl's ring Abnormal thick ridge of uterine muscle between upper and lower segment with lower segment thinning.

Bartholin's glands Vulvovaginal glands.

BBT Basal body temperature, a means to identify the time ovulation occurs.

bilirubin Yellowish pigment that is a breakdown product of hemoglobin.

bizarre symptoms Inappropriate behavior.

blastula Stage of ovum development in which an outer layer of cells encloses a hollow cavity.

BOA Abbreviation for born out of asepsis, meaning when birth occurs outside a delivery room.

Braxton Hicks' contractions Intermittent uterine contractions during pregnancy.

breech Presentation in which the buttocks precede the head.

bregma Area of the anterior fontanel of the fetus.

caput The head.

caput succedaneum Swelling of the tissue on the presenting part of the head from birth trauma.

catamenia Menses.

caudal Tail.

cephalohematoma Collection of blood under the periosteum of any area of the cranial bones from birth trauma.

cephalic Pertaining to the head end of the body.

cephalopelvic disproportion (CPD) Baby's head of such size, shape, or position that it cannot pass through the mother's pelvis.

cervix Lower narrow mouth of the uterus.

cesarean birth Delivery of the fetus by way of an incision through the abdominal wall and the uterus.

Chadwick's sign Violet color of the vaginal mucous membrane during pregnancy.

cholasma Blotchy facial pigmentation, the mask of pregnancy.

chorion Outer of the two membranes forming the sac that encloses the fetus in the uterus.

chorionic villi Terminal, fernlike, microscopic projections of chorionic tissue, each of which contains a loop of placetal capillary that projects into the maternal blood sinuses of the uterus.

chromosomes Minute structures within the germ cells that contain the heredity-determining genes.

circumcision Surgical removal of the foreskin of the penis.

climacteric Period of time that marks the end of reproductive function.

clitoris Female organ that is similar to the male penis.

coitus Sexual union or copulation.

colostrum Serumlike secretion of the breasts during pregnancy and after delivery until the true milk comes in.

conception Union of the sperm and ovum.

concurrent sterilization Method of formula preparation in which all the ingredients are sterilized before mixing.

congenital Existing at birth.

conjunctivitis Inflammation of the membrane lining the eyelids and covering the eyeball.

contraception Prevention of conception.

contraction ring See *Bandl's ring*.

Coombs' test Test for Rh-positive antibodies.

copulation Sexual intercourse.

corpus luteum Yellow body formed in a ruptured graafian follicle of an ovary after the escape of a mature ovum.

Credé's prophylaxis Instillation of 1% silver nitrate solution or antibiotic ointment in the eyes of newborn infants to prevent ophthalmia neonatorum.

crowning Stage at which the fetal head can be seen at the vaginal orifice.

curettage Scraping the uterine lining.

cyanosis Blueness of the skin caused by insufficient oxygen in the blood.

cystocele Herniation of the bladder into the vagina.

decidua Thick, spongy lining of the uterus during pregnancy.

desquamation Shedding or peeling of skin or mucous membrane.

dilation Stretching of an opening.

disseminated intravascular coagulation (DIC) A life-threatening clotting disorder that causes widespread bleeding.

dry labor Amniotic fluid escapes too soon.

ductus arteriosus Fetal blood vessel extending from the pulmonary artery to the aorta.

ductus venosus Continuation of the umbilical vein that passes directly to the vena cava.

dyscrasia Literally means "bad mixture," referring to fetal and maternal blood incompatibility.

dysmature infant Poorly developed infant from any cause.

dystocia Excessively painful or slow labor or delivery.

ecchymosis Bruises, bleeding into tissue.

eclampsia Severe form of gestosis during which there are convulsions and coma.

ectopic pregnancy Implantation of the fertilized ovum outside the uterine cavity.

effacement Thinning and shortening of the cervix during labor.

effleurage Gentle stroking used in massage.

embolus Any material that is carried by the blood to another part of the body and obstructs a blood vessel.

embryo Developing baby before it is 5 weeks old.

endocrine glands Ductless glands that secrete complex chemicals called *hormones* into the lymph and blood.

endometritis Infection of the endometrium.

endometrium Inner lining of uterus.

engagement Entrance of fetal presenting part into superior pelvic strait.

engorgement Vascular congestion of breasts that precedes true lactation.

episiotomy Incision of the perineum toward the end of the second stage of labor to facilitate delivery.

Erb's paralysis Paralysis of the newborn's arm and shoulder caused by birth injury of the fifth and sixth cervical nerves.

estriol A by-product of estrogen metabolism.

excoriation Abrasion of the skin from physical or chemical causes.

expulsion Expelling or pushing out.

extrauterine pregnancy Ectopic pregnancy; one in which the fertilized ovum implants itself outside the uterine cavity.

fallopian tubes Oviducts or uterine tubes.

false labor Contractions that do not produce cervical dilation and do not become regular or longer than 20 seconds.

family A group of people bound together by blood or ideology.

fertility Ability to reproduce.

fetal death Death of the fetus after 20 weeks of gestation.

fetal distress Evidence that the fetus is having difficulty, such as a change in the fetal heartbeat or activity.

fetus Developing baby after 5 weeks of gestation until birth.

fimbriated Fringed, such as the ends of the two oviducts.

fissure Open crack or groove in tissue.

fistula Abnormal tube that forms between two normal cavities.

flaccid Complete relaxation with loss of muscle tone.

fontanel Space formed when two or more sutures of the fetal skull come together.

footling, breech One or both feet of fetus present on perineum at birth.

foramen ovale Opening between the auricles of the fetal heart that normally closes after birth.

forceps Double-bladed instrument to grasp fetal head for delivery.

fourchette Tense band of mucous membrane at posterior angle of vagina that connects the posterior ends of the labia minora.

fraternal twins Nonidentical twins who come from different fertilized ova.

full-term infant Born at 38 to 42 weeks of gestation.

fundus Dome-shaped upper portion of the uterus.

funic souffle Muffled sound of the blood rushing through the umbilical vessels, beating in time with the fetal heart.

gavage Feeding by means of a stomach tube.

gender role Expected social behavior of men or women.

gene Heredity determiner located on the chromosomes.

gestation Period of intrauterine fetal development.

glycosuria Presence of glucose (sugar) in the urine.

gonad Sex gland; ovary or testis.

Goodell's sign Softened cervix.

graafian follicle Fully developed ovarian cyst that contains the ripe ovum and a clear liquid.

gravid Pregnant.

gravida Pregnant woman.

Hegar's sign Softening of the lower uterine segmen.

hematoma Abnormal pooling of blood in tissue.

hemolysis Destruction of red blood cells.

heterozygous Indicating two dissimilar genes at the same site or locus on paired chromosomes.

high risk Infant or pregnancy in which there is a likelihood of disease or death.

homozygous Indicating two similar genes at the same locus on paired chromosomes.

hydramnios Excessive amounts of amniotic fluid.

hydrocele Collection of fluid in the sac that surrounds the testicle, causing the scrotum to swell.

hydrocephalus Excessive amounts of cerebrospinal fluid in the infant's skull.

hydrops fetalis Massive edema of a fetus; usually caused by Rh incompatibility.

hymen Membranous fold that partly closes the vaginal orifice.

hyperemesis gravidarum Excessive vomiting.

hypertension High blood pressure.

hypotensive drugs Drugs that help lower the blood pressure.

icterus neonatorum Jaundice of the newborn baby; usually meaning normal physiological jaundice.

idiogram An artist's drawing of chromosomes.

impotence Inability to complete coitus.

in utero Within the uterus.

induction of labor Starting labor by artificial means.

inertia, uterine Weakness or absence of uterine contractions in labor.

infertility Decreased capacity to conceive.

infiltration Process in which a substance is deposited within the tissue, such as a local anesthetic.

intrathecal Within the subarachnoid space.

intrauterine device (IUD) Inert plastic form placed in the uterus to prevent implantation of the ovum.

introitus Entrance into a canal such as the vagina.

inversion Turning inside out, such as inversion of the uterus when it turns inside out.

involution Return of the uterus to its normal size after childbirth.

karyotype Schematic arrangement of chromosomes to demonstrate their numbers and morphology.

Kegel's exercises Contraction of the muscles of the pelvic floor.

laceration Tearing, as of the perineum during delivery.

lactation Secretion of milk.

lactogenic hormone Gonadotropin produced by pituitary gland that promotes breast tissue growth and lactation; prolactin; luteotropin.

lanugo Fine hair covering the body of the fetus during the early months of gestation; usually disappears before birth.

leukorrhea Whitish discharge of the vagina; known as "whites."

lie Relationship of the long axis of the baby to the long axis of the mother; transverse lie means that the baby is lying crosswise in the mother's abdomen; longitudinal lie means that the baby is lying lengthwise.

ligation To suture, sew, or tie shut.

lightening Dropping of the uterus caused by the settling of the fetal head into the pelvis in the last weeks before delivery.

linea nigra Black line of darker pigmentation that appears along the midline of the abdomen of some women during pregnancy.

lithotomy position Position in which the patient lies on her back with her knees flexed and her thighs drawn up toward her chest.

live birth Fetus, regardless of age, that breathes, shows any heartbeat, or displays voluntary movement when born.

lochia Vaginal discharge after delivery that lasts for 3 to 6 weeks.

luteotropic hormone (LTH) Pituitary hormone; also called *prolactin* or *lactogenic hormone*.

maceration Softening and wasting of fetal skin by prolonged exposure to amniotic fluid.

mammary glands The breasts.

mask of pregnancy Brownish pigmentation of the facial skin during pregnancy; cholasma.

mastitis Inflammation or infection of the breasts.

meconium Greenish black stools of the newborn baby composed of mucus, bile, and skin cells.

menarche Occurrence of first menstrual period.

menopause Occurrence of final menstrual period.

menstruation Periodic discharge of a bloody fluid from the uterus; menses or menstrual period.

mentum Chin.

midwife Person, traditionally female, who practices art of aiding the mother during the birthing process.

milia Tiny white plugs of sebaceous gland secretion seen in the pores of the nose and face of some newborn babies.

miscarriage Lay term for spontaneous abortion.

missed abortion Retention of the products of conception for weeks after the fetus dies.

mitosis Indirect cell division in which a single cell divides but both of the new cells have the same number of chromosomes as the first.

molding Shaping of the baby's head to conform to the shape and size of the mother's birth canal.

mongolian spots Bluish, pigmented areas, especially of the back and buttocks, often found on dark-skinned newborn babies.

Montgomery's glands Small sebaceous glands of the nipple that secrete oil.

morbidity State of being diseased.

mortality Death rate.

morula Stage of development of the fertilized ovum in which there is a solid mass of cells resembling a mulberry.

mucous membrane Specialized lining of passage and cavities.

mucus Substance secreted by the mucous membrane.

multipara Woman who has had two or more pregnancies in which the fetuses reached viability, without regard to their being alive or dead at the time of birth.

multiple pregnancy Presence of more than one fetus in the uterus at the same time.

natal Pertaining to birth.

neonate Newborn baby.

nidation Implantation of the fertilized ovum in the endometrium.

nullipara Woman who has not yet delivered a viable fetus.

obstetrics Branch of medicine devoted to the childbearing woman and unborn child.

occiput Back part of the skull.

omphalocele Congenital defect resulting from failure of closure of abdominal wall.

oophorectomy Surgical removal of an ovary.

operculum Mucous plug that fills the cervical canal during pregnancy.

ophthalmia neonatorum Severe, purulent gonorrheal infection of the conjunctiva of the newborn baby.

orifice Normal opening.

ovulation Discharge of the ovum from the ovary.

ovum Female gamete or reproductive cell.

oxytocics Drugs that cause the uterus to contract.

palpation Examination performed by touching with the fingers or hands.

Papanicolaou smear Specially prepared microscopic slide using scrapings from the cervix or other mucous membranes to reveal early cancer cells; also called a *Pap test*.

parametritis Infection of the connective tissue around uterus.

parenteral Administration of food, fluids, or drugs other than by way of the digestive tract.

parturition Act of giving birth.

pelvimetry Measurement of the pelvis.

perineum Space between the vagina and the rectum.

peritoneum Strong serous membrane that lines the abdominal cavity.

peritonitis Infection of the pelvic cavity.

pessary Instrument placed inside the vagina or cervical canal.

phenylketonuria (PKU) Rare metabolic abnormality in which phenylketones are excreted in the urine; if left untreated, severe mental retardation results.

phimosis Tightness of the foreskin of the penis.

phlebitis Inflammation of a vein.

physiological jaundice Jaundice caused by a normal reduction in the number of red blood cells.

placenta Specialized vascular structure within the pregnant uterus that is connected to the fetus by the umbilical cord.

placenta accreta Invasion of the uterine muscle by the placenta, thus making its separation from the muscle nearly impossible.

polyhydramnios Excessive amounts of amniotic fluid.

position Relation of the baby's presenting part to the mother's birth canal.

positive sign of pregnancy Feeling fetal parts or motion, hearing fetal heart tones, or seeing fetal skeleton on an x-ray film.

postterm infant Born after 42 weeks of gestation.

precipitate Hasty or sudden; said of a labor or delivery.

preeclampsia Toxic condition that precedes convulsive stage (eclampsia); characterized by edema, hypertension, and albuminuria.

pregnancy-induced hypertension High blood pressure caused by toxic state. Also called *toxemia* and *preeclampsia-eclampsia*.

premature infant Born before 38 weeks of gestation; preterm.

prenatal Occurring before birth.

prepuce Foreskin of the penis.

presentation Part of the fetus that enters the pelvis first; cephalic, breech, or shoulder.

pressure edema Edema of the lower extremities caused by pressure of the heavy uterus against the large veins.

presumptive signs Evidence that suggests pregnancy but that is not absolutely positive.

primigravida Woman who is pregnant for the first time.

primipara Woman who has been delivered of her first child.

projectile vomiting Forceful, expulsive vomiting.

prolapsed cord Presence of the umbilical cord beside or ahead of the presenting part.

prophylactic Preventive.

proteinuria Excretion of albumin, a protein, in the urine.

pseudocyesis False pregnancy; pseudopregnancy.

pseudopregnancy Appearance of the symptoms of pregnancy although there is no pregnancy.

psychoprophylaxis Method of painless childbirth.

puberty Period of life in which the reproductive organs become functional.

pudendal block anesthesia Injection of an anesthetizing drug at the pudendal nerve root to produce numbness of the genitalia.

puerperal sepsis Postpartum infection of the pelvic organs; childbed fever.

puerperium Period of time following delivery until complete involution of the organs.

quickening First perceptible movements of the fetus.

regurgitate To spit up or to vomit.

relinquishment Type of adoption using a licensed agency.

residual urine Urine that remains in the bladder after urination.

retained placenta Condition in which all or part of the placenta remains in the uterus after delivery.

retrolental Behind the crystalline lens of the eye.

Rh factor Substance in the blood that is capable of causing antibodies to form against it.

rhythm method Coitus at the infertile period in the menstrual cycle to avoid conception.

saddle block anesthesia Type of spinal anesthesia.

sebaceous glands Oil-secreting glands of the skin.

serology Science of studying blood serum for the purpose of diagnosing disease.

serosanguineous Containing both serum and blood.

sexual response cycle Four phases: excitement, plateau, orgasm, and resolution.

siblings Children who have one or both of the same parents.

Skene's glands Two glands opening just within the meatus of the urethra.

smegma Thick, cheesy secretion found under the foreskin in boys and the labia minora in girls.

sperm Male reproductive cell or gamete.

spina bifida A birth defect of the vertebrae.

spontaneous abortion Abortion that occurs of itself.

station Depth to which the presenting part has descended into the pelvis.

STDs Sexually transmitted diseases.

sterile Free of all bacteria; unable to reproduce offspring.

stillbirth Death of the fetus before birth.

striae gravidarum Scars left from rapid stretching of the layers of the skin.

suture Junction between bones of the skull; also refers to sewing together an incision.

teratogenic agent Any agent that can cause malformations in the fetus.

tetany, uterine Prolonged uterine contraction.

thrombus Blood clot that remains at the place it was formed.

TORCH diseases Toxoplasmosis, Other, Rubella, Cytomegalovirus, and Herpes genitalis; conditions that cause adverse maternal, fetal, and neonatal effects.

toxemia Term used for gestosis or preeclampsia/eclampsia.

TPAL system Term-preterm-abortion–living children; used for a woman's obstetrical history.

trauma Wound or injury.

trimester Three-month period of time.

trophoblast Outer layer of cells of the blastodermic vesicle.

umbilicus Navel.

urinary frequency Frequent need to void.

urinary meatus Opening of the urethra.

uterine souffle Sound made by the blood in the arteries of the pregnancy uterus; the mother's pulse.

vaginitis Infection of the vagina.

varicose Swollen and distended veins.

venous Pertaining to the veins.

vernix caseosa Thick, white, pasty sebaceous secretion found on the baby's skin.

version Turning the infant within the uterus.

vertex Top of the head.

viable Living; refers to a fetus when it is able to live outside the uterus.

vulva External female genitalia.

vulvitis Infection of the vulva.

well-child clinics Clinics that offer medical supervision to healthy children; often free or for partial payment.

Wharton's jelly Jellylike substance surrounding the umbilical vessels within the cord.

zona pellucida Membrane covering the ovum.

zygote Cell formed by the union of the sperm and ovum; the fertilized ovum.

Appendix

Activity intolerance
Activity intolerance, potential
Adjustment, impaired
Airway clearance, ineffective
Anxiety
Aspiration, potential for
Body image disturbance
Body temperature, altered, potential
Breastfeeding, ineffective
Breathing pattern, ineffective
Cardiac output, decreased
Communication, impaired verbal
Constipation
Constipation, colonic
Constipation, perceived
Coping, family: potential for growth
Coping, ineffective family: compromised
Coping, ineffective family: disabling
Coping, ineffective individual
Decisional conflict (specify)
Denial, ineffective
Diarrhea
Disuse syndrome, potential for
Diversional activity deficit
Dysreflexia
Family processes, altered
Fatigue
Fear
Fluid volume deficit (1)
Fluid volume deficit (2)
Fluid volume deficit, potential
Fluid volume excess
Gas exchange, impaired
Grieving, anticipatory
Grieving, dysfunctional
Growth and development, altered
Health maintenance, altered
Health seeking behaviors (specify)
Home maintenance management, impaired

Hopelessness
Hyperthermia
Hypothermia
Incontinence, bowel
Incontinence, functional
Incontinence, reflex
Incontinence, stress
Incontinence, total
Incontinence, urge
Infection, potential for
Injury, potential for
Knowledge deficit (specify)
Mobility, impaired physical
Noncompliance (specify)
Nutrition, altered: less than body requirements
Nutrition, altered: more than body requirements
Nutrition, altered: potential for more than body requirements
Oral mucous membrane, altered
Pain
Pain, chronic
Parental role conflict
Parental role, compromised
Parenting, altered
Parenting, altered, potential
Personal identity disturbance
Poisoning, potential for
Posttrauma response
Powerlessness
Rape-trauma syndrome
Rape-trauma syndrome: compound reaction
Rape-trauma syndrome: silent reaction
Role performance, altered
Self-care deficit: bathing/hygiene
Self-care deficit: dressing/grooming
Self-care deficit: feeding
Self-care deficit: toileting
Self-esteem disturbance

From the Proceedings of the Eighth National Conference of the North American Nursing Diagnosis Association held in St. Louis, Missouri, March 13-16, 1988.

(Continued)

NORTH AMERICAN NURSING DIAGNOSIS ASSOCIATION (NANDA) APPROVED NURSING DIAGNOSES, 1988—cont'd

Self-esteem, chronic low
Self-esteem, situational low
Sensory-perceptual alterations (specify) (visual, auditory, kinesthetic, gustatory, tactile, olfactory)
Sexual dysfunction
Sexuality patterns, altered
Skin integrity, impaired
Skin integrity, impaired, potential
Sleep pattern disturbance
Social interaction, impaired
Social isolation
Spiritual distress (distress of the human spirit)

Swallowing, impaired
Thermoregulation, ineffective
Thought processes, altered
Tissue integrity, impaired
Tissue perfusion, altered (specify type) (renal, cerebral, cardiopulmonary, gastrointestinal, peripheral)
Trauma, potential for
Unilateral neglect
Urinary elimination, altered patterns
Urinary retention
Violence, potential for: self-directed or directed at others

INDEX